S. Sasayama · H. Suga (Eds.)

Recent Progress in Failing Heart Syndrome

With 159 Figures

Springer-Verlag
Tokyo Berlin Heidelberg
New York London Paris
Hong Kong Barcelona

SHIGETAKE SASAYAMA, M.D.
Professor of Medicine, The Second Department of Internal Medicine, Toyama Medical and Pharmaceutical University, 2630 Sugitani, Toyama, 930-01 Japan

HIROYUKI SUGA, M.D., D.M. SC.
Professor of Physiology, Okayama University Medical School, 2-5-1, Shikata-cho, Okayama, 700 Japan

ISBN 4-431-70073-0 Springer-Verlag Tokyo Berlin Heidelberg New York
ISBN 3-540-70073-0 Springer-Verlag Berlin Heidelberg New York Tokyo
ISBN 0-387-70073-0 Springer-Verlag New York Berlin Heidelberg Tokyo

Library of Congress Cataloging-in-Publication Data
Recent progress in failing heart syndrome / S. Sasayama, H. Suga (eds). p. cm. Compilation of scientific results of a three year project for research on heart failure organized by the Japanese Circulation Society from 1988 to 1991. Includes bibliographical references and index. ISBN (invalid) 4-431-70073-0. — ISBN (invalid) 3-540-70073-0. — ISBN (invalid) 0-387-70073-0. 1. Congestive heart failure. 2. Heart failure. I. Sasayama, Shigetake, 1937– . II. Suga, H. (Hiroyuki), 1941– . III. Nihon Junkanki Gakkai. [DNLM: 1. Heart—physiopathology. 2. Heart Failure, Congestive. 3. Myocardial Contraction. WG 370 R295] RC685.C53R43 1991, 616.1′29—dc20, DNLM/DLC, for Library of Congress 91-5067

Typesetting, printing, and binding: Best-set Typesetter, Ltd., Hong Kong

Preface

Heart failure is a syndrome caused by a heart dysfunction that leads to insufficient blood in the peripheral tissues for their metabolic demands. This syndrome still remains an obscure clinical entity and even its definition is disputed. It has become increasingly apparent that heart failure may relate not only to cardiac dysfunction but also to other physiological alterations involved in the maintenance of circulatory homeostasis.

In 1988, the Japanese Circulation Society organized a three-year project for research on heart failure. The research group consisted of ten investigators, all relatively young but well recognized internationally for their research accomplishments.

This book represents a compilation of the achievements by this group during the past three years which have led to new insights into the pathophysiologic mechanisms of heart failure, and diagnosis, evaluation and treatment of this syndrome. Contents include research into the cellular biology of congestive heart failure, and a framework of pressure-volume relationships enabling assessment of ventricular contraction energetics or coupling of ventricular properties and arterial load. This conceptual framework is of vital significance, particularly when we consider the failing heart as an energy-depleted state. An understanding of the neuroendocrine responses to explain the pathophysiology of congestive heart failure is perhaps the most important advance, and has led to new developments in therapy.

This book also includes an analysis of mechanical factors, including both regional, and global ventricular functions, and this is related to the understanding of the pathophysiology of congestive heart failure.

With such an increase in knowledge concerning the biological and physiological bases of congestive heart failure, its management has become more complex than before. The therapeutic implications of selective stimulation of high-affinity β_1-receptors are outlined, as well as use of the left ventricular assist system as a viable alternative.

The materials presented in this book summarize the latest knowledge on heart failure syndrome, from basic science to treatment. We hope this book will describe the current state of research on heart failure in Japan and serve as a stimulus for further investigation.

S. Sasayama
H. Suga

Table of Contents

List of Contributors

1

Reconstitution of Actin-Myosin Interaction In Vitro: Its Application to Cardiac Physiology

Seiryo Sugiura[1], Hiroshi Yamashita[1], Takashi Serizawa[1], Masahiko Iizuka[2]

Summary. Recently, biochemical studies have revealed that heart muscle can change the structure of contractile protein under various physiological or pathophysiological conditions. To examine the functional significance of these changes at the molecular level, we applied an in vitro motility assay technique and measured the sliding velocity of cardiac myosin in vitro.

First, various methods to assay in vitro motility are reviewed. These techniques enabled us to study the mechanical aspect of acto-myosin interaction under controlled conditions and thus showed many intriguing results.

Secondly, our preliminary results using rabbit cardiac myosin are presented. We used an assay system in which polystyrene beads coated with cardiac myosin obtained from either normal or hyperthyroid rabbit were made to slide on actin cables of an alga *Nitellopsis obtusa* in the presence of Mg-ATP. The movement observed under photomicroscope was smooth and its velocity was related to the biochemical characteristics of myosin. The velocity changed under various experimental conditions, suggesting that the sliding observed in this system is physiological in nature.

We consider that in vitro motility assay techniques can help us understand the relation between biochemistry and physiology.

Key words: Cardiac myosin — In vitro motility assay — Sliding velocity

Introduction

While recent advances in biochemistry and biotechnology have attracted the interest of researchers studying heart muscle [1, 2], less attention has been paid to the physiological aspect of this field. Of course, continuous efforts have

[1]The Second Department of Internal Medicine, Faculty of Medicine, University of Tokyo, Bunkyo-ku, Tokyo, 113 Japan
[2]The First Department of Internal Medicine, Dokkyo University, School of Medicine, Mibu, Tochigi, 321 Japan

been made towards complete understanding of the mechanical properties [3–6] and energetics [7] of the muscle, but most of these studies are still within the conceptual framework of the "cross-bridge theory" which was first proposed in 1957 [8] and later revised.

This theory has been used for many years to account for experimental results but recently, serious challenges have been made against its basic assumptions. Researchers are now questioning whether one cross-bridge cycling is rigidly coupled to one ATP hydrolysis cycle, and whether a single cross-bridge always exerts a constant force under any loading conditions.

This drastic change in thinking was made possible by the development of in vitro motility assays which allow visualization of the interaction of contractile proteins using light microscopy [9–18]. Direct visualization of acto-myosin interaction eliminates the complex deduction process by providing us with direct results on the fundamental mechanisms of muscle contraction.

In this article, we will review the techniques and results of in vitro motility assays and the application of these techniques in cardiac physiology. Finally, the significance and future direction of these techniques in cardiology will be discussed.

Motility Assay Using Algae

Historical Overview

The first version of the in vitro motility assay was developed independently by Sheetz and Spudich in 1983 [17] and Shimmen and Yano in 1984 [18]. This type of assay is characterized by use of the algae *Characeae*, of which the species *Chara* and *Nitella* are well known. These algae consist of cylindrical internodal cells, about 1 mm in diameter and several cm in length, that are connected in series. The inner surface of the cell wall is covered with well-organized rows of chloroplasts running longitudinally, and the endoplasm inside (sol phase) streams actively (sometimes the rate is as fast as 100 μm/s).

As a mechanism for cytoplasmic streaming, Kamiya and Kuroda proposed that the shear stress was generated by the interaction of the cytoplasm and the inner surface of the chloroplast rows (sol-gel interface) [19]. Interestingly, this discovery coincided with the publication of the cross-bridge theory. Later research identified bundles of actin filaments running on the chloroplast rows [20]. These filaments can be decorated with heavy meromyosin (HMM) to form arrow heads. The direction of cytoplasmic streaming is opposite to the pointed end which is similar to the relative sliding of acto-myosin in muscle sarcomeres. Currently, molecular motors are classified into two categories: actin-based and microtubule-based [21]. In the actin-based molecular motor, myosins are coupled. Indeed, Kato and Tonomura [22] isolated myosin from *Nitella flexilis*. Furthermore, small bodies having myosin-like activities (ATPase activity, generating motive force for the sliding movement) were found to exist on the endoplasmic organelles [23].

These results strongly suggest that cytoplasmic streaming is based on the sliding of myosin on actin bundles fixed on the chloroplast rows. Inspired by this fact, groups of researchers succeeded in reconstituting actin-myosin sliding using skeletal muscle myosin [17, 18], which was actually the first direct evidence for the sliding filament theory.

One of the concerns about this assay system is that Algae actins are not biochemically determined. However, the highly conserved primary structure of actin throughout evolution [24] suggests that the movement may not be influenced significantly by the different species from which actins are derived.

Assay Method

The assay technique is composed of four parts:

1. Washing out of the endoplasm and exposure of the actin bundles
2. Isolation of myosin and attachment to the marker
3. Introduction of myosin onto the actin bundles
4. Observation of movement using a light microscope

Since actin-myosin sliding takes place only in water, as in the cell, we must use a light microscope to visualize the movement, using some kind of marker. An outline is presented below.

Algae, *Nitella axillaris*, *Chara australis*, *or Nitellopsis obtusa*, are cultured in water containing nutrients under illumination by fluorescent lamps. Prior to each experiment, an internodal cell is trimmed free of branches and rinsed.

The two groups of researchers developed quite different techniques to expose the actin bundles. Sheetz and Spudich [17] opened the cell with a transverse cut in a dissection buffer containing EGTA, Mg-ATP, and KCl. By doing this, the cytoplasm was washed away. Shimmen and Yano [18] used a procedure called intracellular perfusion, in which both ends of the internodal cell were cut open and the cell was perfused with a medium containing EGTA to disintegrate the intracellular membranous structure. Next, by perfusing with a medium containing EDTA, the remaining cytoplasm was inactivated and effused out. In either method, the remaining internodal cell can be used as an actin donor cell.

Myosin is isolated by the usual method. To observe active movement, myosin should be fresh, but myosin stored at −20°C in a 50% glycerol solution is usable. In research following these two pioneer studies, myosin from various species (rabbit skeletal [17, 18], siphon muscle of squid [25], adductor muscle of scallop [25], anterior byssus retractor muscle of blue mussel [26], amoeba myosin [27], gizzard smooth muscle of turkey [28], organelles of lily [29], etc.) have been tested.

Small beads are used as markers. In one assay system [17], fluorescent Covaspheres MX (0.7 μm in diameter) were incubated with myosin solution on ice. In another assay [18], latex beads (2 μm in diameter) were first covered with poly (L-lysine) and then suspended in a solution of soluble myosin. By decreasing the ionic strength of the solution, filamentous myosin bound to the beads, and filamentous aggregation around the bead was confirmed either by Nomarski microscopy or electron microscopy.

Myosin-coated beads are suspended in a medium containing Mg-ATP, EGTA, and KCl and then exposed to actin cables by either direct application to the opened cell surface or cell perfusion. The contents of the medium can be altered according to the purpose of the experiment.

The movement of the beads are observed under a light microscope. Since actin bundles are arranged in parallel along the whole length of the cell, the movement is always linear. Linear movement greatly facilitates the measurement of velocity.

Findings

When myosin-coated beads are exposed to the internodal cell, those close to the actin bundles move smoothly at a constant rate over a long distance. However, others floating in the medium (the density of the beads is close to that of the medium) show only Brownian motion. In the internodal cell, there is a narrow bare zone (lacking chloroplast rows) running in a spiral form, and this is called the indifferent line. On each side of this indifferent line the polarity of the actin filament is reversed (indicated by the decoration with HMM), and so is the direction of cytoplasmic streaming [17, 18]. The fact that the direction of bead movement is reversed on each side of the indifferent line supports that this movement is active in nature. Sometimes the beads aggregate without affecting the velocity [27].

For the myosin from rabbit skeletal muscle (fast muscle), the velocity ranged from 3–6 μm/s [27], 0.5–10 μm/s [17], and 0.5–2.5 μm/s [18] at room temperature, and for turkey gizzard myosin (smooth muscle), from about 0.2–0.4 μm/s [28]. Other studies using myosins from various types and species also indicate that the velocity of bead movement is dependent on the intrinsic property (probably ATPase activity) of myosin. These values are comparable to that of the relative sliding of acto-myosin in muscle sarcomere. One problem not yet solved is the disproportionately high rate of cytoplasmic streaming (50–100 μm/s). This could be due to the very high ATPase activity (not yet determined), or configuration of the myosin molecules on the organelles.

Other factors which modify the velocity of the movement have also been examined for skeletal muscle myosins [27]. When the pH of the medium was varied, there was a sharp decline in velocity under acidic conditions. Under alkaline conditions however, the decline was more gradual. The activation energy was estimated from the temperature dependence of velocity, and was found to be close to that of actin-activated ATPase activity. These results suggest that the velocity of movement is tightly coupled with the actin-activated ATPase activity of myosin. However, with regard to dependence on the ATP concentration, movement was found to be ATP dependent at lower concentrations, but the velocity was nearly constant about 100 μM of ATP, which is much higher than that of actin-activated ATPase activity in vitro. As Sheetz et al. discussed [27], this is probably because of the interaction among myosin molecules, i.e., myosin molecules lacking ATP make rigor bonds, exerting a drag on the movement. The velocity of the beads is an expression of the actin-activated ATPase activity but factors which cannot be studied using myosin solution may play important roles in determining the velocity.

Further Development

Following the above reports, Shimmen and Yano [30] introduced Ca^{2+} sensitivity to this assay system by adding troponin-tropomyosin complex obtained from rabbit skeletal muscle to the actin bundles of *Chara*. In this report, no movement was observed in the absence of Ca^{2+} in the medium. The threshold level of Ca^{2+} for the movement was pCa = 7–5, which was close to that under in vivo conditions. One thing to be noted, however, was that the maximal velocity was about 50% of that without troponin-tropomyosin complex.

Motility Assay Using Native Actin

Although the motility assay using algae actin bundles is reproducible and exhibits physiological responses to various alterations in the medium, the use of biochemically undefined actin may raise questions about the nature of movement observed. To overcome this problem, investigators have developed several types of assay systems using both muscle myosin and actin.

Yano and Shimizu [31] described a system called the stream cell, which is composed of a pair of concentric cylinders attached to a base-plate. Between the two cylinders, there is a narrow slit. F-actins were fixed on both walls of the slit, and the slit was filled with a solution containing HMM, ATP, and ions. Steady and uniform streaming was observed under physiological conditions.

They also developed an actomyosin motor [11], which has a rotor, with three blades made of mica, on one side of which is a teflon coating. This teflon layer is further coated with poly (L-lysine) and F-actin is anchored on it with a specific polarity. When the rotor was placed in a medium containing Mg-ATP and HMM, it began to rotate spontaneously in one direction, as determined by the polarity of the F-actin. Furthermore, they could introduce Ca^{2+} regulation by attaching troponin-tropomyosin complex to the F-actin. Subfragment-1 could also induce rotation in this assay system.

Spudich et al. [12] observed the movement of myosin-coated beads on a synthetic actin array. The actin array was reconstituted by binding the barbed end of the actin filaments to the electron-microscope grid by a protein having high affinity to the barbed end. These actin filaments were then placed in a flow cell so that the pointed ends were oriented downstream. Myosin-coated beads moved on these actin filaments at a rate similar to that observed on algae actin bundles.

More recently, a simplified version of the motility assay that uses muscle myosin and actin has been developed. In this assay fluorescent-labeled actin filaments slide on a layer of myosin coated on a glass surface. Since the first report by Kron and Spudich [10], many important findings have been revealed by this assay [9, 15, 32–35]. As this assay system is currently used widely, its methodology and findings are described in detail.

Method

A fluorescent dye, phalloidin-tetramethyl-rhodamine (PHDTMR), is used to visualize the actin filaments. This dye is suitable for observation of actin movement because it binds to F-actin without affecting its physiological properties. Purified G-actin is incubated with PHDTMR to form labeled F-actin. Labeled single actin filament can be observed under a microscope equipped with epifluorescence optics. Since the PHDTMR binds F-actin with a 1:1 stoichiometry, the length of the actin filament can be estimated beyond the resolution of the photomicroscopy (0.2 μm). Although the strong illumination required for fluorescent microscopy causes photobleaching and protein denaturation, this can be overcome by removing oxygen with reducing agents in the medium. Myosin (or its subfragment) is coated on the surface of coverslips to act as the substratum for the actin filaments to slide on. Myosin is attached to the glass surface directly, by silicone coating, or by nitrocellulose coating. In this way, the myosin is arranged randomly. For smooth movement to be observed, myosin is packed maximally to form a single layer with a very smooth surface. If not, the filament will stop or detach from the surface and will be blown away.

Fluorescent-labeled actin filaments in a medium containing Mg-ATP is applied on the myosin coated surface and the movement is observed. The movement is recorded on video tape and analyzed later.

Findings

In the presence of ATP, actin filament moved smoothly but followed a winding path reflecting the random arrangement of myosin filaments on the glass surface. According to Harada et al. [9] the rate of movement was not dependent on the length of the actin filament. The rate of movement for skeletal muscle myosin was 5.5 μm/s [9] or 3.5 μm/s [10], and for smooth muscle myosin 0.25 μm/s [32]. These values are close to those of the beads' movement on algae actin bundles.

Warshaw et al. [32] examined the parameters affecting velocity for the smooth muscle myosin. The velocity was maximal between pH7.0 and 7.5 and decreased under both acidic and alkaline conditions. The velocity was constant with sufficient ATP and the concentration for the half maximal velocity was 29 μM. Concerning the temperature dependence, the apparent Q_{10} was 2.1. For skeletal muscle myosin, Harada et al. [9] reported a Q_{10} value of 2.4.

Other intriguing findings have also been reported. In addition to intact myosin, one-headed myosin [33], HMM [34], and subfragment-1 (although the velocity was slightly low) [34] could bear the sliding of actin filament. Furthermore, actin filament can slide in either direction on myosin filament despite its polarity [35]. These results are serious challenges against the validity of the cross-bridge theory, since it assumes a structural change in myosin molecules (rotation of the head portion) is the origin of force.

Energetic considerations also raise an important question. Yanagida et al. [9] estimated the minimum value of the sliding distance during one ATP hydrolysis cycle under unloaded conditions. According to their calculations, actin filament can slide on myosin under zero load conditions for at least 150 nm during one ATP hydrolysis cycle. Prior to this study, they directly measured the sliding distance using a single sarcomere from which Z-lines had been removed by protease [16]. In that experiment the actin slid at least 60 nm on the average. These values are much larger than predicted by the cross-bridge theory in which the sliding distance should be as long as the size of myosin head (about 10 nm). From these results, the very basic assumption of the cross-bridge theory (1:1 coupling of the mechano-chemical transduction) is now in question.

Force Measurement

In the preceding sections, in vitro motility assays measuring the velocity under zero-load conditions were reviewed. Since, however, muscle contracts under a certain amount of load in physiological conditions, an assay system is needed with which we could observe the acto-myosin sliding under known load or with which we could measure the force the cross-bridge generates.

Kishino and Yanagida [15] measured the force generated by a single actin filament sliding on a glass surface covered with myosin or its subfragment obtained from skeletal muscle. They used a compliant glass microneedle (elastic coefficient 1.5–10 pN/1 μm) calibrated by bending against the glass needle of known compliance. By coating the tip of the glass microneedle with denatured myosin, actin could attach to the microneedle rigidly in the presence of ATP. When the actin filament slides on the myosin layer, the filament pulls the needle and bends it. Since the elastic coefficient is known, the force can be calculated from the displacement. Measured force was proportional to the length of the actin-filament reflecting the number of cross-bridges working. Considering the density of myosin (or subfragment-1), they estimated the force which a single cross-bridge can generate is 0.2–1 pN. This value is comparable to the force produced in isometrically contracting muscle.

Chaen et al. [14] recorded the movement of a myosin-coated glass microneedle with algae *Nitellopsis* actin cables. The tip of the microneedle was first coated with poly (L-lysine) and then coated with myosin of skeletal muscle. When the myosin-coated tip came in contact with the inner surface of the opened internodal cell, the microneedle began to bend and finally stopped where the force of acto-myosin interaction and the elastic force of the microneedle balanced. Since the movement of well-organized actin bundles is linear, the velocity and the simultaneous force (calculated from the displacement) could be easily determined. The obtained force-velocity relation was convex upward. The researchers considered that this shape was due to the auxotonic contraction (increasing force as the myosin bends the needle) observed in this study.

The steady-state force-velocity relation of the actin-myosin interaction (interaction proceeding under constant load) was also studied. Oiwa et al. [36] observed the movement of myosin-coated beads on *Nitella actin* cables under constant load by applying centrifugal force. Polystyrene beads (specific gravity = 1.3) were coated with myosin of skeletal muscle and introduced into the internodal cell of *Nitella* by intracellular perfusion. The prepared cell was mounted on the stage of a centrifugal microscope. This is a light microscope equipped with a rotating stage and a stroboscopic light source. By rotating the stage at a certain rate, a steady centrifugal force can be applied to the bead in the cell. The observed force-velocity relation deviated from hyperbola in the high load region resulting in a double hyperbola which is analogous to that of single muscle fiber. In addition to the characteristic shape in the force-velocity relation, this result suggested an interesting property of the muscle contraction. In this study, the maximal force was in the range 1.9–39 pN which corresponded to 2–40 myosin heads. This implies that a single myosin molecule can modulate the velocity and force according to the load imposed. Furthermore, the force muscle produces may not be entirely controlled by the number of cross-bridges but the property of the unit force generator.

Why in Cardiology?

We have reviewed the novel findings elucidated by in vitro motility assays. These findings may introduce drastic changes in thinking on the mechanism of muscle contraction or cell motility. However, do these findings have any significance in cardiology, especially in its clinical aspect? In the following paragraph, we will discuss some questions which might be answered by in vitro motility assay techniques.

The diversity of cardiac myosin isozymes and their expression in response to various mechanical or humoral stimuli have been well recognized [1, 2]. Biochemical studies have revealed that V_1 isoform (homodimer of α-myosin heavy chain (α-MHC) has higher ATPase activity than V_3 isoform (homodimer of β-myosin heavy chain (β-MHC)) [37]. Its functional meaning has also been studied using either papillary muscle [3, 4], ventricular trabeculae [38], or isolated myocytes [39]. These studies have demonstrated that the shortening velocity under zero load correlates with the content of V_1 or α-MHC. In these specimens, however, the complex cellular structure is preserved and so is the excitation-contraction process. Since muscle contraction is the final expression of these subcellular mechanisms, nobody can be sure that only the alteration in myosin isoform is responsible for the change in shortening velocity observed. Indeed, recent studies suggested that cellular components other than myosin also change under various conditions [40]. Interaction among cross-bridges may also be important. In vitro motility assays in which only the interaction between actin and myosin is examined (even single component interactions) can give a useful clue to these questions. The energetics of cardiac muscle have attracted the interest of cardiologists. To assure good prognosis for patients with heart failure, efficiency in chemo-mechanical transduction is believed to be important. In animal experiments, it has been shown that papillary muscle or ventricle rich in V_1 isoform has poor efficiency [7]. Generally speaking, muscles shortening slowly seem to have high efficiency. Based on the cross-bridge theory, changes in cross-bridge cycling are suggested as the underlying mechanism. However, findings provided by in vitro motility assays may require re-consideration on this subject.

Contractility, its origin and regulation, is of great importance in cardiology. So far it has been generally believed that the force generated by muscle is proportional to the number of cross-bridges formed or that the force is regulated by the number of myosin heads attached to actin filament assuming a constant force per cross-bridge under any loading conditions. Furthermore, the force-velocity relation is the reflection of change in number. It is also well known that the number of cross-bridges is primarily determined by the intracellular concentration of calcium ions and its affinity to troponin-C resulting in the release of inhibition exerted by troponin-tropomyosin complex [41]. Most inotropic agents currently used in clinical settings are believed to exert their effects by increasing calcium levels. However, measurement of the force produced by acto-myosin interaction strongly suggested that each cross-bridge can regulate force generation according to the load applied. The possibility that different myosin or acto-myosin coupling may produce different levels of force cannot be denied either.

Application to Cardiology

As discussed in the preceding section, in vitro motility assays may also reveal interesting findings in cardiology. In this section, we will present some data from our initial attempt to study the properties of cardiac acto-myosin interaction [42]. We applied the method developed by Shimmen and Yano and measured the sliding velocity of beads coated with myosin from rabbit cardiac muscle on *Nitellopsis* actin cables. We also examined the effect of pH, ATP concentration, myosin isoforms and others on velocity.

Materials and Methods

Preparation of Myosin

Heart muscle was obtained from the left ventricle of adult Japanese white rabbits. Myosin was extracted with Guba-Straub solution and purified by repeated precipitation and dissolving. Finally, ultra-centrifugation was performed for two and a half hours at 100,000 g to remove the actin. All procedures were carried out at 4°C and dithiothreitol and E64-C were added to the solution.

Purity of myosin was confirmed using sodium dodecyl sulphate polyacrylamide gel electrophoresis.

Bead Preparation

Small latex beads (Dow Chemical Company, Uniform Latex Particles, 2 μm in diameter) were incubated with 5 mg/ml poly (L-lysine) (Sigma, M.W. 70,000–150,000) in 400 mM KOH for 3 h, and washed three times with a medium (400 mM KCl and 5 mM N-2-hydroxyethylpiperazine-N′-2-ethanesulfonic acid (HEPES)-KOH, pH 7.5). By this procedure, the beads were coated with poly (L-lysine). These beads were mixed with myosin dissolved in a high ionic strength medium (400 mM KCl, 10 mM imidazole-HCl, pH 7.0). As the ionic strength of the solution was decreased, filamentous myosin attached around the beads. After unbound myosin was removed by centrifugation, the myosin-coated beads were suspended in Mg-ATP medium (1 mM ATP, 5 mM ethyleneglycol-bis(β-aminoethylether) N,N,N′,N′-tetraacetic acid (EGTA), 6 mM $MgCl_2$, 70 mM KOH, 30 mM piperazine-N,N′-bis(2-ethanesulfonic acid) (PEPES), 200 mM sorbitol, pH 7.0). This bead suspension was used for the motility assay.

Actin Donor Cell Preparation

The fresh water green alga *Nitellopsis* obtusa was cultured in a bucket containing soil and mold and filled with tap water. The bucket was illuminated from above by fluorescent lamps (20 W) in a 14-hour light 10-hour dark cycle at 25°C. Prior to the experiment, long straight cells were selected and all the branches were cut. These individual internodal cells were stored in artificial pond water (0.1 mM each of KCl, NaCl and $CaCl_2$, pH about 5.6). From these cells, actin donor cells were prepared by cutting open both ends of the internodal cell and replacing the cell sap by cellular perfusion with Mg-ATP medium. After this procedure, the cell was kept on the perfusion bench in a moist chamber for twenty minutes to avoid damage by drying. After the cell was taken out from the moist chamber, the cell content was effused out and the second perfusion was performed with a medium (5 mM ethylenediaminetetraacetic acid (EDTA), 1 mM ATP, 71 mM KOH, 30 mM PIPES, 200 mM sorbitol). When Mg^{2+} was depleted by EDTA treatment, the endoplasm lost its ability to generate motive force for the cytoplasmic streaming but the actin bundles preserved their physiological properties. This EDTA-treated cell was placed in the moist chamber for a minute and then again cell content was replaced by Mg-ATP medium by cell perfusion. Finally, the internodal cell was ready for use for the motility assay as an actin donor.

Motility Assay

Myosin-coated beads were suspended in Mg-ATP medium and introduced into the actin donor cell by cell perfusion. Then both ends were ligated with polyester threads to isolate the environment around the myosin-coated bead and actin cables. The cell was immersed in medium (0.1 mM K_2SO_4, 1 mM NaCl, 0.1 mM $CaCl_2$ 150 mM sorbitol) on a slide glass. The movement of the bead or bead aggregate was observed with a photomicroscope (Labophoto-2 Nikon, Japan) and recorded on a videocassette by a video camera (KV-24 Hitachi Denshi, Japan) and a videocassette recorder (HR D-23 JVC Japan) system. The magnification of the objective used was × 40 and the final magnification on the monitor screen was × 900. Velocity was measured on a monitor screen by replaying the cassette tape. Since the movement was always linear, reflecting the well-arranged actin bundles of the *Nitellopsis* cell, the measurement was very easy to perform. The average velocity over at least 10 μm was taken for analysis. The same internodal cell could be used for as long as 30 min, by which time most of the beads or bead aggregates ceased moving. Standard assay was performed at a temperature between 21°C and 23°C. To control temperature, a brass plate perfused with temperature-controlled water was placed on the stage. The temperature was measured by a thermistor placed as close as possible to the internodal cell. The content of the Mg-ATP medium was altered according to the purpose of the experiment.

Induction of Myosin Isoform Redistribution

To examine the relationship between myosin isoform and the sliding velocity, hyperthyroidism was induced in adult rabbit [7]. L-thyroxine (0.2 mg/kg-wt per day) was injected subcutaneously for 14 days. If the body weight became 80% of the initial value, the injection was omitted on that day. The content of myosin isoform was determined by pyrophosphate gel electrophoresis and scanning at 550 nm [37]. The content of α-MHC was calculated by adding half of the area under the V_2 isozyme (α, β-heterodimer) peak to that of the V_1 isoform.

Myosin ATPase activity was determined by measuring the amount of inorganic phosphate liberated by ATP hydrolysis. Protein concentration was determined by a modified version of Lowry's method.

Results

The Nature of the Sliding Movement

A number of beads or bead aggregates were observed in the internodal cell. However, only those located close to the chloroplast layer moved smoothly along the rows of actin bundles. Others floating in the core portion of the cylindrical cell (not attached to actin bundles) exhibited only Brownian motion. The velocity was constant over a long distance (>100 μm), and independent of the size of the bead aggregate. The direction of the movement was opposite on each side of the indifferent line of the internodal cell (Fig. 1) reflecting the reversal of the polarity of actin filament. These findings are the evidence for the active movement. We recorded 5–15 beads or bead aggregates in one internodal cell depending on its length.

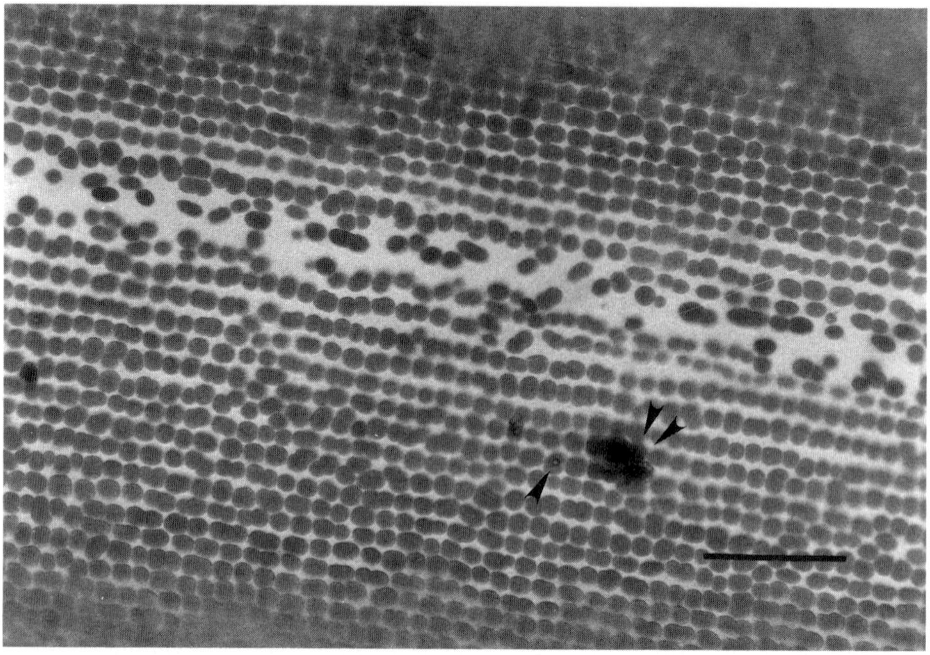

Fig. 1. A micropraph showing a single bead (*single arrow head*) and a bead aggregate (*double arrow heads*) sliding on the actin bundles (not visible). The bare zone in the middle is the indifferent line. The *bar* represents 50 μm

Velocity of Movement

The sliding velocity was fairly consistent when bead movement was observed in one internodal cell. Furthermore, the velocity was also reproducible in different cells when the myosin from one animal was studied. For myosin prepared from one animal, the coefficient of variability (standard deviation/mean) was less than 0.20. However, significant variation was observed among different animals. The velocity distribution collected from different animals is shown in Fig. 2. The distribution is fairly broad, probably because this is the sum of multiple groups each corresponding to each animal. The average velocity of movement for adult rabbit cardiac myosin was 0.30 ± 0.10 μm/s.

Effect of Physiological Interventions

When ATP was depleted from the medium, no movement was observed. However, for an ATP concentration of about 50 μM, the velocity was constant. Half maximal velocity was attained at about 30 μm.

When the pH of the Mg-ATP medium was changed, the velocity fell sharply on the acidic side (pH < 7.0). In contrast, we observed a fairly gradual decline in velocity on the alkaline side. The optimum was between 7.0 and 7.5.

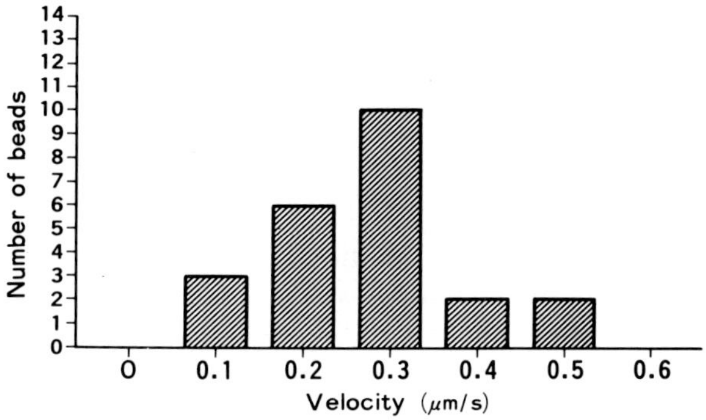

Fig. 2. Velocity distribution for myosin from control rabbits

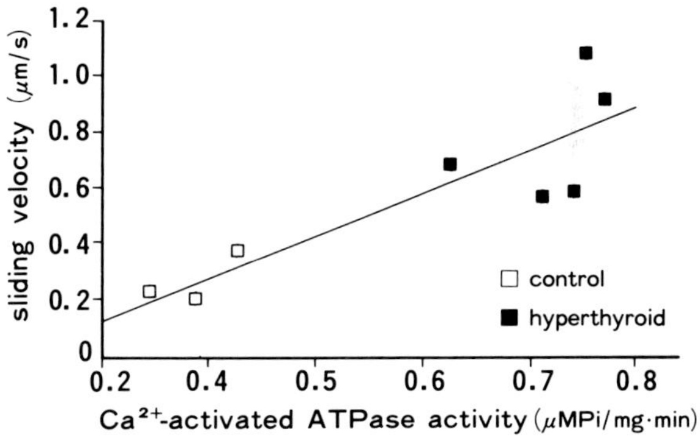

Fig. 3. Relation between sliding velocity and myosin Ca^{2+}-activated ATPase activity. Sliding velocity is plotted as a function of Ca^{2+}-activated ATPase activity for control and hyperthyroid rabbit myosin

Relation Between Myosin Isoform and Velocity

Induction of hyperthyroidism by L-thyroxine treatment increased the V_1 or α-MHC content in adult rabbits (relative content of α-MHC (%α-MHC): control 21 ± 13%, hyperthyroid 75 ± 16%). Similarly, Ca^{2+}-activated activity increased from 0.39 ± 0.04 μM Pi/mg · min (control) to 0.72 ± 0.06 μM Pi/mg · min (hyperthyroidism). As for the sliding velocity, it also increased from 0.31 ± 0.10 μm/s (control) to 0.73 ± 0.25 μm/s (hyperthyroidism). When the sliding velocity was plotted as a function of Ca^{2+}-activated ATPase, there was a significant correlation between them (Fig. 3).

Discussion

We applied an in vitro motility assay system developed by Sheetz and Spudich [17] and Shimmen and Yano [18], and studied the properties of cardiac myosin. It proved to be a reproducible and quantitative assay system.

Nature of the Sliding Movement

The movement of the beads coated with cardiac myosin was similar to that observed with skeletal muscle myosin. Smooth movement along the chloroplast rows, reversal of the direction on each side of the indifferent line, and ATP dependence all point to the fact that this movement is active and coupled with ATP hydrolysis [17, 18, 27]. We also observed that the velocity is sensitive to temperature [27].

Velocity of the Movement

According to the calculation by Sheetz et al. [27], the force required to move a bead in water is much less than that which a single cross-bridge can generate. This implies that the sliding velocity observed in this assay system is an estimate of load-free shortening velocity (V_{max}) which has been studied with various species and techniques. Sheetz et al. [27] reported the sliding velocity of beads coated with skeletal muscle myosin to be 2–6 μm/s. It has also been suggested that the velocity depends on myosin ATPase activity. Considering that the actin-activated ATPase activity of rabbit cardiac myosin was one-fifth to one tenth that of skeletal myosin [43], the velocity observed in this study was in the expected range. Comparison with V_{max} measured in intact muscle is difficult because it varies depending on the types of preparations, experimental techniques used, and the experimental conditions. If we assume that a muscle contracts uniformly throughout its length and that the length of a half sarcomere is approximately 1.0 μm, the sliding velocity observed in this study (0.31 μm/s) corresponds to 0.31 length/s. Pagani and Julian [4], using rabbit ventricular papillary muscle, estimated the V_{max} to be between 0.4 and 0.8 length/s at 25°C. Considering the temperature dependence of shortening velocity, the sliding velocity of myosin-coated beads observed was in a reasonable range.

Effect of Physiological Interventions

The ATP dependence of the sliding velocity was similar to that of skeletal muscle myosin. As Sheetz et al. pointed out [27], this result presents one of the very important properties of motility assay. The estimated ATP concentration at which half maximal velocity was attained was much higher than that for the ATPase activity. This was probably because the myosin heads lacking ATP form rigor bonds and become drag to the working cross-bridges. This kind of phenomenon can never be revealed by biochemical assay in which all myosin molecules are behaving independently (Fig. 4).

The depressive effect of acidosis on cardiac function has been well recognized. Although multiple factors have been proposed for cardiac dysfunction, an abnormality at the cross-bridge level is also suggested from this study. The optimal condition for movement was between pH 7.0 and pH 7.5 which is close to intracellular pH level. The response to pH was similar to that of skeletal myosin in a similar assay [27], but a bit different from that observed in an assay using fluorescent actin [10].

Relation Between Myosin Isoform and Velocity

As expected from the previous studies comparing myosins from different types of muscles, the sliding velocity of cardiac myosin in vitro was dependent on

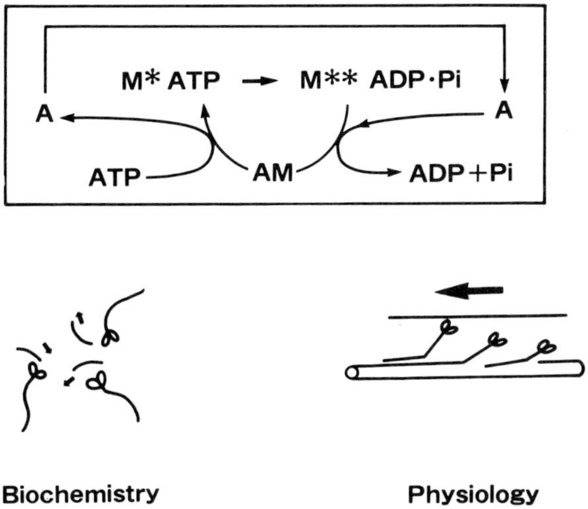

Fig. 4. Actomyosin-interaction. Proposed scheme for acto-myosin interaction. Biochemical assay (*lower left*): each myosin molecule interacts with actin independently. Motility assay (*lower right*): myosin molecules interact among them

the content of isoforms or ATPase activity. The velocity ratio between control and hyperthyroidism was about 2.4 which was close to the value obtained in intact muscle.

Whether there is a linear relation between α-MHC and velocity is questionable. Although the curvature of this relation was not clear in this study because of the lack of data points in the mid range, previous reports demonstrated negative results. The velocity of mixture of skeletal muscle myosin (high ATPase activity) and smooth muscle myosin (low ATPase activity) was studied by Sellers et al. [28] (myosin-coated beads) and Warshaw et al. [32] (fluorescent labeled actin filament). Both groups of researchers showed that the relation between the relative amount of skeletal muscle myosin and the velocity is non-linear. As Warshaw proposed [32], slow myosin may be a drag to fast myosin. This is another property which cannot be revealed by biochemical study. As for cardiac energetics this internal load should be taken into consideration when different isoforms coexist.

Future Direction

Although in vitro movement assays have already revealed many important findings, their application to cardiac physiology has just been initiated. Studies into not only the velocity but also the force of the acto-myosin interaction at molecular level are now being undertaken.

So far, the cardiac myosin-actin interaction has been estimated from the input-output relation of the muscle or whole heart (black box approach). However, the in vitro motility assay provides us with direct evidence for it. By this type of approach, we hope that the understanding of cardiac physiology will be greatly advanced.

References

1. Izumo S, Lompré AM, Matsuoka R, Koren G, Schwartz K, Nadard-Ginard B, Mahdavi V (1987) Myosin heavy chain messenger RNA and protein isoform transition during cardiac hypertrophy: interaction between hemodynamic and thyroid hormone-induced signals. J Clin Invest 79;970–977
2. Lompré AM, Nadard-Ginard B, Mahdavi V (1984) Expression of cardiac ventricular α- and β-myosin heavy chain genes is developmentally and hormonally regulated. J Biol Chem 259:6437–6446
3. Schwartz K, Lecarpentier Y, Martin JL, Lompré AM, Mercadier JJ, Swynghedauw B (1981) Myosin isozymic distribution correlates with speed of myocardial contraction. J Mol Cell Cardiol 13:1071–1075
4. Pagani ED, Julian FJ (1984) Rabbit papillary muscle myosin isozymes and the velocity of muscle shortening. Circ Res 54:586–594
5. Maughan D, Low E, Litten III R, Brayden J, Alpert N (1979) Calcium-activated muscle from hypertrophied rabbit hearts: mechanical and correlated biochemical changes. Circ Res 44:279–287
6. Hamrell BB, Low RB (1978) The relationship of mechanical V_{max} to myosin ATPase activity in rabbit and marmot ventricular muscle. Pflugers Arch 377: 119–124
7. Alpert NR, Mulieri LA (1983) Thermomechanical economy of hypertrophied hearts. In: Alpert NR (ed) Myocardial hypertrophy and failure. Raven Press, New York, pp 619–630 (Perspective in cardiovascular research, vol 7)
8. Huxley AF (1957) Muscle structure and theories of contraction. Prog Biophys Chem 7:255–318
9. Harada Y, Sakurada K, Aoki T, Thomas DD, Yanagida T (1990) Mechanochemical coupling in actomyosin energy transduction studied by in vitro movement assay. J Mol Biol 216:49–68
10. Kron SJ, Spudich JA (1986) Fluorescent actin filaments move on myosin fixed to a glass surface. Proc Natl Acad Sci USA 83:6272–6276
11. Yano m, Yamamoto Y, Shimizu H (1982) An actomyosin motor. Nature 299: 557–559
12. Spudich JA, Kron SJ, Sheetz MP (1985) Movement of myosin-coated beads on oriented filaments reconstituted from purified actin. Nature 315:584–586
13. Yanagida T, Nakase M, Nishiyama K, Oosawa F (1984) Direct observation of motion of single F-actin filaments in the presence of myosin. Nature 307:58–60
14. Chaen S, Oiwa K, Shimmen T, Iwamoto H, Sugi H (1989) Simultaneous recordings of force and sliding movement between a myosin-coated glass microneedle and actin cables in vitro. Proc Natl Acad Sci USA 86:1510–1514
15. Kishino A, Yanagida T (1988) Force measurements by micromanipulation of a single actin filament by glass needles Nature 334:74–76
16. Yanagida T, Arata T, Oosawa F (1985) Sliding distance of actin filament induced by a myosin cross-bridge buring one ATP hydrolysis cycle. Nature 316:366–369
17. Sheetz MP, Spudich JA (1983) Movement of myosin-coated fluorescent beads on actin cables in vitro. Nature 303:31–35

18. Shimmen T, Yano M (1984) Active sliding movement of latex beads coated with skeletal muscle myosin on *Chara* actin bundles. Protoplasma 121:132–137
19. Kamiya N, Kuroda K (1956) Velocity distribution of the protoplasmic streaming in *Nitella* cells. Bot Mag Tokyo 69:544–554
20. Kamitsubo E (1966) Motile protoplasmic fibrils in cells of *Characeae*. II. Linear fibrillar structure and its bearing on protoplasmic streaming. Proc Jap Acad 42: 640–643
21. Scholey JM (1990) Multiple microtubule motors. Nature 343:118–120
22. Kato T, Tonomura Y (1977) Identification of myosin in *Nitella flexilis*. J Biochem (Tokyo) 82:777–782
23. Nagai R, Hayama T (1979) Ultrastructure of the endoplasmic factor responsible for cytoplasmic streaming in Chara internodal cells. J Cell Sci 36:121–136
24. Korn ED (1982) Actin polymerization and its regulation by proteins from non-muscle cells. Physiol Rev 62:672–737
25. Vale RD, Szent-Gyorgyi AG, Sheetz MP (1984) Movement of scallop myosin on *Nitella* actin filaments: regulation by calcium. Proc Nat Acad Sci USA 81:6775–6778
26. Yamada A, Ishii N, Shimmen T, Takahashi K (1987) Thick filaments isolated from a molluscan smooth muscle show ATPase and sliding activities. Cell Struct Funct 12:620
27. Sheetz MP, Chasan R, Spudich JA (1984) ATP-dependent movement of myosin in vitro: characterization of a quantitative assay. J Cell Biol 99:1867–1871
28. Sellers JR, Spudich JA, Sheetz MP (1985) Light chain phosphorylation regulates the movement of smooth muscle myosin on actin filaments. J Cell Biol 101:1897–1902
29. Kohno T, Shimmen T (1988) Accelerated sliding of pollen tube organelles along *Characeae* actin bundles regulated by Ca^{2+}. J Cell Biol 106:1539–1543
30. Shimmen T, Yano M (1985) Ca^{2+} regulation of myosin sliding along Chara actin bundles mediated by tropomyosin. Proc Jap Acad (B) 61:86–89
31. Shimizu H Yano M (1978) Studies of the chemo-mechanical conversion in artificially produced streaming. J Biochem 84:1087–1092
32. Warshaw DM, Desrosiers JM, Work SS, Trybus KM (1990) Smooth muscle myosin cross-bridge interactions modulate actin filament sliding velocity in vitro. J Cell Biol 111:453–463
33. Harada Y, Noguchi A, Kishino A, Yanagida T (1987) Sliding movement of single actin filaments on one-headed myosin filaments. Nature 326:805–808
34. Toyoshima YY, Kron SJ, McNally EM, Niebling KR, Toyoshima C, Spudich JA (1987) Myosin subfragment-1 is sufficient to move actin filaments in vitro. Nature 328:536–539
35. Toyoshima YY, Toyoshima C, Spudich JA (1989) Bidirectional movement of actin filaments along tracks of myosin heads. Nature 341:154–156
36. Oiwa K, Chaen S, Kamitsubo E, Shimmen T, Sugi H (1990) Steady-state force-velocity relation in the ATP-dependent sliding movement of myosin-coated beads on actin cables in vitro studied with a centrifuge microscope. Proc Natl Acad Sci USA 87:7893–7897
37. Hoh JFY, McGrath PA, Hale PT (1977) Electrophoretic analysis of multiple forms of rat cardiac myosin: effects of hypophysectomy and thyroxine replacement. J Mol Cell Cardiol 10:1053–1076
38. Ebrecht G, Rupp H, Jacob R (1982) Alterations of mechanical parameters in chemically skinned preparations of rat myocardium as a function of isoenzyme pattern of myosin. Basic Res Cardiol 77:220–234

39. Josephson RA, Spurgeon HA, Lakatta EG (1990) The hyperthyroid heart. An analysis of systolic and diastolic properties in single rat ventricular myocytes. Circ Res 66:773–781
40. Dieckman LJ, Solaro RJ (1990) Effect of thyroid status on thin-filament Ca^{2+} regulation and expression of troponin I in perinatal and adult rat hearts. Circ Res 67:344–351
41. Katz AM (1977) Physiology of the heart. Raven Press, New York
42. Sugiura S, Yamashita H, Serizawa T, Iizuka M, Shimmen T, Sugimoto T (to be published) Active movement of cardiac myosin on *Characeae* actin cables.
43. Delcayre C, Swynghedauw B (1975) A comparative study of heart myosin ATPase and light subunits from different species. Pflugers Arch 355:39–47

2
Molecular Basis for Cardiac Adaptation to Overload

Yoshio Yazaki[1], Masahiko Kurabayashi[1], Issei Komuro[1]

Summary. The process of enlargement of the heart due to overload involves a significant reconstitution of the organ, including myocytes and intracellular constituents. We demonstrated the distribution of two types of cardiac myosin heavy chains (HCα and HCβ) in the human heart using monoclonal antibodies. The ventricle comprised mainly of HCβ has low ATPase activity, whereas the atrium was predominantly composed of HCα and has high ATPase activity. We also demonstrated isozymic transition of HCα to HCβ in the human atrium and ventricle by hemodynamic overload, regarded as a compensatory mechanism to meet an increased demand in work.

To examine the possibility that this isozymic transition of HCs due to overload is associated with the expression of the genes, we have isolated human HCα and HCβ cDNA clones from a fetal heart cDNA library. Comparison of the nucleotide and amino acid sequences deduced from these cDNA clones showed 91 and 96% homology, respectively. Using HCα and HCβ gene-specific sequences, we demonstrated that the transition of HCα to HCβ in the overloaded human heart was induced by the expression of HCβ gene.

To determine the role of cellular oncogenes in the process of cardiac growth and hypertrophy, we examined the expression pattern of eight cellular oncogenes during the developmental stage and pressure-overloaded hypertrophy of the rat heart by Northern blot analysis. c-*fos*, c-*myc* and c-Ha-*ras* were expressed in the heart in response to pressure overload and in a stage-specific manner, suggesting that these cellular oncogenes participate in the normal developmental process and hypertrophy of the heart. We also cloned the genes of which the expression level was rapidly changed by pressure overload by a differential hybridization technique. Our results suggest that clone 4 may be involved in the development of cardiac hypertrophy due to overload.

[1]Third Department of Internal Medicine, The Faculty of Medicine, University of Tokyo, Bunkyo-Ku, Tokyo, 113 Japan

Finally, we examined the molecular mechanisms by which mechanical stimuli induce cardiac hypertrophy and specific gene expression. For this purpose, we cultured rat neonatal cardiocytes in deformable dishes and imposed mechanical load by stretching the adherent cells. Myocyte stretching increased total cell RNA content and mRNA levels of c-*fos* and skeletal α-actin. The transfected chloramphenicol acetyltranferase gene linked to upstream sequences of the *fos* gene indicated that sequences containing a serum response element were required for efficient transcription by stretching.

The accumulation of c-*fos* mRNA by stretching was suppressed by protein kinase C inhibitors at the transcriptional level. Moreover, myocyte stretching increased inositol phosphate levels. We concluded from these data that mechanical stimuli might directly induce cardiac hypertrophy and specific gene expression, possibly via protein kinase C activation.

Key words: Cardiac hypertrophy — Cardiac myosin — Inositol phosphate — Protein kinase — Transactivating factor AP2

Introduction

During the process of enlargement of the heart due to overload, a significant reconstitution of the organ occurs, including myocytes and intracellular constituents, as well as cellular hypertrophy induced by increased synthesis of cellular components in order to meet an increased work demand. This adaptational phenomenon can be defined at the molecular level in terms of altered transcription of specific genes.

To analyze the molecular mechanism of the adaptive response of the heart to overload, one must be able to identify individual types of muscle proteins and their specific genes. Since analysis of cardiac myosin isoforms, whose enzymatic activities regulate both contractility and energy efficiency for contraction of the muscle, can provide insight into the process of cardiac hypertrophy, we developed monoclonal antibodies specific for two types of cardiac myosin and characterized these isoforms by immunofluorescence study. We mainly investigated human materials to obtain clinical implications from our observations. Furthermore, we cloned specific genes encoding the heavy and light chains of these cardiac myosin isoforms from the human cDNA library and demonstrated the regulation of their expression in the overloaded human heart. We also examined experimentally the transcriptional regulation of specific genes of which the early expression was observed in the heart after acute overloading, such as the cellular oncogenes, to investigate the mechanism of cardiac hypertrophy in vivo.

However, in the in vivo experiments of cardiac hypertrophy due to overload, we could not rule out the participation of humoral factors, such as norepinephrine and angiotensin II, which have recently been reported to induce hypertrophy in cardiac myocytes. From this point of view, to address the question of whether mechanical load directly regulates gene expression and increases protein synthesis in cardiac myocytes, we cultured cardiac myocytes in deformable silicone dishes and imposed a mechanical load on them by stretching. Using this method, we elucidated the signal transduction pathway of mechanical loading on cardiac myocytes. Furthermore, we analyzed the promotor function of the cardiac myosin alkali light chain gene, to elucidate how signals inducing cardiac hypertrophy are transmitted to gene regulation systems.

Redistribution of Cardiac Myosin Isozymes in the Human Heart Due to Overload

Enzymatic [1–4], electrophoretic [5–7], and immunochemical [8–10] analyses have shown the existence of two distinct cardiac myosin heavy chains, HCα and HCβ. However, it has not been conclusively determined that isoforms are present in human cardiac myosin, since nondenaturing pyrophosphate gel electrophoretic analysis failed to separate individual isozymes of human cardiac myosin. On electrophoretic gels, human cardiac myosin is composed of a single band, which appears to be very close to the rat V_3 isomyosin.

In order to discriminate between human cardiac HCα and HCβ, we prepared monoclonal antibodies specific for the heavy chains of either type HCα or HCβ. Anti-myosin monoclonal antibodies were produced by hybridomas obtained by fusion of myeloma cells (P3 × 63Ag8U1) with isolated spleen cells of BALB/c mice immunized with bovine atrial or human ventricular myosin as HCα or HCβ antigen, respectively, essentially by the method of Kohler and Milstein [11]. Two clones (CMA19 and HMC14) of hybrid cells secreting anti-myosin antibodies were selected for discriminating the antigenic difference between HCα and HCβ by ELISA tests [12, 13]. The distribution of myosin isozymes in human atrial and ventricular myocardium was investigated by immunofluorescence assay using these monoclonal antibodies. Human myocardial specimens were obtained from the patients with or without valvular disease during open heart surgery or at autopsy. Cryostat tissue sections were stained with the indirect immunofluorescence procedure.

Our immunofluorescence study using two types of monoclonal antibodies demonstrates (a) the existence of two types of myosin isozymes in the human myocardium, (b) a striking difference in their distribution between atrial and ventricular myocardium, and (c) significant regional variation in the number of ventricular myocytes containing HCα [12–14]. HCβ is the predominant myosin heavy chain isoform in the ventricle, whereas the main isoform is HCα in the atrium (Fig. 1). Considering that ventricular pressure is much higher than atrial pressure, and that HCβ appears to be suited for pressure work, the difference in the distribution of myosin isozymes between atrial and ventricular myocardium is regarded as a physiological adaptation to their loaded hemodynamic work.

Evidence has been accumulated that the relative proportions of the two basic isoforms of myosin change in rat and rabbit ventricles during development [8,

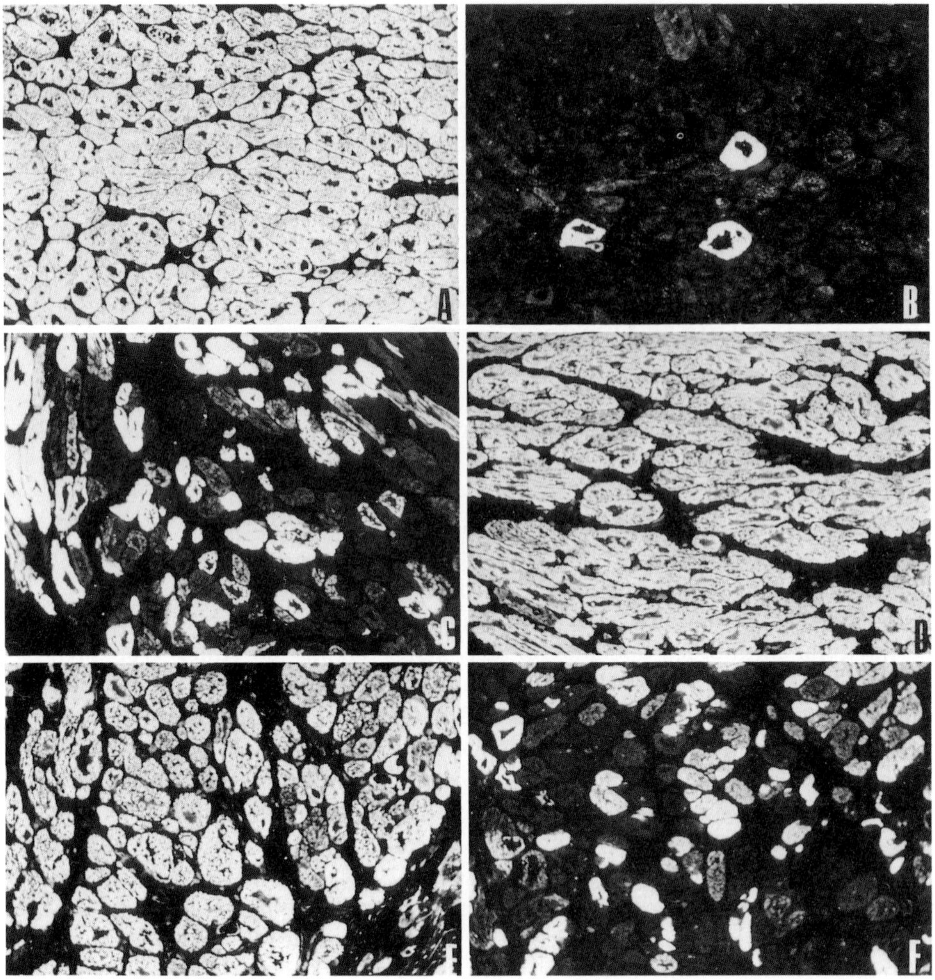

Fig. 1. Distribution of cardiac myosin in human atrial and ventricular tissues. **A** Cryostat section of normal human ventricle stained by HMC14. All fibers reacted strongly and uniformly. **B** as **A**, except that the muscle fibers were stained by CMA19. A small number of fibers were reactive. **C** Cryostat section of normal human atrium stained by HMC14. The staining intensity was highly variable. **D** as **C**, except that the myofibers were stained by CMA19. Almost all fibers were strongly reactive. **E** Cryostat section of a pressure-overloaded atrium stained by HMC14. The specimen was obtained from a patient with mitral stenosis and regurgitation. Almost all fibers became reactive. **F** as **E**, except that the myofibers were stained by CMA19. Unreactive fibers were significantly increased [12]

9, 15–17] and cardiac overload [18–21]. To confirm whether or not redistribution of these isozymes occurs in the overloaded human myocardium, we performed a further immunohistochemical study using monoclonal antibodies, CMA19 and HMC14.

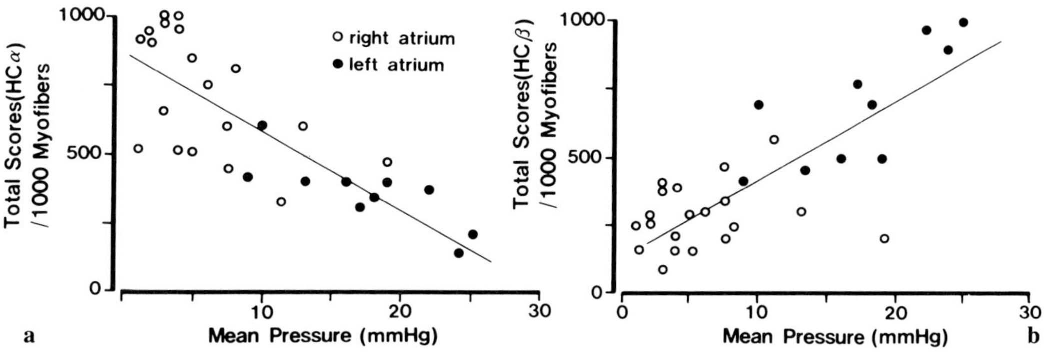

Fig. 2. Correlation between isozymic distribution of cardiac myosin and pressure-overload in human atrial tissues. The total scores per 1000 myofibers of HCα (**a**) or HCβ (**b**) plotted against the mean atrial or pulmonary capillary wedge pressure. (From [12] with permission)

When pressure-overloaded atria obtained from patients with mitral stenosis and/or regurgitation or tricuspid regurgitation during open heart surgery were stained by each antibody, a striking reversal of the staining pattern was observed (Fig. 1). The number of the myocytes reactive with HMC14 was increased significantly, while that of the myocytes reactive with CMA19 showed a corresponding decrease. To demonstrate the changes in the amount of each myosin isozyme more quantitatively, we counted the number of myocytes which reacted with each antibody and the total scores per 1000 myocytes were calculated in each specimen and plotted against each mean atrial pressure or mean pulmonary wedge pressure (Fig. 2). This observation revealed that the degrees of HCα decrement and HCβ increment correlated well with the mean atrial pressure [12]. We also observed a decrease in the number of myocytes reactive with CMA19 in the left ventricular specimen obtained from patients with mitral and/or aortic valvular disease according to the increment of peak left ventricular pressure [22]. These results showed that pressure overload may play a major role in the isozymic transition of cardiac myosin.

The isozymic redistribution in pressure overloaded myocardium may have a physiological implication. Since the low ATPase activity related to low velocity of shortening improves the efficiency of contraction for an equivalent amount of work as previously described [23–26], HCβ appears to be a physiological myosin isozyme for performing pressure work. Overloaded atrial myocytes may promote synthesis of HCβ instead of HCα in order to improve the efficacy of contraction. Thus, the isozymic redistribution can be considered as a physiological adaptive mechanism to meet increased pressure overload. Isozymic transition from HCα to HCβ in the overloaded atrium presented in our study may participate in a compensatory mechanism by which mechanical function of the atrium changes from volume work to pressure work. In the ventricular myocardium, normal myosin isozyme pattern has already been an exclusively HCβ-dominant one. Therefore, the physiological importance of isozymic

```
Glu Ala Val Asn Ala Lys Cys Ser Ser Leu Glu Lys Thr Lys His Arg Leu Gln Asn Glu Ile Glu Asp Leu Met Val Asp Val Glu Arg
GAG GCT GTT AAT GCC AAA TGC TCC TCA CTG GAG AAG ACC AAG CAC CGG CTA CAG AAT GAG ATA GAG GAC TTG ATG GTG GAC GTA GAG CGC   90
                            --- --G --- --- --- --- --- --- --- --- --- --- --C --- --- --- --- --- --- --- --- ---
                            --- --- --- --- --- --- --- --- --- --- --- --- --- --- --- --- --- --- --- --- --- ---

Ser Asn Ala Ala Ala Ala Ala Leu Asp Lys Lys Gln Arg Asn Phe Asp Lys Ile Leu Ala Glu Trp Lys Gln Lys Tyr Glu Glu Ser Gln
TCC AAT GCT GCT GCT GCT GCT CTG GAC AAG AAG CAG AGG AAC TTT GAC AAG ATC CTG GCC GAG TGG AAG CAG AAG TAT GAG GAG TCG CAG  180
--- --- --- --- --- --- --- --- --- --- --- --- --- --- --C --- --- --- --- --- --- --- --- --- --- --- --- --- --- ---
--- --- --- --- --- --- --- --- --- --- --- --- --- --- --- --- --- --- --- --- --- --- --- --- --- --- --- --- --- ---

Ser Glu Leu Glu Ser Ser Gln Lys Glu Ala Arg Ser Leu Ser Thr Glu Leu Phe Lys Leu Lys Asn Ala Tyr Glu Glu Ser Leu Glu His
TCT GAG CTG GAG TCC TCA CAG AAG GAG GCT CGC TCC CTC AGC ACA GAG CTC TTC AAG CTC AAG AAC GCC TAC GAG GAG TCC CTG GAG CAC  270
--G --- --- --- --- --G --- --- --- --- --- --- --- --- --- --- --- --- --A --- --- --- --- --T --- --- --- --- --A --T
--- --- --- --- --- --- --- --- --- --- --- --- --- --- --- --- --- --- --- --- --- --- --- --- --- --- --- --- --- ---

Leu Glu Thr Phe Lys Arg Glu Asn Lys Asn Leu Gln Glu Glu Ile Ser Asp Leu Thr Glu Gln Leu Gly Glu Gly Gly Lys Asn Val His
CTA GAG ACC TTC AAG CGG GAG AAC AAG AAC CTT CAG GAG GAA ATC TCG GAC CTT ACT GAG CAG CTA GGA GAA GGA GGA AAG AAT GTG CAT  360
--G --- --- --- --- --- --- --- --A --- --G --- --- --G --- --C --- T-G --- --- --- T-G --T TCC A-C --- --- -C- A-C ---
--- --- --- --- --- --- --- --- --- --- --- --- --- --- --- --- --- --- --- --- --- --- --- Ser Arg --- --- Thr Ile ---

Glu Leu Glu Lys Val Arg Asn Gln Leu Glu Val Glu Lys Met Glu Leu Gln Ser Ala Leu Glu Glu Ala Glu Ala Ser Leu Glu His Glu
GAG CTG GAG AAG GTC CGA AAC CAG CTG GAG GTG GAG AAG ATG GAG CTG CAG TCA GCC CTG GAG CAG GCA GAG GCC TCC CTG GAG CAC GAG  450
--- --- --- --- --- --- --G --- --- --- -CC --- --- --- --- --- --- --- --- --- --- --- --C --- --- --- --- --- --- ---
--- --- --- --- --- --- Lys --- --- --- Ala --- --- --- --- --- --- --- --- --- --- --- --- --- --- --- --- --- --- ---

Glu Gly Lys Ile Leu Arg Ala Gln Leu Glu Phe Asn Gln Ile Lys Ala Glu Ile Glu Arg Asn Val Ala Glu Lys Asp Glu Glu Met Glu
GAG GGC AAG ATC CTC CGG GCC CAG CTA GAG TTC AAC CAG ATC AAG GCA GAG ATC GAG CGG AAC GTG GCA GAG AAG GAC GAG GAG ATG GAA  540
--- --- --- --- --- --- --- --- --G --- --- --- --- --- --- --- --- --- --- --- --- *-- --- --- --- --- --- --- --- ---
--- --- --- --- --- --- --- --- --- --- --- --- --- --- --- --- --- --- --- --- --- --- --- --- --- --- --- --- --- ---

Gln Ala Lys Arg Asn His Gln Arg Val Val Asp Ser Leu Gln Thr Ser Leu Asp Ala Glu Thr Arg Ser Arg Asn Glu Val Leu Arg Val
CAG GCC AAG CGC AAC CAC CAG CGG GTG GTG GAC TCG CTG CAG ACC TCC CTG GAT GCA GAG ACA CGC AGC CGC AAC GAG GTC CTG AGG GTG  630
--- --- --- --- --- --- -T- --- --* --- --- --- --- --- --- --- --- --C --- --- --- --- --- --- --- --- -C- --- --- ---
--- --- --- --- --- --- Leu --- --- --- --- --- --- --- --- --- --- --- --- --- --- --- --- --- --- --- Ala --- --- ---

Lys Lys Lys Met Glu Gly Asp Leu Asn Glu Met Glu Ile Gln Leu Ser His Ala Asn Arg Met Ala Ala Glu Ala Gln Lys Gln Val Lys
AAG AAG AAG ATG GAA GGA GAC CTC AAT GAG ATG GAG ATC CAG CTC AGC CAC GCC AAC CGC ATG GCT GCC GAG GCC CAG AAG CAA GTC AAG  720
--- --- --- --- --- --- --- --- --- --- --- --- --- --- --- --- --- --- --- --- --- --C --- --- --- --- --- --- --- ---
--- --- --- --- --- --- --- --- --- --- --- --- --- --- --- --- --- --- --- --- --- --- --- --- --- --- --- --- --- ---

Ser Leu Gln Ser Leu Leu Lys Asp Thr Gln Ile Gln Leu Asp Asp Ala Val Arg Ala Asn Asp Asp Leu Lys Glu Asn Ile Ala Ile Val
AGC CTC CAG AGC TTG CTG AAG GAC ACC CAG ATC CAG CTG GAC GAT GCG GTC CGT GCC AAC GAC GAC CTG AAG GAG AAC ATC GCC ATC GTG  810
--- --- --- --- --- T-- --- --- --- --- --T --- --- --- --- --A --- --- --- --- --- --- --- --- --- --- --- --- --- ---
--- --- --- --- --- --- --- --- --- --- --- --- --- --- --- --- --- --- --- --- --- --- --- --- --- --- --- --- --- ---

Glu Arg Arg Asn Asn Leu Leu Gln Ala Glu Leu Glu Glu Leu Arg Ala Val Val Glu Gln Thr Glu Arg Ser Arg Lys Leu Ala Glu Gln
GAG CGG CGC AAC AAC CTG CTG CAG GCT GAG CTG GAG GAG TTG CGC GCC GTG GTG GAG CAG ACG GAG CGG TCC CGG AAG CTG GCG GAG CAG  900
--- --- --- --- --- --- --- --- --- --- --- --- --- --- --- --- --- --- --- --- --A --- --- --- --- --- --- --- --- ---
--- --- --- --- --- --- --- --- --- --- --- --- --- --- --- --- --- --- --- --- --- --- --- --- --- --- --- --- --- ---

Glu Leu Ile Glu Thr Ser Glu Arg Val Gln Leu Leu His Ser Gln Asn Thr Ser Leu Ile Asn Gln Lys Lys Lys Met Asp Ala Asp Leu
GAG CTG ATT GAG ACT AGT GAG CGC GTG CAG CTG CTG CAT TCC CAG AAC ACC AGC CTC ATC AAC CAG AAG AAG AAG ATG GAT GCT GAC CTG  990
--- --- --- --- --- --- --- --G --- --- --- --- --- --- --- --- --- --- --- --- --- --- --- --- --- --- --C --- --- ---
--- --- --- --- --- --- --- --- --- --- --- --- --- --- --- --- --- --- --- --- --- --- --- --- --- --- --- --- --- ---

Ser Gln Leu Gln Ser Glu Val Glu Glu Ala Val Gln Glu Cys Arg Asn Ala Glu Glu Lys Ala Lys Lys Ala Ile Thr Asp Ala Ala Met
TCC CAG CTC CAG TCG GAA GTG GAG GAG GCA GTG CAG GAG TGC AGA AAC GCC GAG GAG AAG GCC AAG AAG GCC ATC ACG GAT GCC GCC ATG 1080
--- --- --- --- A-T --- --- --- --- --- --- --- --- --- --G --T --T --- --- --- --- --- --- --- --- -*- --- --- --- ---
--- --- --- --- Thr --- --- --- --- --- --- --- --- --- --- --- --- --- --- --- --- --- --- --- --- --- --- --- --- ---

Met Ala Glu Glu Leu Lys Lys Glu Gln Asp Thr Ser Ala His Leu Glu Arg Met Lys Lys Asn Met Glu Gln Thr Ile Lys Asp Leu Gln
ATG GCA GAG GAG CTG AAG AAG GAG CAG GAC ACC AGC GCC CAC CTG GAG CGC ATG AAG AAG AAC ATG GAG CAG ACC ATT AAG GAC CTG CAG 1170
--- --- --- --- --- --- --- --- --- --- --- --- --- --- --- --- --- --- --- --- --- --- --A --- --- --- --- --- --- ---
--- --- --- --- --- --- --- --- --- --- --- --- --- --- --- --- --- --- --- --- --- --- --- --- --- --- --- --- --- ---

His Arg Leu Asp Glu Ala Glu Gln Ile Ala Leu Lys Gly Gly Lys Lys Gln Leu Gln Lys Leu Glu Ala Arg Val Arg Glu Leu Glu Gly
CAC CGG CTG GAC GAG GCC GAG CAG ATC GCC CTC AAG GGC GGC AAG AAG CAG CTG CAG AAG CTG GAA GCG CGG GTG CGG GAG CTG GAG GGT 1260
--- --- --- --- --A --- --- --- --- --- --- --- --- --- --- --- --- --- --- --- --- --- --- --- --- --- --- --- --- AA-
--- --- --- --- --- --- --- --- --- --- --- --- --- --- --- --- --- --- --- --- --- --- --- --- --- --- --- --- --- Asn

Glu Leu Glu Ala Glu Gln Lys Arg Asn Ala Glu Ser Val Lys Gly Met Arg Lys Ser Glu Arg Arg Ile Lys Glu Leu Thr Tyr Gln Thr
GAG CTG GAG GCC GAG CAG AAG CGC AAC GCA GAG TCG GTG AAG GGC ATG AGG AAG AGC GAG CGG CGC ATC AAG GAG CTC ACC TAC CAG ACA 1350
--- --- --- --- --- --- --- --- --- --- --- --- --- --- --- --- --- --- --- --- --- --- --- --- --- --- --- --- --- --G
--- --- --- --- --- --- --- --- --- --- --- --- --- --- --- --- --- --- --- --- --- --- --- --- --- --- --- --- --- ---

Glu Glu Asp Lys Lys Asn Leu Leu Arg Leu Gln Asp Leu Val Asn Lys Leu Gln Leu Lys Val Lys Ala Tyr Lys Gly Gln Ala Glu Glu
GAG GAG GAC AAA AAG AAC CTG CTG CGG CTG CAG GAC CTG GTA AAC AAG CTG CAA CTG AAG GTC AAG GCC TAC AAG GGC CAG GCC GAA GAG 1440
--- --- --- -GG --A --- --- --- --- --- --- --- --- --- G-- --- --- --G --A --- --- --- --- --- --- C-- --- --- --G ---
--- --- --- Arg --- --- --- --- --- --- --- --- --- --- Asp --- --- --- --- --- --- --- --- --- --- Arg --- --- --- ---

Ala Glu Glu Arg Ala Asn Thr Asn Leu Ser Lys Phe Arg Lys Val Gln His Glu Leu Asp Glu Ala Glu Glu Arg Ala Asp Ile Ala Glu
GCG GAG GAG CGA GCC AAC ACC AAC CTG TCC AAG TTC CGC AAG GTG CAG CAT GAG CTG GAT GAG GCA GAG GAG CGG GCG GAC ATC GCT GAG 1530
--- --- --- -A- --- --- --- --- --- --- --- --- --- --- --- --- --C --- --- --- --- --- --- --- --- --- --- --- --C ---
--- --- --- Gln --- --- --- --- --- --- --- --- --- --- --- --- --- --- --- --- --- --- --- --- --- --- --- --- --- ---

Ser Gln Val Asn Lys Leu Arg Ala Lys Ser Arg Asp Ile Gly Ala Lys Lys Met His Asp Glu Glu END
TCC CAG GTC AAC AAG CTT CGA GCC AAG AGC CGT GAC ATT GGT GCC AAG AAA ATG CAC GAT GAG GAG TGA  CACTGCCTCGGGAACCTCACTGCTTG 1619
--- --- --- --- --- --G --G --- --- --- --- --- --- --C A-G --- GGC T-- A-T --G --- T--  CTT  TG-CA-A--TT--T-TG-T-A--GCC
--- --- --- --- --- --- --- --- --- --- --- --- --- --- Thr --- Gly Leu Asn Glu --- END

CCAACCTGTAATAAATATGAGTGCC(A)n
TG-GGTGCC-GC---GCCCCA---TGGAGCCTGTGTAACAGCTCGCTTGGGAGGAAGCAGAATAAAGCAATTTCCTTGAAGCCG(A)n
```

redistribution in the human heart induced by overload seems to be greater in the atrium than in the ventricle, since the content of HCα which could be transformed to HCβ is much larger in the atrial myocardium.

Molecular Cloning and Characterization of Human Cardiac α- and β-type Myosin Heavy Chain cDNA Clones: Regulation of Their Expression During Pressure Overload

To understand the molecular basis of the myosin heavy chain isozyme transition in overloaded human myocardium, we investigated the level of expression of individual myosin heavy chain mRNA in the pressure-overloaded human atrium. For this purpose, we isolated two cDNA clones encoding either HCα or HCβ from a fetal human heart cDNA library and analyzed the different accumulation of these mRNAs in the human heart with Northern blot hybridization using the cDNAs as probes.

Our successful cloning of HCα and HCβ cDNAs has established the existence of the two molecular variants in the human heart [27]. In Fig. 3, the nucleotide sequences of these two types of heavy chain cDNA clones are compared. These cDNAs are quite homologous, exhibiting 96% nucleotide homology within the translated region. Only 77 out of 1596 nucleotides compared in our study are divergent. In contrast, 3′-untranslated regions show extensive sequence divergence.

We examined the expression of these two types of myosin heavy chain genes in the human heart by Northern blot analysis using the cDNAs as probes. Since the nucleotide sequences of these two cDNAs are highly homologous, it is difficult to identify the specific heavy chain mRNA expressed in the myocardium by RNA blot analysis using the cDNA coding sequence. To overcome this difficulty, synthetic oligonucleotide probes complementary to the unique 3′-untranslated regions were used in Northern blot analysis.

Hybridization patterns of atrial mRNA from patients whose atria suffered from pressure overload by valvular disease or pulmonary hypertension are shown in Fig. 4. Nine patients were examined [27]. In the control patient who died from breast cancer, HCα mRNA was predominant in both right and left atria. However, in pressure-overloaded atria, accumulation of HCβ mRNA was observed. In Fig. 4, patient 1 shows the hybridization pattern of atrial

←

Fig. 3. Nucleotide and deduced amino acid sequences of HCα and HCβ clones. Nucleotides are numbered to the right of each line. *Line 1*, amino acid sequence of the HCα clone; *line 2*, nucleotide sequence of the HCα clone; *line 3*, nucleotide sequence of the HCβ clone; *line 4*, amino acid sequence of the HCβ clone. Nucleotides and amino acids are written only where different from those of the HCα clone. The dashed line indicates an identical sequence to that of the HCα clone. The *underlined 26 bases* represent complementary sequences of the oligonucleotides synthesized for probes. *Wavy lines* indicate the polyadenylation signal sequence [27]

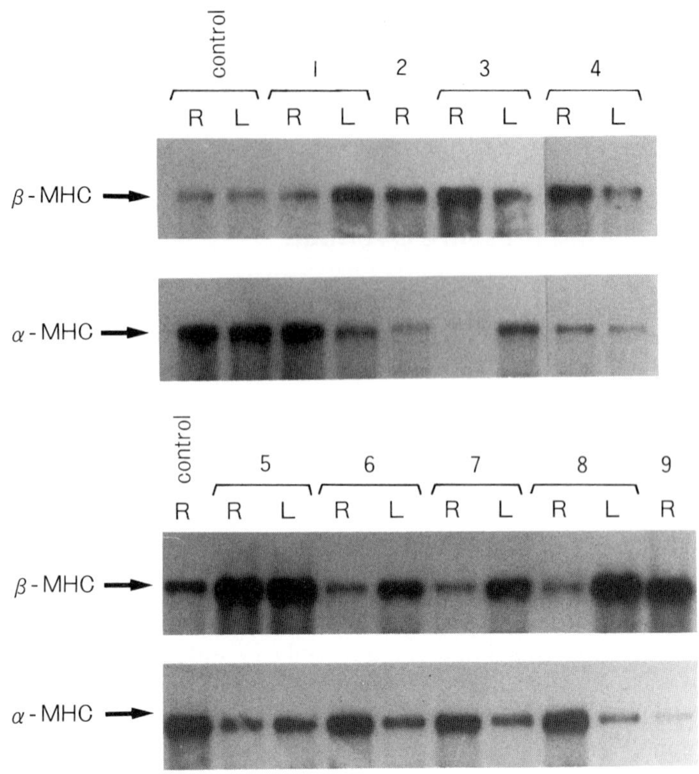

Fig. 4. Detection of HCα and HCβ mRNA in total cellular RNA from normal and diseased human atria. The same RNA blot was sequentially hybridized with labeled oligonucleotides specific for HCβ mRNA, exposure, 24h; HCα mRNA, exposure, 24h. Normal atrial RNA controls are shown in the *left* lanes. The lanes containing right (*R*) and left (*L*) atrial RNA (10μg) from patients 1 to 9 are indicated. The heavy chain mRNA band is marked *β-MHC*, *α-MHC* [27]

mRNA from the patient with mitral regurgitation. The strong hybridization of the left atrial mRNA with the HCβ probe was observed, whereas diminished hybridization with the HCα probe appeared. In this patient, the left atrium suffered from pressure overload. In patient 3, an almost complete reversal hybridization pattern was shown in the right atrial mRNA. Strong hybridization with the HCβ probe but very little hybridization with the HCα probe were observed. This patient suffered from primary pulmonary hypertension. In this case, the right atrium was submitted to pressure overload. The degrees of Northern blot of atrial mRNA with the proves were analyzed by densitometric scanning. The results are summarized in Fig. 5. In overloaded atria, the level of HCβ mRNA was significantly elevated, whereas the level of HCα mRNA was markedly decreased. Our study demonstrated that the HCα and HCβ gene in the human atrium also respond to hemodynamic overload in the same fashion as seen in the hypertrophied rat ventricle.

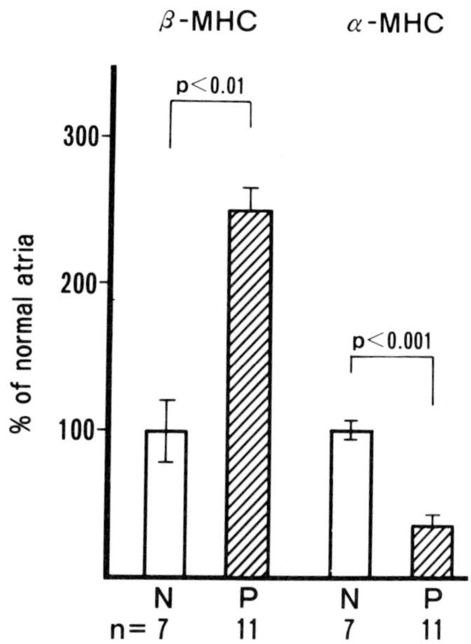

Fig. 5. Steady state mRNA content for HCα and HCβs in normal (*N*, n = 7) and pressure overloaded (*P*, n = 11) atria. Data from each group are presented as mean ± SE. RNA content in each atrium was quantitated by means of densitometric analysis of autoradiograms of Northern blots hybridized with the appropriate ^{32}P-labeled probes. Results are expressed as percentage of values in normal atria. Student's *t*-test indicated the HCβ mRNA level was significantly higher and the HCα mRNA level was significantly lower in pressure-overloaded atria compared with normal atria [27]

From the results of comparative examination by Northern blot hybridization and immunofluorescence staining, changes in the HCα and HCβ mRNA level are in a large part reflected by the changes in their respective proteins. Although immunofluorescence staining is not a quantitative determination, translation and post-translational mechanisms, if present, do not appear to play a major role in the production of heavy chain isozyme switches in response to hemodynamic overload.

It is very interesting to determine whether the same isoform transition occurs in cardiac myosin light chain. In an electrophoretical study [28], Cummins reported that the ventricular-type light chain replaces the atrial-type light chain in overloaded human atria. We have isolated essentially full-length cDNA clones encoding atrial or ventricular alkali light chains from a fetal human heart cDNA library and examined the level of each type of myosin light chain mRNA in overloaded atria by Northern blot analysis [29]. Our data demonstrated the increased level of ventricular light chain mRNA from overloaded atria (Fig. 6), suggesting that ventricular myosin light chain gene expression is upregulated by overload as observed in ventricular heavy chain gene expression. Although the physiological significance of ventricular light chain induction in overloaded atria remains unclear, the concomitant replacement of ventricular-type heavy and light chains should work against pressure overload.

From the data presented here, the following important question remains to be answered. What is the biochemical signal that regulates the HCα and HCβ gene expression in the pressure overloaded condition?

To resolve this question, we examined experimentally the expression of cellular oncogenes which participate in cell proliferation as well as in cell

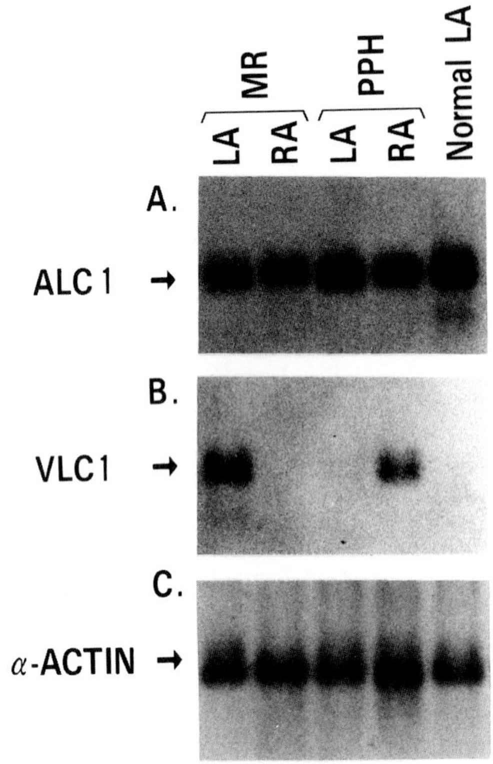

Fig. 6. Northern blot hybridization analysis of RNA from diseased human atria. Total RNA (10 μg) from the left atrium (*LA*) and right atrium (*RA*) of a patient with mitral regurgitation (*MR*), from the left atrium and right atrium of a patient with primary pulmonary hypertension (*PPH*), and from a normal left atrium were analyzed by Northern blotting. Specific ALCI and VLCI mRNA were detected by hybridization with each probe. The same RNA blot was sequentially hybridized with a mouse α-actin cDNA probe to show the integrity of the RNA samples [28]

transformation, using rat ventricular myocardium placed in the pressure overloaded condition due to aortic banding.

Characterization of Genes With Expression Levels Changed by Pressure Overload

Expression of Cellular Oncogenes During Cardiac Hypertrophy

Cellular hypertrophy and isoform switching were thought to be due to an increase in the transcriptional activity. Recently, several peptides were reported to regulate the transcriptional activity of genes. To investigate the molecular mechanism of cardiac hypertrophy and isoform switching, we studied genes with changed expression levels due to pressure overload.

Cellular oncogenes have been presumed to play a role in growth control. This hypothesis is strongly suggested by recent evidence that the products of several cellular oncogenes are either growth factors or growth factor receptors. To investigate the role of cellular oncogenes in the growth of the heart, the expression patterns of eight cellular oncogenes during the developmental stage and pressure-overloaded hypertrophy of rat hearts were examined [30].

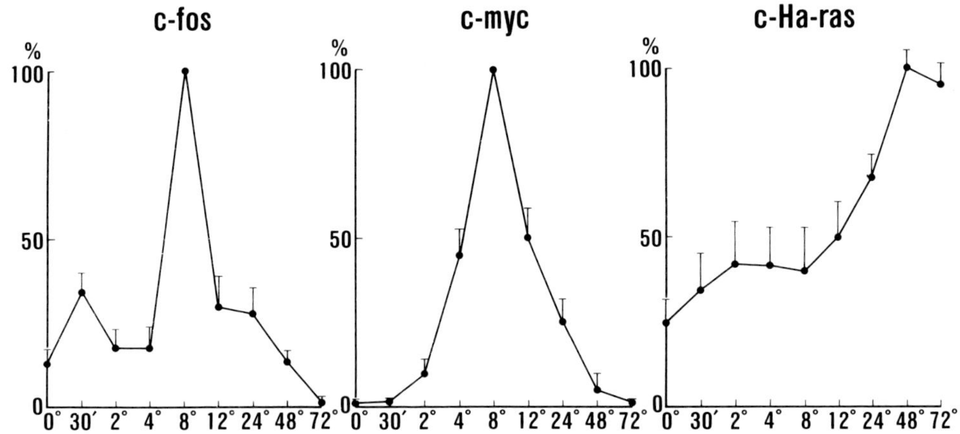

Fig. 7. Relative amounts of c-oncogene expression in pressure-overloaded cardiac hypertrophy. Relative amounts of c-oncogene expression were determined by soft-laser density scanning of the RNA blot autoradiograms. Relative optical density was plotted against time after aortic constriction, and values were expressed as percent to the highest level of expression of a given c-oncogene. Average levels from three separate experiments are shown [30]

To induce pressure-overloaded cardiac hypertrophy, the upper part of the abdominal aorta of 40-day-old male Wistar rats were constricted with a hemoclip. To investigate the developmental changes, hearts of embryos, neonates and adults were examined. After killing, RNA was extracted from the ventricles and 3 μg of poly(A) RNA was separated using 1.2% agarose gels, transferred to a nylon membrane, and mRNA was hybridized with eight oncogene probes (*myc*, *fos*, *sis*, Ha-*ras*, *erbA*, *erbB*, *myb*, *src*). Three oncogenes, c-*myc*, c-*fos*, and c-Ha-*ras*, which are known to play an important role in proliferation, were expressed in the pressure-overloaded hearts. Figure 7 shows the expressed patterns of these three genes. The increased expression of c-*fos*-related sequences were recognized from as early as 30 min after the operation. By densitometric scanning, the peak at 8 h after the operation showed an eight–ten-fold increase over the level of the pre-operative control. The level of expression was gradually decreased thereafter to the baseline at 48 h. The expression pattern of c-*myc* was similar to that of c-*fos*. Its expression was detectable 4 h after the operation, peaked at 8 h, and decreased to the base-line at 48 h. Some c-Ha-*ras*-related sequences were expressed in sham-operated hearts, and increased gradually after pressure overload.

c-*fos* is the cellular homolog of the oncogene of two mouse osteosarcoma viruses, FBJ-MSV and FBR-MSV [31]. All *fos* genes encode nuclear proteins and show a complex pattern of tissue-type, cell-type, and stage-specific expression [32], suggesting a correlation with the cellular differentiation process. In hypertrophic hearts, cellular differentiation should occur actively. For instance the β-myosin heavy chain was expressed 24 h after aortic constriction, and in the other contractile proteins, actin or tropomyosin, fetal isoforms were reported to be expressed in the hypertrophic hearts. So, it is of interest that the expression of c-*fos* showed a peak 8 h after aortic constriction and returned to the uninduced level by 48 h. During development, the level of c-*fos* expression was very low in fetal periods, and gradually increased. Although the role of c-*fos* is unknown, its expression was stage-specific, and these results suggest that c-*fos* might be related to the differentiation process during cardiac hypertrophy and aging.

c-*myc* also encodes nuclear protein, is expressed in relation to the cell cycle, and my play a role in cellular proliferation [33]. Recently, the expression of c-*myc* was reported to be increased in cultured cardiac myocytes hypertrophy induced by α_1-adrenergic agents [34]. In the present study, the c-*myc* gene was also expressed in pressure-overloaded hearts in vivo. Although the α_1-adrenergic mechanism may be activated by aortic constriction, further investigation is necessary to determine the stimuli inducing the expression of the c-*myc* gene and cardiac hypertrophy. The c-*myc* gene was expressed only in the fetal period, which is the proliferative period, suggesting that enhanced expression of the c-*myc* gene may be related to both cardiac cell division and cell hypertrophy.

Ha-*ras* genes encode 21-kDa proteins (p21) that appear to be involved in the control of cellular growth and differentiation [35], and mutations affecting *ras* genes and overproduction of normal p21 can induce a transformed phenotype [36]. Recently, p21 was reported to affect the phosphatidylinositol-4,5-bisphosphate breakdown pathway and the level of inositol-1,4,5-trisphosphate to be elevated in the *ras*-transformed cells [37]. In cultured cardiac myocytes, α_1-adrenergic agonists have been reported to induce hypertrophy via the phosphoinositide/protein kinase C pathway [34]. In this study, mRNA encoding the *ras* gene was highly expressed in the pressure-overloaded heart. These results and observations suggest that enhanced expression of the *ras* gene might be associated with cardiac hypertrophy.

In cardiac hypertrophy, c-*fos* and c-*myc* genes were expressed from the early period, and the expression of c-Ha-*ras* was gradually enhanced, as observed in cellular proliferation. In normal physiological development of the heart, the genes c-*fos*, c-*myc* and c-Ha-*ras* were each expressed in different periods (data not shown).

These results suggest that cellular oncogenes might participate in the normal developmental process and hypertrophy of hearts.

Molecular Cloning of Genes With an Expression Level Rapidly Changed by Pressure Overload

Hypertrophy of the left ventricles was evident 3 days after pressure loading. The isozymic transition of myosin heavy chain from α to β was detected 24 h after the aortic constriction, as determined at the mRNA level by α- and β-heavy chain specific oligo probes. Taken together, these results indicate that the genes with rapidly changed expression might produce 'signal peptides' for cardiac hypertrophy or isoform switching.

To clarify which genes had expression levels that changed as rapidly as 0.5–4h after aortic banding, we isolated their clones using a differential hybridization technique [38]. A rat heart cDNA library was hybridized with mRNA of normal and pressure-overloaded hearts using reverse transcriptase. The clones with expression levels changed by 8h pressure overload were isolated and subcloned to a plasmid vector. Four clones were selected and designated clones 2, 4, 5, and 6. The expression of clone 2 rapidly increased after the operation, and decreased thereafter. In the case of clone 4, in addition to the increased expression level, the distinctive isoform was expressed. The expression level of clone 5 decreased gradually, and a decrease of clone 6 was recognized at 8–12h.

In the embryonic period, hearts grow by cell proliferation as mentioned above. The expression of these clones were examined during the developmental stage. The expression pattern in embryonic hearts was similar to that of the hypertrophic hearts. The degree of expression of clones 2 and 4 was high in fetal and neonatal periods, and that of clones 5 and 6 was low in the fetal heart. The isoform of clone 4 was also recognized during the fetal period.

What mechanism induced the expression of clone 4? We examined this problem by the injection of cycloheximide, a protein synthesis inhibitor. The expression of its isoform was not inhibited by cycloheximide but was induced at 4h after injection, which suggested that this isoform was suppressed in normal adult hearts by some proteins. Furthermore, taken together with the previous results, the suppressive proteins were thought to be decreased in growing hearts, both hypertrophic hearts and embryonic hearts.

However, since these studies were performed in the heart in vivo, we could not rule out the participation of humoral factors, such as norepinephrine and angiotensin II, in the process of the protooncogene and early-response gene expression and hypertrophy in the overloaded myocardium.

To address the question of whether mechanical load directly regulates gene expression, or how mechanical stimuli are converted into intracellular signals of gene regulation, we imposed mechanical stress directly on myocytes by using deformable culture dishes, and examined gene expression.

Mechanical Load Stimulates Expression of the c-*fos* and Skeletal α-actin Genes

We devised deformable culture dishes to impose mechanical stimuli directly on cardiac myocytes. Whole culture dishes were made of silicone, with a 1-mm-thick dish bottom. The dish was highly transparent because no inorganic filler was used. We mechanically expanded the dishes with a plastic frame to increase their length uniaxially. Following expansion, attached cardiac myocytes were stretched. The resting length of the myocytes was increased parallel to the axis of expansion by the same percent length as the dish [39].

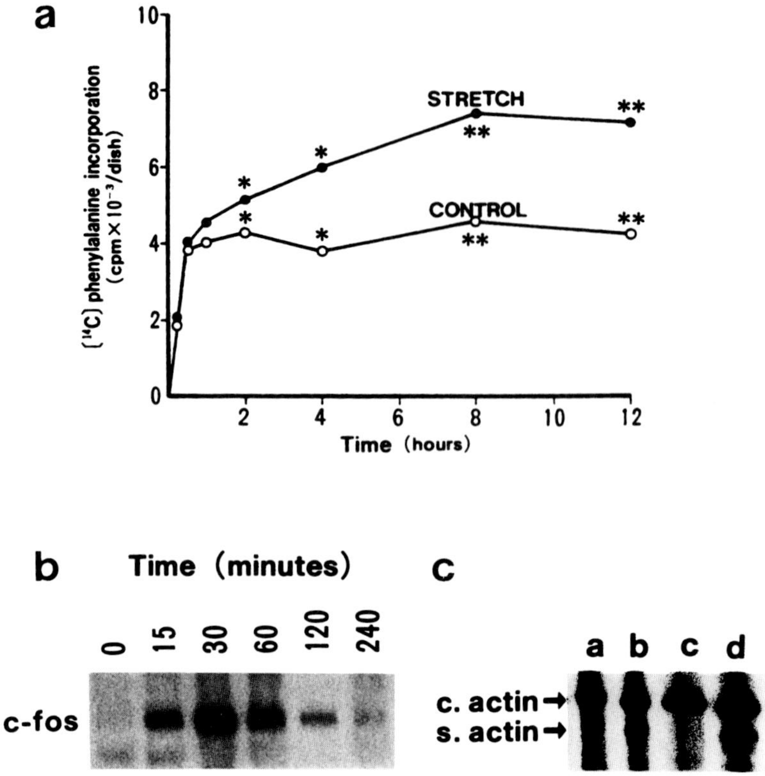

Fig. 8. Stimulation of amino acid uptake and c-*fos* and skeletal α-actin gene expression by myocyte stretching. **a** after 2 days maintained in a serum-free medium, culture dishes were stretched by 10% in length along a single axis and 1 μCi/ml ^{14}C-phenylalanine was added for 30 min prior to processing the cells for intracellular trichloroacetic-acid-insoluble radioactivity. Each point represents the mean ± SE from three experiments performed in duplicate. *, $P < 0.05$, **, $P < 0.01$. **b** cardiac myocytes were stretched by 10% for 30 min. RNA was extracted and 10 or 20 μg of total RNA (indicated in *parentheses*) was analyzed by Northern blot hybridization using a 0.8-kb *AccI* fragment of human c-*fos* as a probe. **c** cardiac α-actin (*c. actin*) and skeletal α-actin (*s. actin*) were separated by a primer extension technique. RNA was extracted from neonatal cardiocytes cultured for one (*a*, *b*) or two (*c*, *d*) days with (*b*, *d*) or without (*a*, *c*) stretching

This method allowed us to carry out more detailed analyses, such as quantitative assessment of mRNA levels, because we could obtain larger scaled samples.

We prepared primary cultures of cardiac myocytes from the ventricles of 1-day-old Wistar rats. A cardiac myocyte-rich fraction was obtained by the preplating method. Myocytes not attached to the preplated dishes were plated onto laminine-coated silicone dishes at a field density of 1×10^5 cells/cm^2. A nonmuscle-cell-rich fraction was obtained by preplating the cells onto silicone dishes for the first hour.

The effect of myocyte stretch on amino acid incorporation into cardiac proteins is shown in Fig. 8a. To avoid the effect of serum, we performed this experiment after 2 days in the serum-free, chemically defined medium. Myocytes were stimulated by 10% of linear length stretch of the attached dishes. At this point, more than 90% of cells were beating. The incorporation of ^{14}C-phenylalanine was significantly increased 2 h after stretch and the stimulation was maintained for over 12 h. This finding suggests that mechanical stress stimulates cardiac cellular hypertrophy.

To ascertain whether mechanical stress induces specific genes, such as protooncogenes and fetal-type isogenes of contractile proteins as observed in the heart in vivo, we examined the expression of c-*fos* and skeletal α-actin genes. Northern blot analysis revealed that c-*fos* was rapidly and transiently expressed by stretching in myocytes. The level of c-*fos* mRNA was increased as early as 15 min after the passive stretch of myocytes, and reached the maximum level at 30 min, followed by a decline to an undetectable level (Fig. 8b). The kinetics of this c-*fos* expression by stretching is the same as those when cells are stimulated with serum or growth factors. This protooncogene expression was observed abundantly in the cardiac myocyte-rich fraction rather than in the nonmuscle cell-rich fraction. This result confirmed that the stimulation of c-*fos* gene expression by stretching occurred in cardiac myocytes. The induction of c-*fos* mRNA depended on the stretch-length of the dishes. The stimulation of c-*fos* gene expression was recognized by 5% of linear length stretch of the dishes. The maximum stimulation was obtained by 20% of stretch.

Skeletal α-actin mRNA also accumulated after the passive stretch of myocytes. Skeletal α-actin mRNA was significantly increased 4 h after stretching, and gradually accumulated up to 2 days during stimulation (Fig. 8c). Because it has been known that acute pressure overload induces cardiac hypertrophy and gene expression, such as expression of protooncogenes and fetal-type isogenes of contractile proteins in the heart in vivo, our observations revealing the expression of c-*fos* and skeletal α-actin gene by myocyte stretching suggested that stretching cardiac myocytes in vitro could substitute for hemodynamic overload in vivo.

Transcriptional Regulation of the c-*fos* Gene by Myocyte Stretching

To examine whether c-*fos* gene expression by myocyte stretching was regulated at the transcriptional level or post-transcriptional level, we analyzed its promoter function using the CAT assay method [40]. We linked the 5′ flanking region of the *fos* gene, including its promoter, to the 5′ end of the chloramphenicol acetyltransferase (CAT) encoding sequences in a plasmid. The plasmid was transfected into primary cultures of neonatal rat cardiac myocytes and the CAT activity of the cell extracts was measured. The pSVO CAT construct containing the entire coding sequences of the procaryotic

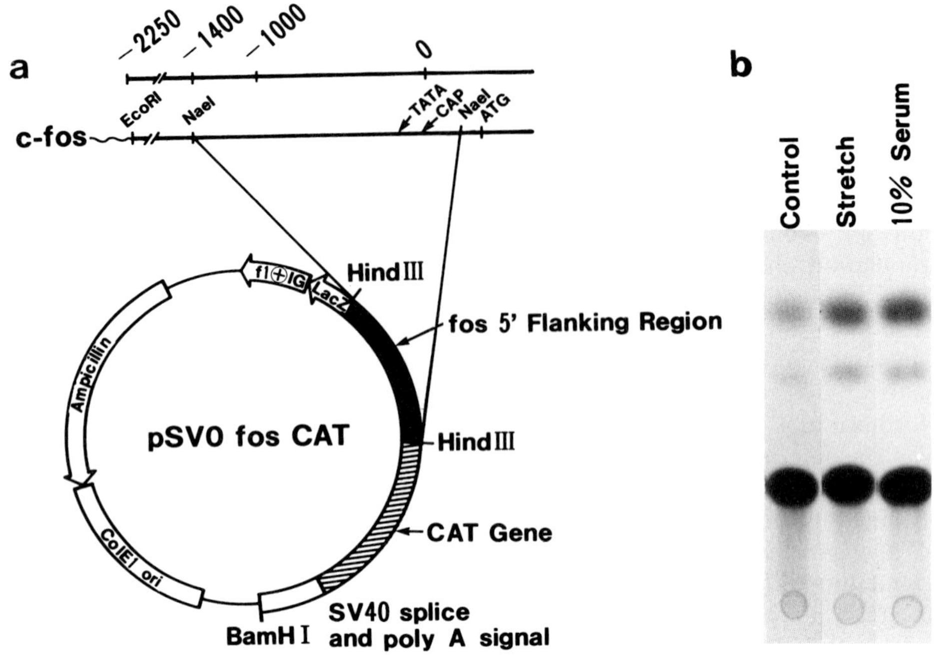

Fig. 9. Cardiocyte stretch responsiveness of CAT activity in transfected cells. **a** construction of recombinant plasmid pSV0fosCAT, containing the c-*fos* upstream and promoter region linked to the CAT coding sequence. A 1.4-kb *Nae*I fragment was cloned into the unique *Hin*dIII site in the pSV0CAT vector. **b** cultured cardiocytes were stretched by 10% 48 h after transfection with the plasmids pSV0fosCAT into primary 1-day-old rat heart myocytes. Autoradiograms of thin layer chromatograms using the assay mixture after 1 h of incubation are demonstrated. *Control*, unstretched cells; *stretch*, stretched cells; *10% serum*, cells incubated with 10% serum [39]

CAT gene minus its promoter showed very little CAT activity in either the absence or presence of stretch stimulation. By contrast, when pSVO *fos* CAT, which contained the 5′ c-*fos* flanking region, was introduced into the system, myocytes stretching reproducibly for 48 h showed more than a seven-fold increase in CAT activity, but there was little activity without stretching (Fig. 9). When the pSV2CAT construct, which contained SV40 enhancer and early promotor sequences, was introduced into myocytes, a large amount of CAT activity was observed. However, additional activity was not obtained after stretching. Furthermore, the run-on study using myocyte nuclei also revealed the accumulation of c-*fos* mRNA by stretching. These results suggested that the c-*fos* gene expression by stretching was regulated at the transcriptional level and that the stretch response element was located in the 5′ flanking region of the c-*fos* gene.

These results revealed that mechanical stress markedly induced the expression of the c-*fos* protooncogene without the participation of humoral factors.

Therefore, hemodynamic overload itself seems to be one of the main factors to stimulate the expression of the c-*fos* gene in the heart in vivo. Recently, Fos, the protein which the *fos* gene encodes, was found to be localized in the nucleus and to bind to the 12-0-tetradecanoylphorbol-13-acetate-responsive elements of some genes, followed by the activation of their gene transcription in cooperation with the transcription factor AP-1. These observations suggest that some early responsive gene products like Fos may stimulate other subsequent gene expressions in the heart under conditions of hemodynamic overload.

To identify the sequences essential for the transcription of the *fos* gene induced by stretching, we analyzed effects of deletion of the 5′ flanking region of the gene on CAT activity.

Mechanism of c-*fos* Gene Expression by Myocyte Stretching

Deletion mutagenesis of the 5′ flanking region of the c-*fos* gene indicated that the sequences between −227 and −404 base pairs were required for the efficient transcription of the *fos* gene by myocyte stretching (Fig. 10) [40]. Since it is known that there are serum and cAMP responsive elements in this region, we hypothesized that three known factors, cAMP, protein kinase C and tyrosine kinase, are involved in c-*fos* gene stimulation by stretching.

We therefore carried out a desensitization study to determine which protein kinase system plays a central role in the signal transduction induced by mechanical stress. We pretreated myocytes with either phorbol esters (TPA), epidermal growth factor (EGF) or forskolin for 24 h to down-regulate individual protein kinases, C kinase, tyrosine kinase or A kinase, respectively, and then treated again with one of these inducers. We assessed the mRNA level of c-*fos* using Northern blot analysis 30 min after treatment. Our results showed that, after pretreatment with TPA, c-*fos* stimulation was not obtained only with TPA. Again, the pretreatment with EGF or forskolin induced desensitization against only EGF or forskolin, respectively. The most important observation was that only the pretreatment with TPA desensitized myocytes against stretch (Fig. 11a). These results suggest that the induction of the c-*fos* gene by myocyte stretching might be caused by the activation of protein kinase C.

To confirm this possibility, we examined the effect of protein kinase C inhibitors on the expression of c-*fos* by myocyte stretch. H-7 strongly inhibited c-*fos* mRNA induction by stretching, whereas H-1004 inhibited it weakly, depending on their K_i value for protein kinase C. Staurosporin also strongly inhibited c-*fos* induction (Fig. 11b). Furthermore, the treatment of myocytes with TPA induced both c-*fos* and skeletal α-actin mRNA.

Finally, to examine the mechanism for the activation of protein kinase C by myocyte stretching, we measured phosphatidyl inositol turnover after myocyte stretch. Immediately after stretching, the activation of phosphatidyl inositol turnover was observed in myocytes. Inositol monophosphate and bisphosphate significantly increased 1 min after stretching, and reached about two-fold

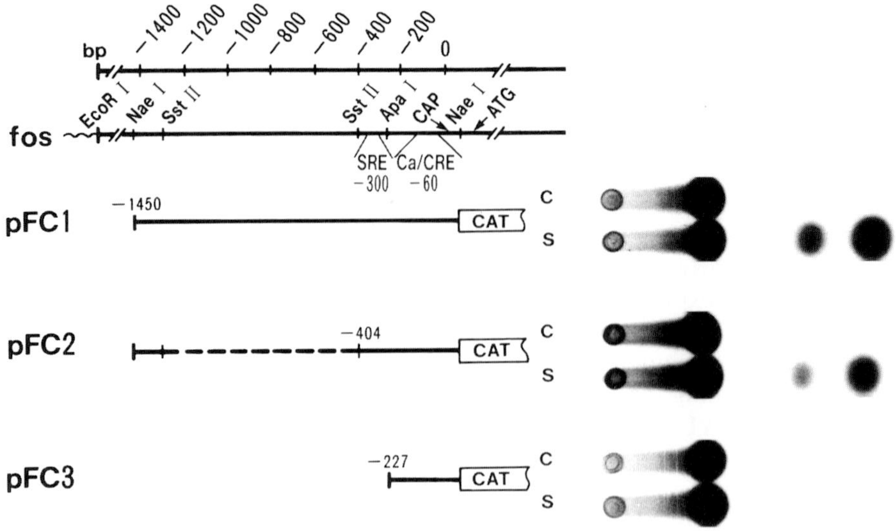

Fig. 10. CAT activity of c-*fos* recombinants containing deletions in the 5′ flanking region. Cardiac myocytes were transfected with 1 μg of DNA per dish and stretched for 2 h. Cell extracts were prepared and assayed for CAT activity. *C*, control cells; *S*, stretched cells; *SRE*, serum response element; *Ca/CRE*, calcium/cAMP response element [40]

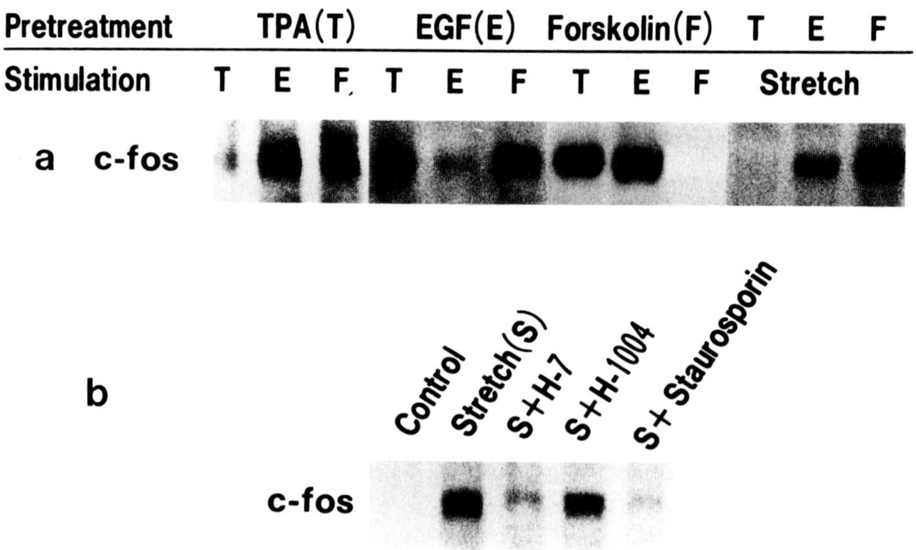

Fig. 11. Desensitization, down-regulation, and pharmacological study of c-*fos* induction. **a** myocytes were pretreated with 10 ng/ml TPA (*T*), 10 ng/ml epidermal growth factor (*EGF E*), or 1 μM forskolin (*F*) for 4 h, then stimulated by the same doses of these inducers or stretching for 30 min. **b** cells were stretched in the presence and absence of the indicated inhibitors for 30 min. RNA was extracted, run on a gel, and transferred to the filters. The filters were hybridized with the c-*fos* probe. *S*, stretched cells [40]

Fig. 12. Effect of stretching on the levels of inositol phosphates. Myocytes were incubated for 24 h in Dulbecco's modified Eagle's medium containing myo-[2-^{3}H]inositol and stretched 10% for the indicated times. The water-soluble inositol phosphates were separated by column chromatography. Each histogram represents the average percentage of control from five experiments performed in duplicate (mean ± SE). Control values (cpm × 10^{-2}/dish) were as follows: inositol monophosphate (IP_1), 160–350; inositol bisphosphate (IP_2), 30–42; inositol trisphosphate (IP_3), 62–93. Statistical significance was determined by analysis of variance [40] * $P < 0.05$, ** P, 0.01

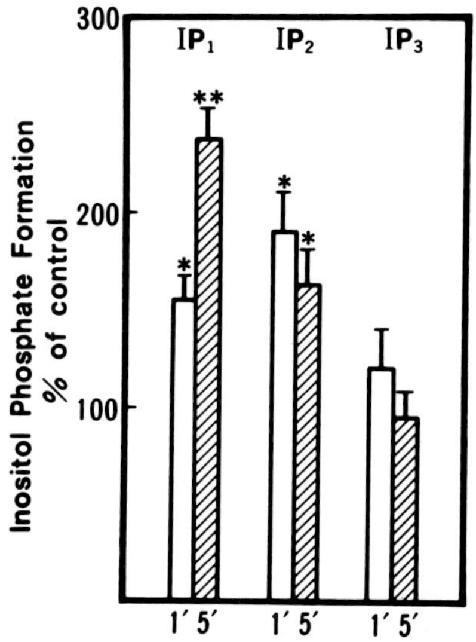

levels of the control after 5 min (Fig. 12). We could not detect the elevation of inositol trisphosphate levels at either time point. However, these results suggest that mechanical stress might stimulate protein kinase C activity via phospholipase C activation in cardiac myocytes. Recently, mechanical stress has been reported to induce prostaglandin production in skeletal and endothelial calls via the phospholipase C pathway. These reports might support our hypothesis. However, further investigation is necessary to elucidate the precise molecular mechanisms of how mechanical load activates phospholipase C or protein kinase C [40].

Molecular Bases for the Transcriptional Stimulation of the Cardiac Myosin Alkali Light Chain Gene: the Involvement of Protein Kinase Activation

To elucidate how signals inducing cardiac hypertrophy may directly regulate the transcription level of specific cardiac genes, we analyzed the promoter function of the ventricular myosin alkali light chain (VLCI) gene in relation to the activation of protein kinases [41]. Recently, we [29] and Cummins [28] have reported that VLCI mRNA was selectively induced in the pressure-overloaded human atria. Therefore, we considered the expression of the human VLCI gene a good model for studies of the hypertrophic response of the contractile protein genes in the heart.

Our myocyte-stretch experiments revealed that mechanical stress directly induced the expression of specific genes, such as the protooncogene, c-*fos*, the fetal type isogene, and the skeletal α-actin gene, as well as an increase in protein synthesis. Furthermore, our analysis of the promoter function of the c-*fos* gene stimulated by the passive stretch of myocytes suggested that the activation of protein kinase systems may be associated with the regulation of the gene expression induced by mechanical load.

On the other hand, evidence has been accumulated that the stimulation of α- or β-adrenoceptors by catecholamines induces cardiac hypertrophy and the expression of protooncogenes. Simpson et al. [42] have shown that the activation of protein kinase C induced by α_1-adrenoceptor stimulation might play an important role in the cellular hypertrophy of rat neonatum cardiac myocytes. Xenophontos et al. [43] have also reported that the elevation of cAMP content in perfused adult rat hearts by forskolin accelerates the protein synthesis rate. These observations suggest that the activation of protein kinase systems, including both protein kinase C and protein kinase A, may be involved in the regulation of gene expression during the process of cardiac hypertrophy induced by catecholamines.

Consequently, to examine the possibility that protein kinase systems directly regulate the transcriptional level of specific cardiac genes, we analyzed the promoter function of the VLCI gene by CAT assay. We fused the 5′ flanking region of the VLCI gene to the CAT gene in the plasmid and introduced this plasmid to rat neonatal myocytes. After transfection, the CAT activity of the cell extracts was measured. As predicted, phorbor esters and forskolin significantly increased CAT activity of the transfected myocytes. Deletion mutagenesis of the 5′ flanking region of the VLCI gene revealed the presence of positive and negative regulatory elements in the region up to −300 base pairs from the cap site. The proximal region located between −150 to −40 base pairs appears to determine the cell-type-specific high level expression of the VLCI gene in muscle cells. This region contains specific sequence elements, reffered to as a CArG box, the Myo D binding site and TC II motif (the SV40 enhancer element). When the TC II motif was deleted from the plasmid, neither cAMP nor forskolin could stimulate the expression of the VLCI gene. The TC II motif has been shown to be a binding site of the transcription factor AP2, which is identified as a mediator of signal transduction systems involving both protein kinase C and protein kinase A. Therefore, together with the observations that mechanically-induced and hormone-stimulated hypertrophy of cardiac myocytes might be associated with the activation of protein kinase systems, our results suggest that AP2 may be involved in the mechanism for the enhanced transcriptional activity of myofibrillar proteins during the hypertrophic process.

Acknowledgements. This investigation was supported in part by Grant-in-Aid for Scientific Research from the Ministry of Education, Science and Culture of Japan, grants from the Ministry of Welfare and Uehara Memorial Foundation, and for Basic Research on Cardiac Hypertrophy from the Vehicle Racing Commemorative Foundation.

References

1. Yazaki Y, Raben MS (1974) Cardiac myosin adenosine triphosphatase of rat and mouse: distinctive enzymatic properties compared with rabbit and dog cardiac myosin. Circ Res 35:15–23
2. Yazaki Y, Raben MS (1975) Effect of thyroid state on the enzymatic characteristic of cardiac myosin: a difference in behaviour of rat and rabbit cardiac myosin. Circ Res 36:208–215
3. Yazaki Y, Ueda S, Nagai R et al. (1979) Cardiac atrial myosin adenosine triphosphatase of animals and humans: distinctive enzymatic properties compared with cardiac ventricular myosin. Circ Res 45:522–527
4. Mercadier JJ, Bouveret P, Gorza L et al. (1983) Myosin isozymes in normal and hypertrophied human ventricular myocardium. Circ Res 53:52–62
5. Hoh JFY, McGrath PA, Hale PJ (1978) Electrophoretic analysis of multiple forms of rat cardiac myosin: effect of hypophysectomy and thyroxine replacement. J Mol Cell Cardiol 10:1053–1976
6. Flink IL, Raber JH, Morkin E (1979) Thyroid hormone stimulates synthesis of a cardiac myosin isozyme: comparison of the two-dimensional electrophoretic patterns of the cyanogen bromide peptides of cardiac myosin heavy chains from euthyroid and thyrotoxic rabbits. J Biol Chem 254:3105–3110
7. Chizzonite RA, Everett AW, Clark WA et al. (1982) Isolation and characterization of two molecular variants of myosin heavy chain from rabbit ventricle: change in their content during normal growth and after treatment with thyroid hormone. J Biol Chem 257:2056–2065
8. Sartori S, Gorza L, Pierobon-Bormioli S et al. (1981) Myosin types and fiber types in cardiac muscle. I. Ventricular myocardium. J Cell Biol 88:226–233
9. Clark WA Jr, Chizzonite RA, Everett AW et al. (1982) Species correlations between cardiac isomyosins: a comparison of electrophoretic and immunological properties. J Biol Chem 257:5449–5454
10. Gorza L, Sartore S, Schiaffino S (1982) Myosin types and fiber types in cardiac muscle. II. Atrial myocardium. J Cell Biol 95:838–845
11. Kohler G, Milstein C (1973) Continuous cultures of fused cells secreting antibody of predefined specificity. Nature 256:495–497
12. Tsuchimochi H, Sugi M, Kuro-o M et al. (1984) Isozymic changes in myosin of human atrial myocardium induced by overload: immunohistochemical study using monoclonal antibodies. J Clin Invest 74:662–665
13. Yazaki Y, Tsuchimochi H, Kuro-o M et al. (1984) Distribution of myosin isozymes in human atrial and ventricular myocardium: comparison in normal and overload heart. Eur Heart J 5(Suppl F):103–110
14. Kuro-o M, Tsuchimochi H, Ueda S et al. (1986) Distribution of cardiac myosin isozymes in human condition system: immunohistochemical study using monoclonal antibodies. J Clin Invest 77:340–347
15. Lompre AM, Mercardiar JJ, Winsewsky C et al. (1979) Myosin isozyme redistribution in chronic heart overload. Nature 282:105–107
16. Schwartz K, Lompre AM, Bouveret P et al. (1982) Comparison of rat cardiac myosin at fetal stages in young animals and in hypothyroid adults. J Biol Chem 257:14412–14418
17. Chizzonite RA, Everett AW, Prior G et al. (1984) Comparison of myosin heavy chains in atria and ventricles from hyperthyroid, hypothyroid, and euthyroid rabbits. J Biol Chem 259:15564–15571

18. Gorza L, Pauletto P, Pessina AC et al. (1981) Isomyosin distribution in normal and pressure-overloaded rat ventricular myocardium: an immunohistochemical study. Circ Res 49:1003–1009
19. Mercadier JJ, Lompre AM, Wisnewsky C et al. (1981) Myosin isozymic changes in several models of rat cardiac hypertrophy. Circ Res 49:525–532
20. Litten RZ, Martin BJ, Low RB et al. (1982) Altered myosin isozyme patterns from pressure-overloaded and thyrotoxic hypertrophied rabbit hearts. Circ Res 50: 856–864
21. Rupp H (1982) Polymorphic myosin as the common determinant of myofibrillar ATPase in different hemodynamic and thyroid states. Basic Res Cardiol 77:34–46
22. Kawana M, Kimata S, Taira A et al. (1986) Isozymic changes in myosin human ventricular myocardium induced by pressure overload. Circulation 74:11–82
23. Alpert NR, Murieri LA (1982) Increased myothermal economy of isometric force generation in compensated cardiac hypertrophy induced by pulmonary artery constriction in the rabbit. Circ Res 50:491–500
24. Ebrecht G, Rupp H, Jacob R (1982) Alteration of mechanical parameters in chemically skinned preparations of rat myocardium as a function of isoenzyme pattern of myosin. Basic Res Cardiol 77:220–234
25. Pagani ED, Julian FJ (1984) Rabbit papillary muscle myosin isozymes and the velocity of muscle shortening. Circ Res 54:586–594
26. Holubarsch C, Goulette RP, Litten RZ et al. (1985) The economy of isometric force development, myosin isozyme pattern, and myofibrillar ATPase activity in normal and hypothyroid rat myocardium. Circ Res 56:78–86
27. Kurabayashi M, Tsuchimochi H, Komuro I et al. (1988b) Molecular cloning and characterization of human cardiac α and β-form myosin heavy chain cDNA clones: regulation of expression during development and pressure overload in human atrium. J Clin Invest 82:524–531
28. Cummins P (1982) Transition in human atrial and ventricular myosin light-chain isozymes in response to cardiac pressure-overload-induced hypertrophy. Biochem J 205:195–204
29. Kurabayashi M, Tsuchimochi H, Komuro I et al. (1988a) Molecular cloning and characterization of human atrial and ventricular myosin alkali light chain cDNA clones. J Biol Chem 263:13930–13936
30. Komuro I, Kurabayashi M, Takaku F, Yazaki Y (1988) Expression of cellular oncogenes in the myocardium during the developmental stage and pressure-overloaded hypertrophy of the rat heart. Circ Res 62:1075–1079
31. Curran T, Teich NM (1982) Candidate product of the FBJ murine osteosarcoma virus oncogene: characterization of a 55,000-dalton phosphoprotein. J Virol 42: 114–122
32. Muller R, Muller D, Guilbert L (1984) Differential expression of c-*fos* in hematopoietic cells: correlation with differentiation of monomyelocytic cells in vitro. EMBO J 3:1887–1890
33. Campici J, Gray HE, Pardee AB (1984) Cell-cycle control of c-*myc* but not c-*ras* expression is lost following chemical transformation. Cell 36:241–247
34. Starksen NF, Simpson PC, Bishopric N et al. (1986) Cardiac myocyte hypertrophy is associated with c-*myc* protooncogene expression. Proc Natl Acad Sci USA 83: 8348–8350
35. Mulcahy LS, Smith MR, Stacey DW (1985) Requirement for ras protooncogene function during serum-stimulated growth of NIT 3T3 cells. Nature 313:241–243

36. Chang EH, Furth ME, Scolnick EM (1982) Tumorigenic transformation of mammalian cells induced by a normal human gene homologous to the oncogene of Harvey murine sarcoma virus. Nature 297:479–483
37. Fleischman LF, Chahwala SB, Cantley L (1986) *Ras*-transformed cells: altered levels of phosphatidylinositol-4,5-bisphosphate and catabolites. Science 231: 407–410
38. Komuro I, Shibazaki Y, Kurabayashi M et al. (1990) Molecular cloning of gene sequences from rat heart rapidly responsive to pressure overload. Circ Res 66(4): 979–985
39. Komuro I, Kaida T, Shibazaki Y et al. (1990) Stretching cardiac myocytes stimulates protooncogene expression. J Biol Chem 265:3595–3598
40. Komuro I, Katoh Y, Kaida T et al. (1991) Mechanical loading stimulates cell hypertrophy and specific gene expression in cultured rat cardiac myocytes. J Biol Chem 266:1265–1268
41. Kurabayashi M, Komuro I, Shibasaki Y et al. (1990) Functional identification of the transcriptional regulatory elements within the promoter region of the human ventricular myosin alkali light chain gene. J Biol Chem 265:19271–19278
42. Simpson P (1985) Stimulation of hypertrophy of cultured neonatal rat heart cells through an α_1-adrenergic receptor and induction of beating through an α_1- and β_1-adrenergic receptor interaction: evidence for independent regulation of growth and beating. Circ Res 56:884–894
43. Xenophontos XP, Watson PA, Chua BHL, et al. (1989) Increased cyclic AMP content accelerates protein synthesis in rat heart. Circ Res 65:647–656

3

Role of Ca^{2+} Overload in Myocardial Contractile Dysfunction

Masatsugu Hori[1], Yukihiro Koretsune[1], Masafumi Kitakaze[1], Hideo Kusuoka[2], Eduardo Marban[2], Michitoshi Inoue[1]

Summary. Despite a paucity of direct evidence, calcium appears in the center of most hypothetical schemes that link ischemia to histological or functional abnormalities. If calcium concentration rises within the cell and remains elevated, a number of unfavorable sequelae can ensue.

Previous studies suggest that intracellular calcium acts as a mediator of injury in reversible contractile dysfunction: low-$[Ca]_o$ reperfusion, pretreatment of hearts with ryanodine, or acidosis during early reperfusion virtually prevent myocardial stunning. Taken together, calcium overload may play a crucial role in the pathogenesis of myocardial stunning. In this chapter, we summarize the role of calcium in myocardial cell injury during ischemia and reperfusion. We also describe the role of calcium overload in the failing heart.

Almost all measurements of intracellular Ca^{2+} concentration ($[Ca^{2+}]_i$) have been performed in superfused muscle or dissociated cells whose responses cannot be assumed to resemble those of the native tissue. In particular, the effects of alterations in coronary perfusion cannot be mimicked in isolated muscle or cells. To check $[Ca^{2+}]_i$ directly in perfused hearts, we used fluorine-19 NMR spectroscopy in a series of studies to measure a Ca^{2+}-sensitive chemical shift of 5,5′-difluoro BAPTA.

Key words: Stunned myocardium — NMR spectroscopy — Heart failure — 5F-BAPTA — Myocardial ischemia

Introduction

Calcium ions play a key role as intermediaries of cell function in cardiac muscle. Such physiological actions are made possible by the low Ca^{2+} concentration normally present within the cells of the myocardium. The cytoplasmic Ca^{2+}

[1] The First Department of Medicine, Osaka University Medical School, Osaka, 553 Japan
[2] Division of Cardiology, Department of Medicine, The Johns Hopkins University, School of Medicine, Baltimore, Md 21205, U.S.A.

concentration ($[Ca^{2+}]_i$) of unstimulated cells is approximately 10^{-7} M, whereas extracellular Ca^{2+} concentration ranges around 10^{-3} M [1]. This chemical gradient for Ca^{2+} is magnified by the normal electronegativity of the interior of the resting cell. It is well known that the influx of Ca^{2+} into the myocardial cell occurs during the plateau phase of the action potential through a set of membrane proteins which are permeable primarily to Ca^{2+}, termed "slow channels" or voltage-dependent calcium channels [2]. The absolute quantity of Ca^{2+} that crosses the sarcolemma during each beat is relatively small and incapable by itself of bringing about full activation of the contractile apparatus in mammalian heart cells [3, 4]. Instead, the major portion of the Ca^{2+} used to activate contraction is stored within the cell, largely in the sarcoplasmic reticulum from which Ca^{2+} is released by the Ca^{2+} which enters the cell through the slow channels (calcium-induced calcium release) [5]. The released Ca^{2+} then diffuses toward the myofibrils and triggers the contractile process by binding to troponin C and enabling the interaction of actin and myosin. The number of activated contractile elements and the resultant force generated are directly related to the quantity of Ca^{2+} present in the vicinity of the myofibrils, which ultimately depends on the influx of Ca^{2+} through the slow channels. Relaxation of cardiac muscle results from a cessation of the inward slow Ca^{2+} current coupled with the uptake of Ca^{2+} by sarcoplasmic reticulum and the extrusion of Ca^{2+} by the sarcolemmal Na^+-Ca^{2+} exchange. Therefore, the abnormal handling of Ca^{2+} in cardiac muscle may lead to dysfunction of contraction and relaxation of the heart. The role of abnormal Ca handling in myocardial dysfunction is discussed in this chapter.

Calcium and Its Role in Myocardial Cell Injury During Ischemia and Reperfusion

Contractile dysfunction in heart muscle after a period of ischemia brief enough to avoid necrosis is defined as "myocardial stunning" [6, 7]. Although the phenomenon has important clinical implications for reperfusion therapy, the cellular mechanisms of the contractile dysfunction after reperfusion remain unclear. Stunned myocardium is responsive to catecholamines [8–10], and to an increase in the extracellular Ca^{2+} ($[Ca]_o$) [11, 12]. However, the maximal response is attenuated [11]. Despite a paucity of direct evidence, calcium appears in the center of most hypothetical schemes that link ischemia to histological or functional abnormalities. If calcium concentration rises within the cell and remains elevated, a number of unfavorable sequelae can ensue. First of all, much of the high energy phosphate supply will be spent in the sequestration of calcium into the sarcoplasmic reticulum and into mitochondria. The sequestration of calcium into mitochondria also decreases oxidative phosphorylation, thereby compounding the imbalance of energy supply and demand [13]. Second, an increase in the intracellular free Ca^{2+} concentration ($[Ca^{2+}]_i$) will activate a number of enzymes that are capable of damaging cell membranes and cytoskeletons. One such Ca^{2+}-activated protease has been proposed as an agent which may destruct the cytoskeletal proteins during myocardial ischemia [14]. Third, calcium can trigger the phosphorylation of a variety of cellular proteins [15] by Ca^{2+}-activated calmodulin-dependent protein kinase, and alter their functions. Fourth, an increase in $[Ca^{2+}]_i$ favors triggered arrhythmias mediated by delayed afterdepolarizations [16]. The notoriety of calcium thus stems from its protean metabolic roles which render it capable of modulating virtually any cellular process.

Previous studies suggest that intracellular calcium acts as a mediator of injury in reversible contractile dysfunction: (a) low-$[Ca]_o$ reperfusion after 15 min of global ischemia at 37°C preserves contractility [11], (b) pretreatment of hearts with ryanodine, an inhibitor of cellular calcium overload, decreases the severity of stunning [17], (c) acidosis during early reperfusion decreases the calcium influx and attenuates the calcium binding to intracellular sites, virtually preventing the stunning [18]. Taken together, calcium overload may play a crucial role in the pathogenesis of myocardial stunning.

Intracellular Ca^{2+} Measurements in Perfused Hearts

Although a change in $[Ca^{2+}]_i$ plays a central role in the regulation of muscular contraction, there is still considerable uncertainty about how $[Ca^{2+}]_i$ is regulated in cardiac muscle cells. The sarcoplasmic reticulum is centrally involved in these processes, and its function has been studied extensively. However, the sarcoplasmic reticulum is not the sole system involved in the regulation of cytoplasmic Ca^{2+} in the muscle cell. In cardiac muscle, the roles of sarcoplasmic reticulum, sarcolemmal Ca^{2+} channels, Na^+-Ca^{2+} exchange, sarcolemmal ATP dependent Ca^{2+} pumps, membrane binding sites, and the mitochondria are also debated.

The application of various techniques to measure $[Ca^{2+}]_i$ in isolated heart muscle and in single cardiac cells [19] has led to considerable advances in our understanding of excitation-contraction coupling and other Ca^{2+}-mediated processes. During each cardiac cycle, $[Ca^{2+}]_i$ rises quickly (within 50 msec) from about 100 nM to values an order of magnitude higher, then decays back to baseline (Fig. 1) [20], and the increase in $[Ca^{2+}]_i$ initiates contraction by removing the inhibitory effect of troponin C on the interaction of actin and myosin. Major conceptual gaps remain, however, particularly regarding the regulation of $[Ca^{2+}]_i$ in hearts perfused via the normal arterial circulation. Almost all measurements of $[Ca^{2+}]_i$ have been performed in superfused muscle or enzymatically dissociated cells whose responses cannot be assumed to resemble those of the native tissue. In particular, the effects of alterations in coronary perfusion can only be crudely mimicked in isolated muscle or cells.

Three strategies have recently been used to estimate $[Ca^{2+}]_i$ in perfused hearts. The first [21] uses the fluorescent Ca^{2+} indicator quin2 [22] or related compounds [23] (Fig. 2). When narrowband UV light is focused on the heart loaded with these indicators, the resultant fluorescent emission varies with a change in $[Ca^{2+}]_i$. This technique potentially has a rapid time resolution [24]

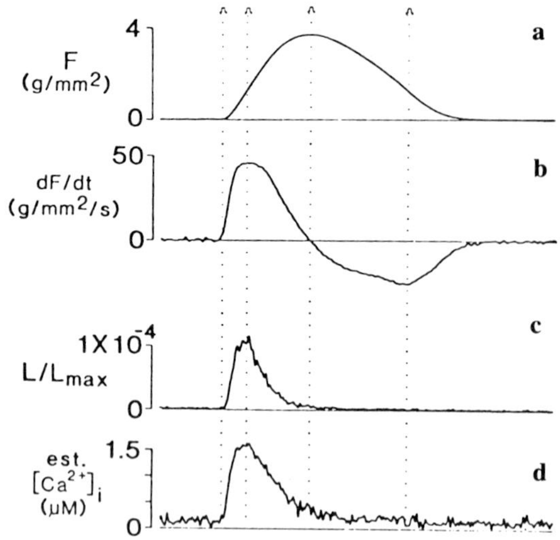

Fig. 1. Developed tension and Ca^{2+} transient measured using the aequorin technique in ferret papillary muscle. **a** developed tension (*F*), **b** rate of rise of tension (d*F*/d*t*), **c** fractional luminescence (L/L_{max}), **d** estimated intracellular [Ca^{2+}] ([Ca^{2+}]$_i$) was calculated from normalized luminescence according to calibration curve. (From [20] with permission)

but is limited by autofluorescence, bleaching, movement artifacts, and other problems which the investigators are careful to acknowledge [21–23]. Another fluorescent indicator is indo-1 [25] (Fig. 2). By using this indicator, motion artifacts can be cancelled by obtaining the ratio of signals at two emission wavelengths. However, the major limitations of indo-1 are the absence of a satisfactory calibration procedure [25] and the intense accumulation of indo-1 in endothelial cells [26] when the hearts are loaded with the cell-permeant form of the indicator, indo-1-AM.

The second approach is chemical loading of the bioluminescent Ca^{2+}-sensitive protein aequorin into perfused hearts [27]. The perfusate is replaced with a low Ca^{2+} solution and aequorin is injected into the interstitium of the epicardium (macroinjection) with a low-resistance glass micropipette under the control of a micromanipulator. After injection, the Ca^{2+} concentration of the coronary perfusate is slowly increased in a stepwise fashion to prevent the calcium paradox. In contrast to the findings of Allen and coworkers who used the microinjection method of aequorin in isolated muscle [28, 29], Kihara et al. [27] reported that anoxia in the presence of glucose always caused a gradual decline in the amplitude of the Ca^{2+} transients in the ferret heart chemically loaded with aequorin. Although the exact source of the discrepancy is not clear, Lee and Allen [29] have argued that the rate of glycolysis may have been changed or that the glycogen reserves may be depleted during the procedure of the chemical loading. This method involves exposing the muscle to very low Ca^{2+} concentrations for long enough periods to allow large molecules of photoprotein to permeate cell membranes. Although the contractile performance of such chemically-loaded preparations is reassuringly robust [27, 30], changes in the metabolic condition of the muscle have not been excluded.

The third strategy uses a fundamentally different principle: NMR spectroscopy is used to measure a Ca^{2+}-sensitive chemical shift. Smith et al. [31]

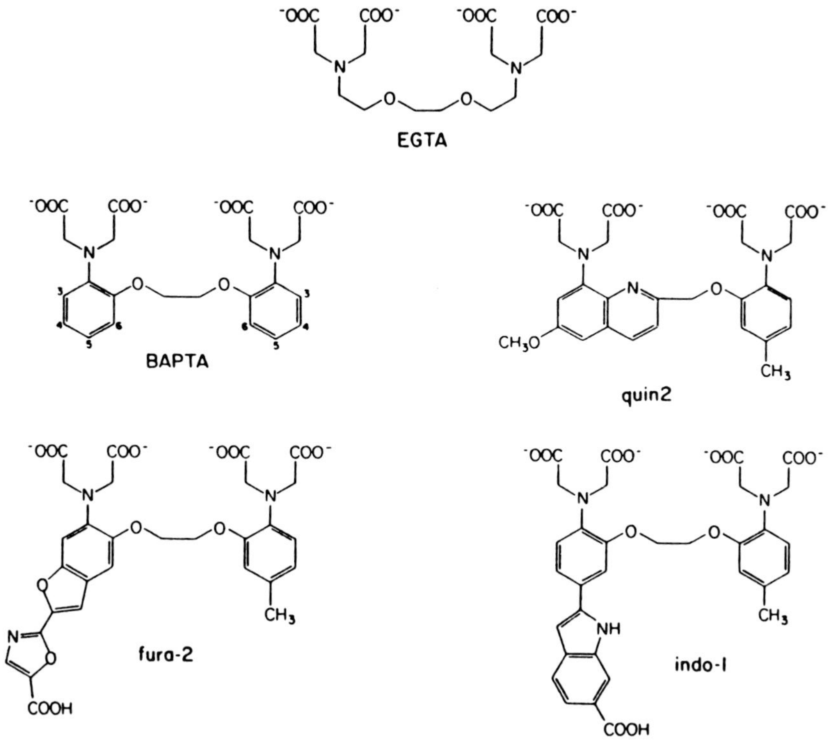

Fig. 2. Structural formulas of EGTA and several related tetracarboxylate indicators. (From [19] with permission)

have developed fluorine-19 NMR-detectable Ca^{2+}-indicators by fluorinating the Ca^{2+}-chelator, 1,2-bis(o-aminophenoxy)ethane-N,N,N′,N′-tetraacetic acid (BAPTA) [19] (Fig. 2). The derivative that appears best-suited for measuring physiological levels of $[Ca^{2+}]_i$ and that has been applied most extensively [31, 32] is 5,5′-difluoro-BAPTA (5F-BAPTA, Fig. 3). The advantages and limitations of this technique are complementary to those of the fluorescence measurements. In contrast to the autofluorescence which complicates quin2 measurements, subtraction of an endogeneous signal is not required. Unlike the other fluorescent indicators which can bleach with time, the concentration of active 5F-BAPTA in cells remains quite stable over the course of an experiment. Since the fluorine-19 chemical shifts and linewidths are distinct for each ion species [31], calcium is distinguished from heavy metals and magnesium which substantially affect the emission of the available fluorescent indicators [33]. Movement artifacts do not plague this technique and thus, this is a particularly favorable property for the study of a beating organ. Although it has been feasible to measure fluorine-19 NMR spectra from rat hearts loaded with 5F-BAPTA [32, 34], the NMR studies using ferret hearts are particularly useful because measurements of $[Ca^{2+}]_i$ are plentiful in isolated ventricular muscle from this species and can be used as bench marks [20, 28, 35, 36].

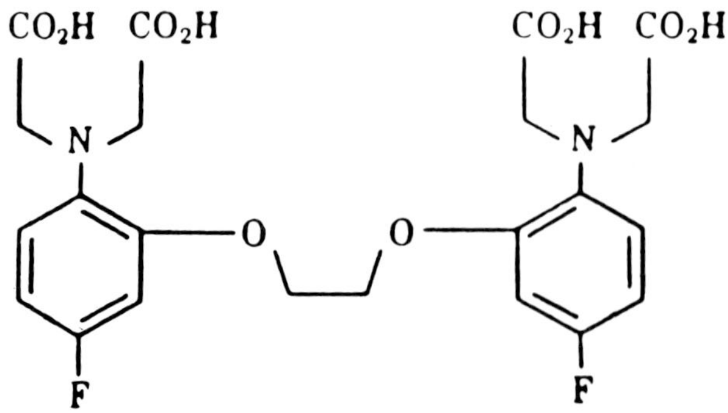

Fig. 3. Structural formula of fluorinated calcium indicator 5,5′-difluoro-BAPTA (5F-BAPTA)

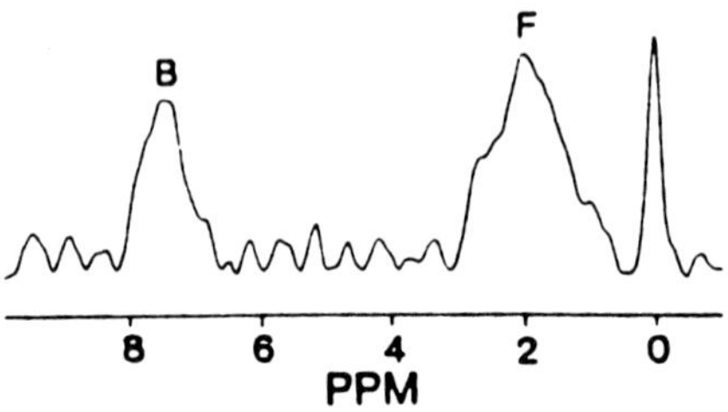

Fig. 4. Spectrum acquired over 5 min from a heart with a relatively low spontaneous heart rate (0.5 Hz), accounting for the low B/F ratio. The signal at 0 ppm arises from 6-fluoro-tryptophan in the ventricular balloon. *B*, indicator bound to Ca^{2+}; *F*, indicator free in the cytoplasm

In studies by Marban and coworkers [37, 38], perfused ferret hearts were placed in a Bruker AM-360 NMR spectrometer (8.46 Tesla; Billerica, Mass) for the simultaneous measurement of NMR spectra and isovolumic left ventricular pressure. External calcium concentration ($[Ca]_o$) was increased by adding 1 M $CaCl_2$ as necessary. The pH was adjusted to 7.4 at 30°C (or 37°C, as indicated), and the perfusate was bubbled with 100% O_2. Loading with the Ca^{2+} indicator 5F-BAPTA was achieved by addition of the cell-permeant acetoxymethyl ester form to the perfusate for 30–60 min [35]. The subsequent NMR data acquisition were gated [38] according to a programmable delay from the time of the pacing stimulus, using two pacemakers; a pacemaker which set the overall cycle length supplied a synchronization signal to the spectrometer and to a second pacemaker which stimulated the heart with no delay. For gated NMR data acquisition, a delay from the pacemaker signal was included in the programmed pulse sequence so that the radiofrequency pulse could be imposed at any time during the cardiac cycle. One pulse was applied during each cycle so that the total interpulse delay approximated 1 s (the exact value depending on the pacing rate). At each point in the cardiac cycle, 100–1200 consecutive gated scans were averaged to achieve an acceptable signal-to-noise ratio. A family of fluorine-19 spectra was obtained throughout the cardiac cycle by sampling sequentially at various delay settings. $[Ca^{2+}]_i$ can be calculated according to the equation $[Ca^{2+}]_i = K_d \times [B]/[F]$, where [B] and [F] represent the concentration of the indicator bound to Ca^{2+} and free in the cytoplasm, respectively. These in turn are proportional to the areas under

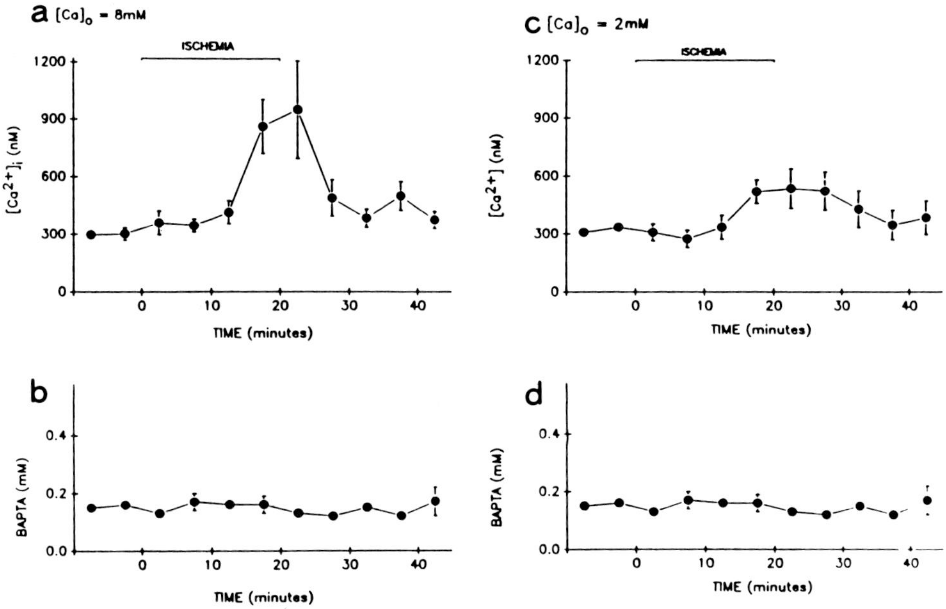

Fig. 5. Pooled data for $[Ca^{2+}]_i$ during ischemia and reperfusion at two extracellular calcium concentrations. **a** means ± SE of serial changes in $[Ca^{2+}]_i$ from 11 hearts perfused with 8 mM [Ca] and subjected to 20 min of global ischemia followed by reperfusion (30°C), **b** serial calculated 5F-BAPTA concentrations during this protocol. Analogous plots are shown in **c** and **d** for another group of hearts (n = 6) perfused with 2 mM [Ca]. (From [40] with permission)

readily-identifiable peaks in the fluorine-19 spectra (Fig. 4). The investigators used a K_d, of 285 nM previously measured at 30°C in EGTA-buffered solution to calibrate the signals [37].

$[Ca^{2+}]_i$ During Ischemia and Reperfusion

Figure 5A displays the average changes in $[Ca^{2+}]_i$ in perfused ferret hearts subjected to 20 min ischemia followed by reperfusion (30°C). In the control period, time-averaged $[Ca^{2+}]_i$ consistently equals about 300 nM. During ischemia, the time-averaged $[Ca^{2+}]_i$ increases, but the changes do not reach statistical significance until the last 5 min of ischemia, when $[Ca^{2+}]_i$ rose about three-fold. $[Ca^{2+}]_i$ remains elevated during the first 5 min after reperfusion, although a significant overshoot of $[Ca^{2+}]_i$ was not detected immediately after reperfusion. After the first 5 min of reperfusion, $[Ca^{2+}]_i$ returned toward the pre-ischemic level. The apparent changes in $[Ca^{2+}]_i$ are unlikely to indicate the leakage of the indicator from the cytosol into the extracellular space; panel B shows the intracellular concentration of 5F-BAPTA calculated by comparing the sum [B]+[F] to the area under the 6F tryptophan standard [37]. The average concentration of 5F-BAPTA remained constant throughout the experiment. After loading of 5F-BAPTA to the extent required for obtaining useful fluorine-19 spectra, the hearts generate only about 10 mmHg in 2 mM $[Ca]_o$ at 30°C [39]. Developed pressure was partially restored by increasing $[Ca]_o$ up to 8 mM [31, 32]. Figure 5C shows the behavior of $[Ca^{2+}]_i$ with the same protocol as in panel A, except that the perfusate calcium was kept at 2 mM throughout. The profile of $[Ca^{2+}]_i$ during ischemia and reperfusion is similar, although the changes are not as great, and there is still a significant increase in $[Ca^{2+}]_i$ in the late period of ischemia and a return to control in early reperfusion. Thus, the observations by Marban et al. [37] that $[Ca^{2+}]_i$ increases after 15 min of ischemia is not an artifact of working in 8 mM $[Ca]_o$. The concentration of 5F-BAPTA in these hearts (Fig. 5D) remained stable throughout the experiments. To check the effect of temperature on the time course of $[Ca^{2+}]_i$, several hearts were studied at 37°C [40, 41]. In this case, $[Ca^{2+}]_i$ was significantly elevated over control values during 10–15 min of ischemia. These results were consistent with previous reports in rat hearts [34]. Despite major technical differences, there is general agreement that $[Ca^{2+}]_i$ rises during reversible ischemia [25, 27, 40].

Although the cellular mechanisms of the increase in $[Ca^{2+}]_i$ have not yet been resolved, previous reports have emphasized the role of Na^+-Ca^{2+} exchange in reperfusion. Since acidosis is known to inhibit Na^+-Ca^{2+} exchange in vesicles [42], Na^+-Ca^{2+} exchange may be relatively inactive during ischemia. The rapid recovery of intracellular pH upon reflow could find the cells loaded with Na, favoring Ca^{2+} influx via the reactivated exchanger. Measurements of total Na and Ca during ischemia and reperfusion are consistent with this idea [43], as are measurements of Na and Ca uptake in chick cell monolayers during hypoxia and reoxygenation [44, 45]. Intracellular Na^+ measurements in ferret hearts reveal that $[Na^+]_i$ increases significantly within the first 5 min of ischemia, and continues to rise progressively thereafter [46]. The increase in $[Ca^{2+}]_i$ apparently lags behind the rise in $[Na^+]_i$ during ischemia, becoming significant only after 15 min at 30°C. The correlation would be much better during early reperfusion when $[Ca^{2+}]_i$ and $[Na^+]_i$ return to normal with a similar time course. These results are consistent with the notion that Na^+-Ca^{2+} exchange is relatively inhibited during ischemia and becomes reactivated upon reflow.

Acidosis itself leads to an increase in Ca^{2+} uptake [47, 48] and to an increase in the amplitude of Ca^{2+} transients [49]. Indeed, the exposure of aequorin-injected ferret papillary muscles to lactic acid (20 mM) suffices to mimic the rise in aequorin luminescence observed during simulated ischemia [50]. Intracellular pH (pH_i) declines almost linearly during ischemia, whereas $[Ca^{2+}]_i$ increases only after 10–15 min. Thus, pH_i does not seem to be the sole determinant of the increase in $[Ca^{2+}]_i$. Depletion of ATP has been cited as the cause of the increase in $[Ca^{2+}]_i$ [51]. This possibility seems unlikely given the observation that $[Ca^{2+}]_i$ returns to control levels after reflow, since [ATP] remains low after reperfusion. The extent of ATP depletion we measured is not itself critical [40], given that perfused hearts can maintain fairly normal function even when ATP depletion is much more severe [52].

Thus, a transient increase in $[Ca^{2+}]_i$ is observed during 20 min of ischemia and reperfusion although the mechanisms have not been completely understood. If the Ca overload during ischemia and reperfusion is involved in the pathogenesis of stunning, the interventions which reduce the increase in $[Ca^{2+}]_i$ could improve myocardial stunning, as discussed later.

Does Low Ca^{2+} Reperfusion or Acidic Reperfusion After a Brief Period of Ischemia Prevent Myocardial Stunning?

A new approach has recently been developed which enables the determination of the maximal Ca^{2+}-activated force (MCAP) in the isolated perfused ferret heart, using tetani elicited by rapid pacing after exposure to ryanodine [53]. This technique was used to study the benefits of reperfusion with low-Ca solution and to elucidate the role of cellular Ca overload in the pathogenesis of stunned myocardium. When the hearts were reperfused stepwise with low-$[Ca]_o$ solutions, first 0.1 mM $[Ca]_o$, then 0.2 and 0.5 mM $[Ca]_o$, and finally with 2 mM $[Ca]_o$ solution, each for 7 min periods, the recovery of twitch responsiveness was significantly higher than that after the abrupt reperfusion with 2 mM $[Ca]_o$ solution ($P < 0.05$). Similarly, the recovery of MCAP was significantly greater than that after abrupt reperfusion [11].

As previously mentioned, prolonged depletion of ATP was observed in stunned myocardium. Then, does the beneficial effect of reperfusion with low $[Ca]_o$ result from a reduction of ATP depletion under these conditions? In the low-$[Ca]_o$ reperfused hearts, [ATP] was comparable with the hearts reperfused with standard solution. The absence of a unique correlation between [ATP] and MCAP is apparent in Fig. 6. These results of Kusuoka et al. [11] indicate that ATP depletion is not the cause of myocardial stunning.

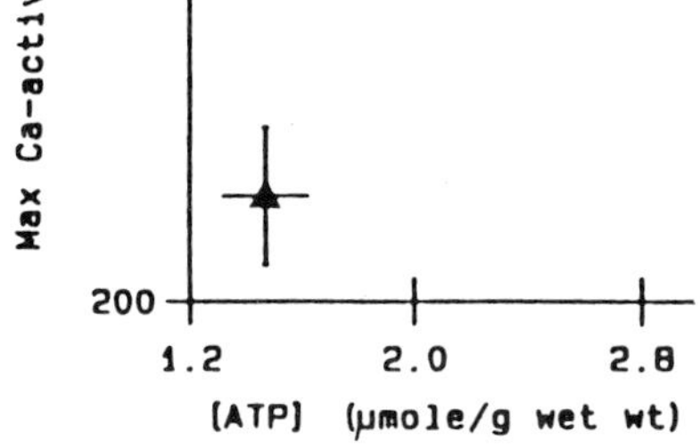

Fig. 6. Relationship between myocardial [ATP] and MCAP. Each point represents the mean ± SEM of [ATP] and MCAP in the initial control phase (*solid square*), after stunning (*solid triangle*), or following low-$[Ca]_o$ reperfusion (*solid circle*). The lack of correlation between [ATP] and MCAP is apparent. (From [11] with permission of the American Society of Clinical Investigation)

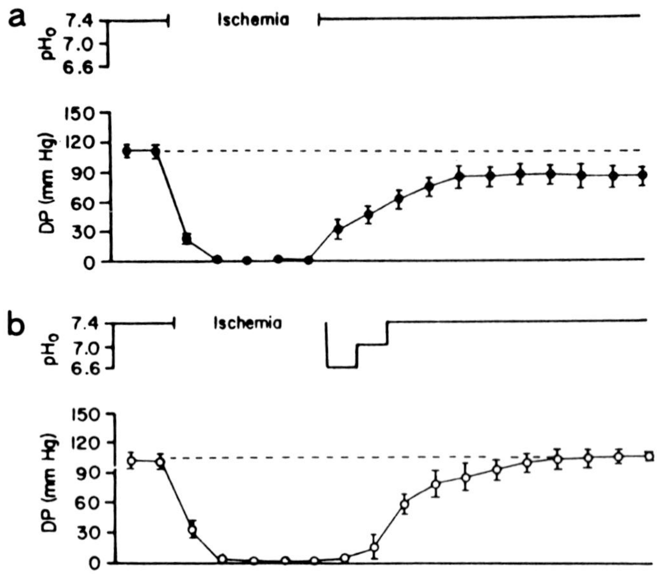

Fig. 7. Serial changes of ventricular function during 15 min of ischemia and reperfusion in two experimental groups. Extracellular pH is indicated above the data for developed pressure in each group. **a** results from the unmodified reperfusion group. After 15 min of ischemia, developed pressure recovers to 68 ± 4% of its initial value, **b** results from the acidic reperfusion group. Hearts reperfused with low pH solutions before return to pH 7.4 show a marked improvement in recovery (to 95 ± 2% of developed pressure before ischemia). (Modified from [18] with permission of the American Society of Clinical Investigation)

An alternative promising intervention may be acidosis, since this intervention is known to blunt Ca^{2+} influx into cells and H^+ compete with Ca^{2+} at the intracellular Ca^{2+} binding sites. If the hearts were reperfused with acidic solutions (pH 6.6 during 0–3 min, pH 7.0 during 4–6 min) before returning to the normal perfusate (2 mM $[Ca]_0$, Hepes-buffered, pH 7.4 bubbled with 100% O_2), ventricular function after 30 min of reperfusion was much greater in the acidic group than in the unmodified group (Fig. 7). Similar differences in developed pressure were found over a broad range of $[Ca]_o$ and during maximal Ca^{2+} activation [18]. A most likely mediator of the effect of H^+ is the Na^+-Ca^{2+} exchange [44, 48], since this ion exchange has been implicated as the pathway primarily responsible for the increase in Ca^{2+} influx upon reperfusion [46, 54]. While acknowledging that the estimate of Ca^{2+} influx via Na^+-Ca^{2+} exchange is technically difficult, a number of investigators have concluded that acidosis inhibits Ca^{2+} transport via this pathway. If $[Na^+]_i$ is elevated during ischemia [55, 56], the rapid restoration of pH_i upon reperfusion may be expected to increase the activity of Na^+-Ca^{2+} exchange and thereby enhance the Ca^{2+} influx. Reperfusion acidosis could slow the pH_i recovery after reperfusion and hence, attenuate the activation of Na^+-Ca^{2+}

exchange. Thus, the driving force for Ca^{2+} entry upon reperfusion may be dissipated before Na^+-Ca^{2+} exchange is fully reactivated. The possibility that acidosis might attenuate injury by decreasing the intracellular Ca^{2+} binding is rendered plausible by other observations [57–59].

Although Ca overload is a plausible factor to cause functional deterioration during stunned myocardium, such Ca overload is not necessarily due to increased Ca entry through traditional voltage-sensitive channels. Non-calcium channel dependent mechanisms [55, 56, 60, 61] are also involved in the increase in $[Ca^{2+}]_i$ during ischemia and reperfusion.

Does Transient Ca Overload Even in the Absence of Ischemia Mimic Myocardial Stunning?

To evaluate the role of calcium as a mediator of injury during myocardial stunning, it is important to determine whether calcium overload per se is sufficient to produce myocardial injury. To determine the contractile, histological, and metabolic sequelae of transient Ca overload, developed pressures in perfused ferret hearts were measured before and 20 min after three 5 min periods of perfusion with a 10 mM $[Ca]_o$, 1 mM $[Mg]_o$ solution (high-Ca group) without ischemia, and in control hearts exposed transiently to the same total divalent cation concentration without a change in $[Ca]_o$ (9 mM $[Mg]_0$, 2 mM $[Ca]_o$) [62]. Developed pressures, measured at various $[Ca]_o$ (0.5 to 5 mM), were depressed in the high-Ca group relative to control (Fig. 8A). The hearts in the control group were histologically normal, whereas foci of "reversible" injury (mitochondrial swelling, glycogen deposition, and clumping of nuclear chromatin) were infrequently observed in hearts from the high-Ca group. MCAP was also decreased in the high-Ca group (Fig. 8B). $[Ca]_o$ sensitivity, determined by normalization of the DP-$[Ca]_o$ relationship to the corresponding MCAP, was shifted to higher $[Ca]_o$ in the high-Ca group (Fig. 8C). Phosphorus NMR spectra were also obtained in high-Ca hearts. [ATP] declined by 30%–40% after exposure to high $[Ca]_o$, but inorganic phosphate, phosphocreatine, and pH remained unchanged. These results of Kitakaze et al. [62] indicate that transient exposure to high $[Ca]_o$ without ischemia leaves behind distinctive contractile, metabolic, and histological sequelae and can mimic stunned myocardium.

There is another analogy of myocardial stunning in the postarrhythmic contractile dysfunction described by Koretsune and Marban [63]. During ventricular fibrillation induced by burst pacing, $[Ca^{2+}]_i$ rose rapidly and dramatically, exceeding by four times the control within 5 min. $[Ca^{2+}]_i$ remained markedly elevated throughout 20 min of fibrillation, but it returned to control values shortly after defibrillation. In the hearts which contract isovolumically with a balloon in the left ventricle, acidosis and high-energy phosphate depletion developed despite the maintenance of normal coronary pressure. Even when the left ventricular volume was decreased during fibrillation to reduce the wall stress to avoid this adverse effect, $[Ca^{2+}]_i$ still increased remarkably

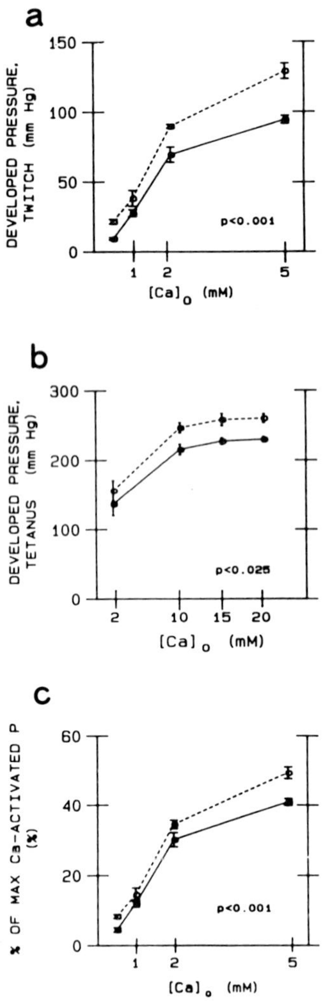

Fig. 8. Characterization of contractile dysfunction in transiently Ca-overloaded hearts. Results from control groups (n = 5) are shown as *open circles*, whereas these from high-Ca hearts (n = 8) are presented as *filled circles*. **a** $[Ca]_o$ responsiveness, **b** developed pressure during tetani (MCAP) in various $[Ca]_o$, **c** Ca_o sensitivity, i.e., Ca_o responsiveness normalized by the corresponding MCAP. (From [62] with permission)

and the hearts mimicked "stunned" since the developed pressure did not recover to the control after defibrillation. Thus, the increase in $[Ca^{2+}]_i$ in post-arrhythmic hearts may cause the contractile dysfunction. It should be noted that the adriamycin-induced heart failure is associated with the increase in $[Ca^{2+}]_i$ even with the perfusion maintained [64]. These lines of evidence strongly suggest that Ca overload per se is sufficient to induce reversible myocardial injury.

Ca Overload in the Failing Heart

Direct measurements of $[Ca^{2+}]_i$ in human heart muscle are very limited. Recently, Morgan et al. [65] reported that intracellular Ca^{2+} handling is abnormal in the human failing cardiac muscle. They measured $[Ca^{2+}]_i$ using aequorin during isometric contraction of myocardium from patients with end-stage heart failure undergoing heart transplantation. Contractions and Ca^{2+} transients of the failing muscle were markedly prolonged and Ca^{2+} transient was biphasic (early peak, L_1; late plateau phase, L_2). In contrast to the control muscle, the failing muscle demonstrated a raised residual component L_2, which probably reflects Ca^{2+} entry through voltage-dependent sarcolemmal channels. Thus, their observations are not incompatible with previous findings that the Ca^{2+} uptake by sarcoplasmic reticulum is depressed in the failing heart [66, 67]. It should be noted that the early peak of the Ca^{2+} transient, L_1, is minimally depressed in the failing heart, suggesting that the release of Ca^{2+} from sarcoplasmic reticulum is not significantly affected. Thus, these results may imply that the dysfunction of Ca uptake by sarcoplasmic reticulum and/or the augmented Ca^{2+} entry through voltage-dependent Ca^{2+} channels mainly cause the Ca overload in the failing cardiac muscle. Ca overload in turn may impair relaxation of the heart, thus decreasing rapid ventricular filling and leading to the low cardiac output during tachycardia. Ca overload also would increase diastolic myocardial stiffness, raising the LV end-diastolic pressure which causes pulmonary congestion. The important results of Morgan et al. [65] may be subject to technical limitations related to the chemical loading method for aequorin; confirmation by other methods is eagerly awaited.

Excessive Ca may induce a number of adverse effects in cardiomyocytes, including activation of Ca^{2+}-sensitive proteases which may disrupt the membranous organellas and cytoskeletons. Recently, we observed that the microtubules of cardiomyocytes are disrupted when extracellular Ca^{2+} concentration is raised to 5 mM and when the cells are treated with calcium ionophores [68].

Given the Ca overload hypothesis, one may raise the possibility that long-term treatment with Ca^{2+} antagonists may be beneficial for patients with chronic heart failure. In a prospective clinical trial, the calcium channel antagonist diltiazem was given to 22 patients with dilated cardiomyopathy in addition to conventional therapy of digitalis, diuretics and vasodilators [69]. The mean survival time was 29 months in the control group, whereas no patient in the diltiazem group died over a mean follow-up period of 15.4 months, and mean LV ejection fraction increased from 0.34 to 0.44 with an improvement of clinical symptoms. Nifedipine is a primarily arteriolar vasodilator and produces an increase in cardiac output due to a decrease in systemic vascular resistance. However, in some patients with severe low cardiac output failure, it worsened ventricular performance through its negative inotropic effect [70]. Although some acute and chronic clinical trials have demonstrated hemodynamic improvement both at rest and during exercise [71–73], favorable results have not been obtained in other studies [70, 74, 75]. Since large scale placebo-controlled studies have not been reported, the clinical efficacy of Ca antagonists in heart failure is still controversial. To clarify the role of Ca antagonists in treatment of chronic heart failure, well-designed, large scale clinical trials are necessary. The underlying mechanism of Ca overload in the failing heart also merits further scrutiny.

References

1. Blinks JR, Prendergast FG, Allen DG (1976) Proteins as biological calcium indicators. Pharmacol Rev 28:1–93
2. Beeler GW, Reuter H (1970) Membrane calcium current in ventricular myocardial fibers. J Physiol (London) 207:191–209
3. New N, Trautwein W (1975) The ionic nature of the slow inward current and its relation to contraction. Pflugers Arch 354:55–74
4. Gibbons WR, Fozzard HA (1975) Slow inward current and contraction in sheep cardiac Purkinje fibers. J Gen Physiol 65:367–383
5. Katz AM (1977) Physiology of the Heart, Raven Press, New York
6. Braunwald E, Kloner RA (1982) The stunned myocardium: prolonged, postischemic ventricular dysfunction. Circulation 60:1146–1149
7. Braunwald E, Kloner RA (1985) Myocardial reperfusion: a double-edged sword? J Clin Invest 76:1713–1719
8. Becker LC, Levine JH, DiPaula AF, Guarnieri T, Aversano TA (1986) Reversal of dysfunction in postischemic stunned myocardium by epinephrine and postextrasystolic potentiation. J Am Coll Cardiol 7:580–589
9. Bolli R, Zhu W, Myers ML, Hartley CJ, Roberts R (1985) Beta-adrenergic stimulation reverses postischemic myocardial dysfunction without producing functional deterioration. Am J Cardiol 56:964–968
10. Ellis SG, Wynne J, Braunwald E, Henscheke CT, Sandor T, Kloner RA (1984) Response of reperfusion-salvaged, stunned myocardium to inotropic stimulation. Am Heart J 107:13–19
11. Kusuoka H, Porterfield JK, Weisman HF, Weisfeldt ML, Marban E (1987) Pathophysiology and pathogenesis of stunned myocardium: depressed Ca^{2+} activation of contraction as a consequence of reperfusion-induced cellular calcium overload in ferret hearts. J Clin Invest 79:950–961
12. Ito BR, Tate H, Kobayashi M, Schaper W (1987) Reversibly injured, postischemic canine myocardium retains normal contractile reserve. Circ Res 61:834–846
13. Kusuoka H, Jacobus WE, Marban E (1988) Calcium oscillations in digitalis-induced ventricular fibrillation: pathogenetic role and metabolic consequences in isolated ferret hearts. Circ Res 62:609–619
14. Steenbergen C, Hill ML, Jennings RB (1987) Cytoskeletal damage during myocardial ischemia; changes in vinculin immunofluorescence staining during total in vitro ischemia in canine hearts. Circ Res 60:478–486
15. Katoh N, Wise BC, Kuo JF (1983) Phosphorylation of cardiac troponin inhibitory subunit (troponin I) and tropomyosin-binding subunit (troponin T) by cardiac phospholipid sensitive Ca^{2+}-dependent protein kinase. Biochem J 209:189–195
16. Marban E, Robinson SW, Wier WG (1986) Mechanisms of arrhythmogenic, delayed, and early afterpolarization in ferret ventricular muscle. J Clin Invest 78: 1185–1192
17. Porterfield JK, Kusuoka H, Weisman HF, Weisfeldt ML, Marban E (1987) Ryanodine prevents the changes in myocardial function and morphology induced by reperfusion after brief periods of ischemia (abstract). Clin Res 35:315A
18. Kitakaze M, Weisfeldt ML, Marban E (1988) Acidosis during reperfusion prevents myocardial stunning in ferret hearts. J Clin Invest 82:920–927
19. Blinks JR (1986) Intracellular $[Ca^{2+}]_i$ measurements. In: Fozzard HA et al. (eds) The Heart and Cardiovascular System. Raven Press, New York, pp 671–701

20. Yue DT (1987) Intracellular [Ca^{2+}] related to rate of force development in twitch contraction of heart. Am J Physiol 252:H760–H770
21. Lattanzio FA, Pressman BC (1986) Alterations in intracellular calcium activity and contractility of isolated perfused rabbit hearts by ionophore and adrenergic agents. Biochem Biophys Res Commun 139:816–821
22. Tsien RY (1980) New calcium indicators and buffers with high selectivity against magnesium and protons: design, synthesis, and properties of prototype structures. Biochemistry 19:2396–2404
23. Grynkiewicz G, Poenie M, Tsien RY (1985) A new generation of Ca^{2+} indicators with greatly improved fluorescence properties. J Biol Chem 260:3440–3450
24. Wier WG, Cannell M, Berlin J, Marban E, Lederer WJ (1987) Cellular and subcellular heterogeneity of $[Ca^{2+}]_i$ in single heart cells revealed by fura-2. Science 235:325–328
25. Lee HC, Mohabir R, Smith N, Franz MR, Clusin WT (1988) Effect of ischemia on calcium-dependent fluorescence transients in rabbit hearts containing indo-1. Correlation with monophasic action potentials and contraction. Circulation 78: 1047–1059
26. Lorell BH, Apstein CS, Cunningham MJ, Schoen FJ, Weinberg EO, Peeters GA, Barry WH (1990) Contribution of endothelial cells to calcium-dependent fluorescence transients in rabbit hearts loaded with indo-1. Circ Res 67:415–425
27. Kihara Y, Grossman W, Morgan JP (1989) Direct measurement of changes in intracellular calcium transients during hypoxia, ischemia, and reperfusion of the intact mammalian heart. Circ Res 65:1029–1044
28. Allen DG, Orchard CH (1983) Intracellular calcium concentration during hypoxia and metabolic inhibition in mammalian ventricular muscle. J Physiol (Lond) 339: 107–122
29. Lee JA, Allen DG (1988) The effects of repeated exposure to anoxia on intracellular calcium, glycogen and lactate in isolated ferret heart muscle. Pflugers Arch 413:83–89
30. MacKinnon R, Gwathmey JK, Morgan JP (1987) Differential effects of reoxygenation on intracellular calcium and isometric tension. Pflügers Arch 409:448–453
31. Smith GA, Hesketh RT, Metcalfe JC, Feeney J, Morris PG (1983) Intracellular calcium measurements by fluorine-19 NMR of fluorine-labelled chelators. Proc Natl Acad Sci USA 80:7178–7182
32. Metcalfe JC, Hesketh TR, Smith GA (1985) Free cytosolic Ca^{2+} measurements with fluorine-labelled indicators using fluorine-19 NMR. Cell Calcium 6:183–195
33. Arslan P, DiVirgilio F, Beltrame M, Tsien RY, Pozzan T (1985) Cytosolic Ca^{2+} homeostasis in Ehrlich and Yoshida carcinomas. J Biol Chem 260:2719–2727
34. Steenbergen C, Murphy E, Levy L, London RE (1987) Elevation in cytosolic free calcium concentration early in myocardial ischemia in perfused rat heart. Circ Res 60:700–707
35. Marban E, Rink TJ, Tsien RW, Tsien RY (1980) Free calcium in heart muscle at rest and during contraction measured with Ca^{2+}-sensitive microelectrodes. Nature 286:845–850
36. Yue DT, Marban E, Wier WG (1986) Relationship between force and intracellular [Ca^{2+}] in tetanized mammalian heart muscle. J Gen Physiol 87:223–242
37. Marban E, Kitakaze M, Kusuoka H, Porterfield JK, Yue DT, Chacko VP (1987) Intracellular free calcium concentration measured with fluorine-19 NMR spectroscopy in intact ferret hearts. Proc Natl Acad Sci USA 84:6005–6009

38. Marban E, Kitakaze M, Chacko VP, Pike MM (1988) Ca^{2+} transients in perfused ferret hearts revealed by fluorine-19 NMR spectroscopy. Circ Res 63:673–678
39. Kirschenlohr HL, Metcalfe JC, Morris PG, Rodrigo GC, Smith GA (1988) Ca^{2+} transient, Mg^{2+}, and pH measurements in the cardiac cycle by fluorine-19 NMR. Proc Natl Acad Sci USA 85:9017–9021
40. Marban E, Kitakaze M, Koretsune Y, Yue DT, Chacko VP, Pike MM (1990) Quantification of $[Ca^{2+}]_i$ in perfused hearts: critical evaluation of the 5F-BAPTA/NMR method as applied to the study of ischemia and reperfusion. Circ Res 66:1255–1267
41. Marban E, Koretsune Y, Corretti M, Chacko VP, Kusuoka H (1989) Calcium and its role in myocardial cell injury during ischemia and reperfusion. Circulation 80:IV17–IV22
42. Philipson ED, Bersohn MM, Nishimoto AY (1982) Effects of pH on Na^{+}-Ca^{2+} exchange in canine cardiac sarcolemmal vesicles. Circ Res 50:287–293
43. Grinwald PM (1982) Calcium uptake during post-ischemic reperfusion in the isolated rat heart: influence of extracellular sodium. J Mol Cell Cardiol 14:359–365
44. Murphy JG, Smith TW, Marsh JD (1988) Mechanisms of reoxygenation-induced calcium overload in cultured chick embryo heart cells. Am J Physiol 254:H1133–1141
45. Kim D, Cragoe EJ, Smith TW (1987) Relations among sodium pump inhibition, Na-Ca and Na-H exchange activities, and Ca-H interaction in cultured chick heart cells. Circ Res 60:185–193
46. Pike MM, Kitakaze M, Marban E (1990) Sodium-23 NMR measurements of intracellular sodium in intact perfused ferret hearts during ischemia and reperfusion. Am J Physiol 259:H1767–H1773
47. Kitakaze M, Weisfeldt ML, Marban E (1988) Acidosis during early reperfusion prevents myocardial stunning in perfused hearts. J Clin Invest 82:920–927
48. Kim D, Smith TW (1987) Altered Ca fluxes and contractile state during pH changes in cultured heart cells. Am J Physiol 253:C137–C146
49. Orchard CH (1987) The role of sarcoplasmic reticulum in the response of ferret and rat heart muscle to acidosis. Pflugers Arch 384:431–449
50. Allen DG, Lee JA, Smith GL (1989) The consequences of simulated ischemia on intracellular Ca^{2+} and tension in isolated ferret ventricular muscle. J Physiol (London) 410:297–323
51. Steenbergen C, Murphy E, Watts J, London R (1988) Cytosolic free calcium changes during ischemia and anoxia in perfused rat heart. J Mol Cell Cardiol 20(supplIII):S.19
52. Hoeter JA, Lauer C, Vassort G, Gueron M (1988) Sustained function of normoxic hearts depleted in ATP and phosphocreatine: a phosphorus-31 NMR study. Am J Physiol 255:C192–C201
53. Marban E, Kusuoka H, Yue DT, Weisfeldt ML, Weir WS (1986) Maximal Ca^{2+}-activated force elicited by tetanization of ferret papillary muscle and whole heart. Mechanism and characteristics of steady contractile activation in intact myocardium. Circ Res 59:262–269
54. Renlund DG, Gerstenblith G, Lakatta EG, Jacobus WE, Kallman CH, Weisfeldt ML (1984) Perfusate sodium during ischemia modifies postischemic functional and metabolic recovery in the rabbit heart. J Mol Cell Cardiol 14:795–801
55. Regan TJ, Broisman B, Haider B, Eaddy C, Oldewurtel HA (1980) Dissociation of myocardial sodium and potassium alterations in mild and severe ischemia. Am J Physiol 238:H575–H580

56. Neubauer S, Balschi JA, Springer CS, Smith TW, Ingwall JS (1987) Intracellular Na^+ accumulation in hypoxic versus ischemic rat heart: evidence for Na^+-H^+ exchange. Circulation 76(supplIV):56
57. Fabiato A, Fabiato F (1978) Effects of pH on myofilaments and the sarcoplasmic reticulum on skinned cells from cardiac and skeletal muscles. J Physiol (Lond) 276:233–255
58. Katz AM, Hecht HH (1969) The early 'pump' failure of the ischemic heart. Am J Med 47:497–502
59. Donaldson SKB, Hermansen L (1978) Differential, direct effects of H^+ on Ca^{2+}-activated force of skinned fibers from the soleus, cardiac and adductor magnum muscle of rabbits. Pflügers Arch 376:55–65
60. Corretti M, Koretsune Y, Zweier JL, Marban E (1990) Intracellular calcium overload and glycolytic inhibition as consequences of exogeneously-generated free radicals in rabbit hearts. Circulation 82(supplIII):700
61. Zweier JL, Flaherty JT, Weisfeldt ML (1987) Direct measurement of free radical generation following reperfusion of ischemic myocardium. Proc Natl Acad Sci USA 84:476–485
62. Kitakaze M, Weisman HF, Marban E (1987) Contractile dysfunction and ATP depletion after transient calcium overload in perfused ferret hearts. Circulation 77:685–695
63. Koretsune Y, Marban E (1989) Cell calcium in the pathophysiology of ventricular fibrillation and in the pathogenesis of postarrhythmic contractile dysfunction. Circulation 80:369–379
64. Kusuoka H, Futaki S, Koretsune Y, Kitabatake A, Suga H, Kamada T, Inoue M (to be published) Alterations of intracellular calcium homeostasis and myocardial energetics in acute adriamycin induced heart failure. J Cardiovasc Pharmacol
65. Gwathmey JK, Copelas L, MacKinnon R, Schon FJ, Feldman MD, Grossman W, Morgan JP (1987) Abnormal intracellular calcium handling in myocardium from patients with end-stage heart failure. Circ Res 61:70–76
66. Lentz RW, Harrison CE Jr, Dewey DA, Barnhorst GK, Danielson GK, Pluth JR (1978) Functional evaluation of sarcoplasmic reticulum and mitochondria in human pathologic states. J Mol Cell Cardiol 10:3–30
67. Lindenmayer GE, Sordahl LA, Harigaya S, Allen JC, Besch HR Jr, Schwartz A (1971) Some biochemical studies on subcellular systems isolated from fresh recipient human cardiac tissue obtained during transplantation. Am J Cardiol 27: 277–283
68. Sato H, Hori M, Iwai K, Kagiya T, Takashima S, Tada M (1990) Ca^{2+} overload disrupts microtubules in cultured rat cardiomyocytes. Circulation 82(supplIII):297
69. Figulla HR, Rechenberg JV, Wiegand V, Soballa R, Kreuzer H (1989) Beneficial effects of long-term diltiazem treatment in dilated cardiomyopathy. J Am Coll Cardiol 13:653–658
70. Agostoni PG, Cesare ND, Doria E, Polese A, Tamborini G, Guazzi MD (1986) Afterload reduction: a comparison of captoril and nifedipine in dilated cardiomyopathy. Br Heart J 55:391–399
71. Bellocci F, Ansalone G, Santarelli P, Loperfido F, Scabbia E, Zecchi P, Manzoli U (1982) Oral nifedipine in the long-term management of severe chronic heart failure. J Cardiovasc Pharmacol 4:847–855
72. Zeng X, Du C, Zhang T, Luo D (1987) Low dose nifedipine therapy for dilated congestive heart failure. Circulation 76(supplIV):70

73. Thomas P, Sheridan DJ (1988) Acute and chronic hemodynamic effects of nicardipine in patients with congestive heart failure. Br J Clin Pharmacol 26:243
74. Metra M, Bonandi L, Canna GL, Nordio G, Nodari S, Raddino R, Guaini T, Danesi R, Cas LD (1988) Acute and chronic hemodynamic effects of nisoldipine in chronic heart failure. Eur Heart J 9(suppl-1):184
75. Tan LB, Murray RG, Litter WA (1987) Felodipine in patients with chronic heart failure: discrepant hemodynamic and clinical effects. Br Heart J 58:122–128

4

Cardiac Oxygen Costs of Contractility (E_{max}) and Mechanical Energy (PVA): New Key Concepts in Cardiac Energetics

HIROYUKI SUGA[1], YOICHI GOTO[2]

Summary. Experimental studies on cardiac mechanoenergetics performed over the last decade in our laboratory are reviewed and the new concepts obtained from them are summarized. We have proposed that the contractile state of the ventricle can be quantified by the end-systolic ventricular maximum volume elastance (E_{max}) and that the total mechanical energy of ventricular contraction can be quantified by the systolic pressure-volume area (PVA). E_{max} is the slope of a linearized end-systolic pressure-volume relation and PVA is the area circumscribed by the end-systolic and end-disatolic pressure-volume relation curves and the systolic pressure-volume trajectory in the ventricular pressure-volume diagram.

We have shown that PVA correlates linearly with ventricular oxygen consumption (Vo_2) regardless of ventricular loading conditions at a stable E_{max} and that the load-independent Vo_2-PVA relation is shifted up or down in a parallel manner with enhancement or depression of E_{max} by various inotropic interventions. These experimental findings can be described by the empirical equations $Vo_2 = a\text{PVA} + b$, and $b = cE_{max} + d$. Coefficient a is the oxygen cost of PVA or mechanical energy, aPVA is the PVA-dependent Vo_2, constant b is the PVA-independent Vo_2, c is the oxygen cost of E_{max} or contractility, and constant d means the PVA-independent Vo_2 at zero E_{max}. The reciprocal of a refers to the efficiency of PVA generation from the PVA-dependent Vo_2, and is called the contractile efficiency. The value for a has been found to be about 1.8×10^{-5} ml O_2/(mmHg ml) or 2.5 (dimensionless) after the units of both Vo_2 and PVA are changed to a common unit of energy (1 ml O_2 = 20 J, 1 mmHg ml = 1.33×10^{-4} J). Therefore, $1/a$ is 0.4 (dimensionless) or 40% on average. We have found that a and c are independent of inotropic interven-

[1] The Second Department of Physiology Okayama University Medical School, Okayama, 700 Japan
[2] Department of Cardiovascular Dynamics, National Cardiovascular Center Research Institute, Suita, Osaka, 565 Japan

tions although *b* changes. However, myocardial stunning slightly decreased *a* and *d* and doubled *c*, and myocardial cooling did not change *a* and *c*. We consider that the behaviors of *a*, *b*, *c* and *d* can characterize the mechanoenergetic changes of hearts under various pathophysiological conditions.

Key words: Cross-bridge — Excitation-contraction coupling — Myocardial energetics — Myocardial mechanics — Pressure-volume area

List of Abbreviations

a: slope of the Vo_2-PVA relation as a measure of the oxygen cost of PVA.
b: Vo_2 intercept of the Vo_2-PVA relation, or unloaded Vo_2.
c: slope of the PVA-independent Vo_2-E_{max} relation as a measure of the oxygen cost of E_{max}.
d: PVA-independent Vo_2 intercept, or zero-E_{max} PVA-independent Vo_2.
E_{max}: maximum volume elastance of the ventricle, determined as the slope of the end-systolic pressure-volume relation.
EW: external mechanical work.
FTI: force-time integral.
PE: mechanical potential energy.
PVA: systolic pressure-volume area, as a measure of the total mechanical energy generated by ventricular contraction. PVA = EW + PE.
PVA(t): PVA developed over the systolic time from the end diastole to a variable systolic time *t*.
r: correlation coefficient.
Vo_2: myocardial oxygen consumption, usually per beat unless otherwise specified.
V_{max}: maximum unloaded shortening velocity

Introduction

The heart maintains its pumping action by converting chemical energy contained in metabolic substrates into mechanical energy and work [1]. Cardiac energy metabolism is normally aerobic, that is, consuming oxygen. Most ATP is produced by oxidative phosphorylation in mitochondria. Cardiac oxygen consumption (Vo_2) is known to be equivalent to the total energy utilization of the heart [2–4]. ATP is the final source of chemical energy for mechanical contraction of the muscle [1–4].

ATP is utilized in myocardium by three major ATPases: Na, K pump ATPase, Ca pump ATPase, and myosin ATPase [5], as shown in Fig. 1. The Na, K pump ATPase is related to the Na^+ and K^+ handling in the electrical activation of the sarcolemma, the Ca pump ATPase is related to the Ca^{2+} handling in the excitation-contraction coupling for the activation of contraction

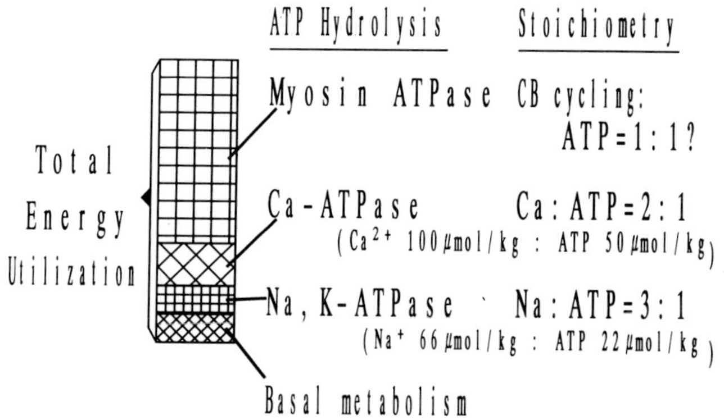

Fig. 1. Total energy utilization of the heart consists of ATP hydrolysis by three major ATPases and basal metabolism. ATP, adenosine 5'-triphosphate. The stoichiometry or coupling ratio of ATP to cross-bridge (*CB*) cycling and Ca^{2+} or Na^{+} is shown. The *question mark* on the *CB* stoichiometry means that this stoichiometry may be variable depending on loading conditions [41]. Ca, Ca^{2+}; Na, Na^{+}; K, K^{+}. Ca^{2+} and Na^{+} concentrations in the parentheses are representative postulated values [5]

and its relaxation, and the myosin ATPase is related to cross-bridge cycling for mechanical contraction [5]. The mechanical loading, excitation rate and contractile state conditions of the heart are known to affect the rate and amount of ATP hydrolysis by these ATPases and hence Vo_2 [2, 3]. However, their quantitative relations remain to be elucidated [6]. When they are fully understood, cardiac ATP and Vo_2 will be accurately predictable from the mechanical loading conditions, heart rate and contractile state of the heart. Until such a time, more efforts are needed for a better understanding of the physiology and pathophysiology of cardiac mechanoenergetics [6].

Empirical approaches so far attempted have not yielded satisfactory results to form a consensus on the determinants of Vo_2 [1, 6, 7]. With this background in mind, we have been continuing our efforts to yield a new determinant of Vo_2 which consistently relates cardiac mechanics and energetics under a variety of experimental conditions. As a result, we have found that the total mechanical energy of ventricular contraction can be quantified by the systolic pressure-volume area (PVA) and that PVA closely correlates with Vo_2 [6, 8], as shown in Figs. 2–5. Our present macroscopic or organ-level view of cardiac mechanoenergetics will eventually be correlated with and accounted for by the myocardial energetics on the microscopic or molecular level which will be elucidated in the future.

In this review, we will summarize our experimental results and new concepts deduced mostly from our own studies [6, 8]. We focus on two key concepts: "oxygen cost of mechanical energy (PVA)" and "oxygen cost of contractility (E_{max})." These two oxygen costs proved to be relatively constant under various physiological conditions but have been shown to be altered under pathophysiological conditions such as myocardial stunning and cooling. We consider that analyses of these two costs will greatly facilitate a better understanding of cardiac mechanoenergetics of normal and failing hearts. We hope that this review will be helpful to cardiologists who wish to better understand the state of the art of cardiac mechanoenergetics.

Brief History

Since the days of Evans and Matsuoka [9], many investigators have extensively studied major factors affecting Vo_2 [2, 3, 6, 10–12]. As a result, the present consensus is that Vo_2 varies considerably with changes in cardiac loading conditions, heart rate, and contractile state. The prevailing concept is that Vo_2 is more directly determined by the afterload, including ventricular or arterial pressure or myocardial tension, than by the preload, including ventricular end-diastolic pressure or volume, and that Vo_2 is increased with heart rate and contractility.

Although the currently available determinants of Vo_2 can be used to make qualitative predictions of Vo_2, they cannot yet provide quantitative predictions of Vo_2 even when all loading conditions, heart rate, and contractility are specified in a given heart [6]. Specifically, the conventional determinants of Vo_2, including cardiac tension and contractile state, are not always sufficient to predict Vo_2 [13–16].

In 1979, Suga proposed the ventricular systolic pressure-volume area (PVA) as a new measure of the total mechanical energy generated by ventricular contraction [17]. Since then, he and his colleagues have endeavored to establish the feasibility of this new measure as a determinant or predictor of Vo_2.

Our results up until 1988 have been summarized in a few review articles written by Suga [6, 8]. Many studies in our laboratory as well as in other laboratories have revealed that PVA is a very promising candidate for a physiologically sound measure of the total mechanical energy generated by ventricular contraction and should be considered as the primary determinant of Vo_2. To contrast PVA, we first briefly comment on the problems of the major conventional determinants of Vo_2.

Conventional Determinants of Myocardial Oxygen Consumption

Conventional determinants of Vo_2 include myocardial tension, mechanical work, shortening, myocardial contractility, stimulation frequency, and basal metabolism [2, 10]. Of these, myocardial tension and contractility are generally considered to be the two most important determinants, and the other terms are relatively minor [10].

Myocardial Tension and Tension-Time Integral

Evans and Matsuoka [9] showed the importance of myocardial tension as a determinant of Vo_2. Later, several research groups including Sarnoff et al. [18]

and Weber and Janicki [19] supported this concept. In particular, these two groups showed that the time integrals of ventricular pressure and myocardial tension primarily determine Vo_2. They showed that external work of shortening or ejection is a secondary determinant of Vo_2.

Since muscular tension has been recognized to be the primary determinant of energy utilization in the skeletal muscle [20], the same has been generally believed to be valid in the cardiac muscle [2, 10, 13]. However, tension is not the only determinant of energetics [20], since shortening is also an important determinant of energetics in the skeletal muscle [21].

In cardiac muscle also, tension development and its maintenance have been shown to be the primary determinants of Vo_2 when the muscle is tetanized for variable durations [12]. Tetanus is an unphysiological contraction in the cardiac muscle. Energy utilization during tetanus is not only for tension maintenance but also for activation (electrical activation and excitation-contraction coupling), the frequency of which is very high. Vo_2 for tension maintenance alone must be removed to quantify the mechanics-dependent Vo_2.

Weber and Janicki [19] explicitly showed that systolic force-time integral uniquely correlated with Vo_2 only in isovolumic contractions but did not uniquely correlate with Vo_2 in ejecting contractions. More recently, we have shown conclusively that neither peak force nor systolic force-time integral consistently correlate with Vo_2 [22].

Contractility

The myocardium is different from the skeletal muscle in that contractile strength of myocardium physiologically varies with various inotropic interventions such as catecholamines and calcium. After finding V_{max} (maximum velocity of unloaded shortening) as an index of contractility, Sonnenblick et al. found that Vo_2 increased with V_{max} despite a constant peak tension [23]. Vo_2 for a given peak tension is greater for a greater V_{max}. Therefore, myocardial tension is not the sole determinant of Vo_2.

However, what contractility means in cardiac mechanoenergetics is a serious question. Does it mean the level of activation or the amount of calcium ions (Ca^{2+}) involved in excitation-contraction coupling? Or does it only mean the speed of shortening or contraction? In those days when the calcium transient (transient time course of cytosolic free Ca^{2+} concentration as monitored by aequorin, fura-2, etc.) [24, 25] was not measured, the mechanism of the Vo_2 determination by V_{max} was unknown.

Recently, when it became possible to analyze the calcium transient under various inotropic interventions [24], a greater amount of Ca^{2+} was suspected to be involved in the excitation-contraction coupling in an enhanced contractile state, and the increase in Vo_2 with contractility is suspected to be caused by an increased amount of total released Ca^{2+}. Although quantitative measurements of total Ca^{2+} released from the sarcoplasmic reticulum are possible by electron-probe microanalysis [25], the relation between total released Ca^{2+} and enhanced contractility has not yet been elucidated in myocardium.

Heart Rate

Vo_2 per min is an increasing function of heart rate per min [23]. However, it is controversial whether Vo_2 per beat increases, decreases or does not change with heart rate. The controversy seems to derive from different experimental conditions among the studies under a variety of cardiodynamic loading conditions. Although Vo_2 per beat was reported to increase with heart rate, the increase proved to be practically insignificant [26].

Conventional Indexes of Vo_2

Combining these major conventional determinants of Vo_2, some investigators have proposed indexes and formulas to predict Vo_2 either retrospectively or prospectively under a variety of loading, contractile and heart rate conditions. However, none of them has been unanimously agreed on as the consistently reliable index or formula of Vo_2 by interested investigators [1–4, 6–8].

Pressure Rate Product or Double Product

This index has been conveniently used for in situ hearts in animal experiments, clinical settings and sports medicine because it is easy to determine non-invasively. However, we have conclusively shown that this index dissociates from Vo_2 when contractility changes [27]. For example, the pressure rate product, which is alternatively called double product, decreases when Vo_2 increases with contractility. Naive application of this index requires caution.

Contractile Element Work

Britman and Levine [28] hypothesized that the total mechanical work as the sum of external and internal mechanical work would be better correlated with Vo_2. The internal work means work performed by the contractile element on the series elasticity in the Hill model of myocardium. It is work performed by the contractile element, but is stored as the elastic potential energy in the series elasticity, unlike external work performed to the outside of the myocardium. This elastic potential energy is both qualitatively (or conceptually) and quantitatively different from what we call the elastic potential energy in the time-varying elasticity (Fig. 2).

Britman and Levine's results showed that the correlation between the contractile element work and Vo_2 was unsatisfactory [28]. Coleman et al. [29] scrutinized the relation between the total work and Vo_2 in papillary muscles. They found that the simple sum of the two types of work did not linearly correlate with Vo_2. To make the correlation linear, internal work must be assumed to have about three times greater oxygen cost of work than the external work. However, according to the cross-bridge models [20], it seems unreasonable that the contractile machinery can differentiate internal work from external work and switch their oxygen costs by three fold.

Moreover, we found that a relaxing ventricle could perform a few times more external work than the internal work [30, 31]. This finding suggests that internal work is not the only mechanical energy stored in the ventricular wall. We consider that any internal work in a damped series elasticity of the myocardium cannot be quantified by the quick release method. Therefore, it is unreasonable to assume that internal work defined in the two element model is the total mechanical potential energy of myocardium as has been assumed conventionally [28, 29].

Graham's Formula

Graham et al. [32] found that Vo_2 for a given peak force increased with indexes of contractility such as V_{max} and maximum d*P*/d*t* when they were increased by various positive inotropic interventions. As a result, they proposed an empirical formula: $Vo_2 = k_1$ (peak force) $+ k_2V_{max} + k_3$, where k_1, k_2 and k_3 are empirical coefficients and constant. However, the number of data points were too small to examine the generality of this linear equation [32]. Nor is there any physiological basis to assume that the relation must be linear. Moreover, the dimensions of k_1 and k_2 must be [length] and [force] [time], respectively. It is not easy to understand the physiological meanings of k_1 and k_2 values with these dimensions.

Bretschneider's E_t Formula

Bretschneider et al. [13] developed a complex equation to predict Vo_2 from various mechanical and nonmechanical parameters of contraction. The sum of these Vo_2 determinants was called total energy demand E_t. The following are the individual terms and their physiological meanings. The mathematical expressions of these terms are omitted here.

E_0 = basal energy demand of the arrested heart

E_1 = energy demand of electrophysiological processes

E_2 = energy demand of maintenance of tension during ejection

E_3 = energy demand of tension development during isovolumic contraction

E_4 = energy demand of relaxation

Baller et al. [13] confirmed E_t to be a good correlate of Vo_2 using many Vo_2-E_t data points, in which each data point was obtained from each subject in a group of either human patients or dogs. However, they did not examine the correlation under varied loading conditions in each individual human or dog heart. When other investigators examined the Vo_2 predictability by this index, their results showed that this index is not superior [14–16].

Rooke and Feigl's Pressure-Work Index

Rooke and Feigl [14] proposed a new index called the pressure-work index. It is the sum of the pressure rate product and external work. They found that this index correlated best with the Vo_2 of several major conventional determinants of Vo_2, including the pressure rate product, external work, triple product, E_t and peak systolic tension. Moreover, they claimed that this index could account for the catecholamine-induced increase in Vo_2 without postulating an oxygen-wasting effect.

Schipke et al. [15] compared this index with the pressure-work index and our PVA under varied afterload and contractility in each dog heart as well as in many dog hearts. They studied prospective predictability of Vo_2 by these predictors using representative coefficients and constants obtained retrospectively. They found that in either a given dog heart or several dog hearts, these three predictors had similar Vo_2 predictabilities. This study was the first that analyzed the Vo_2 predictability of E_t and pressure-work index in individual hearts. They concluded that the predictive power of these three predictors were comparable.

Problems

A major problem with these conventional determinants of Vo_2 is that the mechanical terms and indexes used to predict Vo_2 do not necessarily have dimensions of energy. The non-energy terms do not have dimensionless coefficients. For example, tension has dimensions of [force] and its coefficient to Vo_2 must have dimensions of [energy]/[force] = [force] × [length]/[force] = [length]. What does this [length] dimension mean and what does this length correspond to? The force-time integral has dimensions of [force] × [time] and its coefficient to Vo_2 must have dimensions of [energy]/([force] × [time]) = [length]/[time] = [speed]. What does this speed dimension mean? What does this speed correspond to? To have a dimensionless coefficient, a Vo_2 determinant must have dimensions of energy. When the coefficient of an energy or work term is dimensionless, its meaning is the efficiency of generation of energy or work from Vo_2.

However, it has conclusively been shown that the mechanical work, although it has dimensions of energy, cannot be a candidate for a determinant of Vo_2 because of its poor correlation with Vo_2 [18]. Even what was considered to be the total mechanical work did not closely correlate with Vo_2 [28, 29].

The briefly reviewed history explicitly shows that a unanimously accepted determinant or predictor of Vo_2 does not presently exist. There is ample room to search for better determinants of Vo_2 which can serve as a consistently reliable determinant of Vo_2.

New Determinants of Myocardial Oxygen Consumption

Time-Varying Elastance Model

In 1975, Suga was greatly perplexed by the different oxygen costs of internal and external work in the literature [30], because it was not easily conceivable that the contractile element could discriminate external work from internal work and perform them with different energy costs and efficiencies. In other words, contemporary cross-bridge kinetics do not have a mechanism to change their association and dissociation rate constants in a different manner for internal and external work [20]. There seems to be no mechanism for cross-bridges to know whether the mechanical work performed by cross-bridge cycling is conveyed to the outside of the fiber or stored in the series elasticity within the fiber.

In the mean time, Suga developed the new idea that the time-varying elastance model of the ventricle could help solve this important problem of cardiac energetics [17]. He proposed the time-varying model based on his own ventricular pressure and volume measurements in 1969 in Tokyo (Fig. 2) [8, 33, 34] and developed it together with the late Dr. Kiichi Sagawa in 1971–1978 in the United States [35–38]. Suga's model of the ventricle is conceptually the same as the time-varying capacitance or elastance (elastance = 1/capacitance) models which some cardiovascular modelers had intuitively proposed to simulate cardiac pumping in models of the cardiovascular system [8, 37]. However, Suga was the first who gave a firm physiological basis to the time-variant elastance of the left ventricle [8, 37, 38]. The feasibility and limitations of this model were extensively studied by Suga, Sagawa, Sunagawa, Maughan and their associates [38]. Reference 38 presents the details of the ventricular pressure-volume relation and the time-varying elastance model.

Total Mechanical Energy as Assessed by Ventricular Pressure-Volume Area (PVA)

Suga [17] devised a method to quantify the total mechanical energy which the ventricle generates by contraction based on the time-varying elastance model. The principle is analogous to the mechanical potential energy (strain energy) which is quantified by the area under the force-length (stress-strain) relation curve in the force-length (stress-strain) diagram of a spring [17]. The elastic potential energy is mechanical potential energy in that it can produce mechanical work if the state descends along the stress-strain relation. External work is given by the area under a pressure-volume or force-length (stress-strain) trajectory during the increment in elastance (or spring constant), as shown in Fig. 2. The sum of these two areas, one for the mechanical potential energy (PE) and the other for the external mechanical work (EW) performed during systole, gives the total mechanical energy generated during the systolic increment in elastance in either a spring or a ventricular time-varying elastance model.

Of course, the total mechanical energy generated by contraction could eventually be quantified by the total number of cross-bridge cycles and the thermodynamic efficiency of each cross-bridge hydrolysing ATP [39, 40]. Because the number of cross-bridge cycles per one ATP is considered to be normally 1 [20], the number of cross-bridge cycles can be assumed to be proportional to the number of ATP moles hydrolyzed. However, there is evidence that the

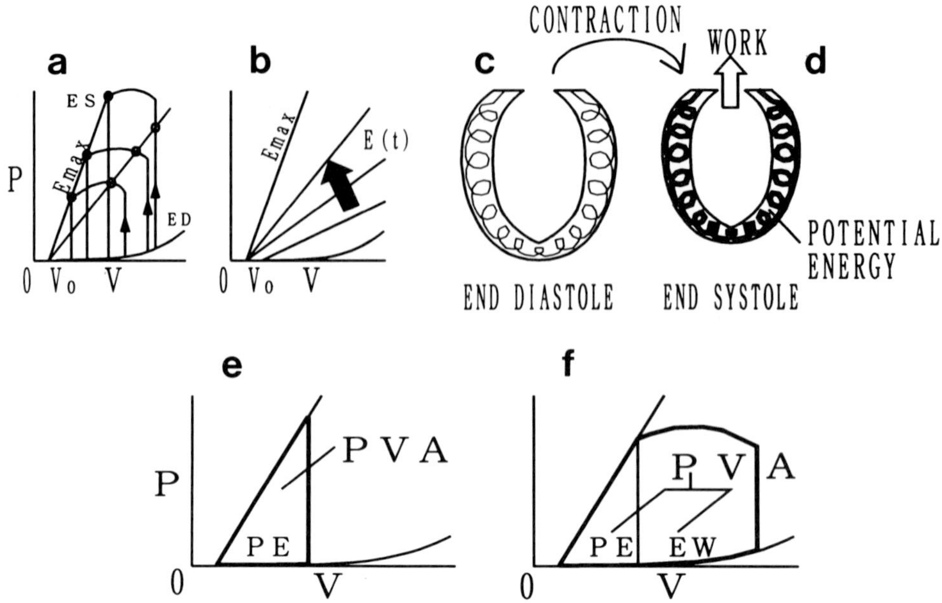

Fig. 2. Instantaneous pressure-volume relations (Panels **a** and **b**), time-varying elastance model of the ventricle (Panels **c** and **d**), and total mechanical energy of ventricular contraction as measured by the systolic pressure-volume area (PVA) (Panels **e** and **f**). *P*, pressure; *V*, volume; *ES*, end-systolic pressure-volume relation line; *ED*, end-diastolic pressure-volume relation curve; E_{max}, slope of the end-systolic pressure-volume relation line; *E*(*t*), time-varying slope of the instantaneous pressure-volume relation; V_0, volume intercept of the end-systolic pressure-volume relation; *PE*, end-systolic mechanical potential energy; *EW*, external mechanical work; $PVA = PE + EW$. In Panel **a**, *solid circles* on the left upper shoulders of the pressure-volume loops are the end-systolic points. The *arrows* indicate the directions of the movement of the loop trajectories. In Panel **b**, the *thick arrow* indicates the direction of the shift of the instantaneous pressure-volume relation. In **Panels c** and **d**, ventricular contraction is simulated by the stiffening of the ventricular chamber elastance from the compliant end-diastolic level to the stiff end-systolic level. The stiffened elastance has performed external mechanical work and increased mechanical potential energy. In Panels **e** and **f**, the areas within the *thick lines* and curves represent PVA of an isovolumic contraction (Panel **e**) and an ejecting contraction (Panel **f**)

coupling ratio between cross-bridge cycling and ATP hydrolysis deviates from unity under certain loading conditions [41]. Therefore, we have to wait until the total mechanical energy can be quantified more precisely from cross-bridge kinetics and thermodynamics. Until then, our PVA method can be utilized to the full extent as a measure of the total mechanical energy of contraction [6, 8]. As explained later in detail, Mast and Elzinga's [42] recent finding is strong evidence that PVA is equivalent to the total mechanical energy of contraction.

We have made some efforts to account for the PVA concept by cross-bridge kinetics. Yasumura and Suga [39] explained PVA by the cumulative number of cross-bridge cycles. Taylor et al. [40] also simulated the relation between PVA and the number of cross-bridge cycles using Huxley's [43] cross-bridge model and Panerai's [44] assumption of myocardial activation function. Their preliminary results [40] show considerable discrepancy between PVA and cross-bridge cycles at different loads, suggesting a yet unknown variable coupling between cross-bridge cycles and ATP hydrolysis.

Vo_2-PVA Relation

Based on his theoretical considerations in 1979, Suga hypothesized that PVA would be somehow correlated with Vo_2 [17]. He searched to see if there were any experimental data which could support that PVA had a close correlation with Vo_2 in a stable contractile state [17], and found some literature with cardiac mechanoenergetics data which supported a close Vo_2-PVA correlation [45].

Greatly encouraged by the preliminary results, Suga decided to perform his own experiments. He and his associates [46] used the same type of excised cross-circulated dog heart preparation as conventionally used for E_{max} studies [36]. The unique feature of this heart preparation, which is often called Suga-Sagawa's heart preparation, compared to the conventional Langendorff-type preparation is that the former can be instituted without any interruption of coronary blood flow.

Moreover, the excised, cross-circulated heart preparation in general has the following advantages:

1. The heart is surgically isolated and denervated, hence independent of neural reflexes including baroreceptor reflex
2. The left ventricle can be opened and fitted with a water-filled balloon for instantaneous absolute volumetry with a volumetric and volume-controlling servo pump [38, 47]
3. Ventricular loading conditions can be widely varied at the experimenter's disposal
4. Total coronary flow and coronary arteriovenous oxygen content difference can be accurately measured
5. Pharmacological intervention of inotropism is easy to do by directly infusing agents into the coronary arterial circulation without significantly affecting the circulatory conditions of the support dog and the inotropism of the support dog's heart
6. Loading conditions can be set on the ventricle independent of inotropic interventions.

There are however a few disadvantages:

1. Elimination of cardiac vagal and sympathetic neural tones by surgical denervation
2. Surgical invasiveness
3. Severance of mitral chordae tendineae.

These factors probably decrease cardiac contractility and coronary vascular tone.

However, the advantages definitely exceed the disadvantages for the purpose of our studies on V_{O_2} and PVA. For this reason, we have been using this heart preparation for nearly two decades.

Load-Independence of the V_{O_2}-PVA Relation

We first investigated extensively the V_{O_2}-PVA relations under different loading contractions in a stable contractile state.

Isovolumic Versus Ejecting

As soon as Suga came across a working hypothesis on the PVA and obtained support from other literature [17], he rushed to examine the V_{O_2}-PVA relation of both isovolumic and ejecting contractions pooled in a stable "baseline" contractile state in dog hearts [46]. "Baseline" means a spontaneously existing level of contractility without any intentional inotropic interventions. In those days, coronary blood flow could be continuously measured but coronary arterial and venous blood were sampled frequently to determine their oxygen contents with an IL 182 CO Oximeter or a Lex-O_2 Con. PVA was determined by manual planimetry on a Polaroid picture showing pressure-volume loops displayed on a storage oscilloscope. The obtained V_{O_2} and PVA data were analyzed for correlation and regression.

The obtained V_{O_2}-PVA relation was consistently linear with a correlation coefficient very close to unity ($r = 0.92$ on average) [46]. After finishing this study at the John Hopkins University Medical School, Suga came back to Japan in 1978 to join the newly opened National Cardiovascular Center (NCVC) Research Institute in Osaka. The following studies were all performed at the NCVC.

To further confirm the load-independence of the V_{O_2}-PVA relation, Suga and his associates started to study more extensively the V_{O_2}-PVA relations of variously loaded contractions in several different ways. One major modification of the experimental system was a switch from the previous method of discrete sampling and oxygen content measurements of coronary arterial and venous blood to continuous measurement of the coronary arteriovenous oxygen content difference. We first used two identical oximeters (Waters Instrument, Rochester, NY, USA, model O-600A), which were calibrated with a Lex-O_2 Con oxygen content meter [48]. These oximeters continuously measured oxyhemoglobin saturation of flowing arterial and venous whole blood. Later we switched to a more direct determination of coronary arterial oxygen content difference with an AVOX Analyzer (AVOX Systems, USA) [49]. Since 1989, we have used our custom-made oximeter (Erma Inc, Tokyo, model PWA-200S), which indicates not only arteriovenous oxygen content difference but also arterial and venous oxyhemoglobin saturations and hemoglobin content

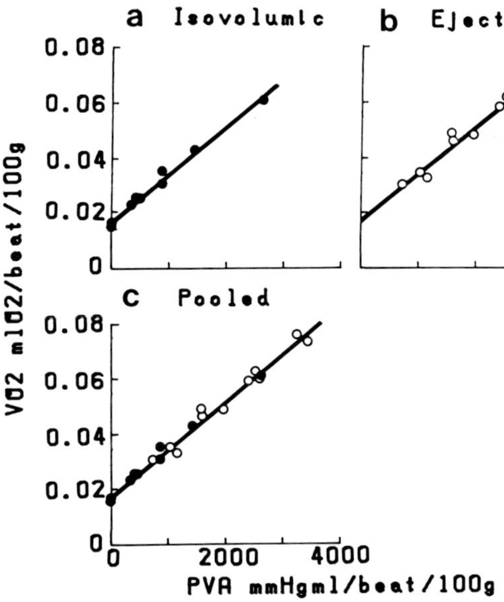

Fig. 3. Left ventricular oxygen consumption per beat (Vo_2) versus systolic pressure-volume area (*PVA*) relations in isovolumic contractions (Panel **a**) and ejecting contractions (Panel **b**) in the same dog heart. Both data are pooled in Panel **c**. From [143] with permission

[50]. These oximeters must be calibrated before each experiment against the IL 182 CO Oximeter or the Lex-O_2 Con oxygen content analyzer.

In our experiments, the Vo_2-PVA relation was first compared between isovolumic and ejecting contractions in each individual dog left ventricle [48]. Fig. 3 compares the Vo_2-PVA relations separately of isovolumic (Panel A) and ejecting (Panel B) contractions. Both of the data are pooled together for a single correlation coefficient and a regression line in Panel C. In either mode of contraction, the relation was linear, very close to unity ($r = 0.96$ on the average). When both are pooled regardless of the mode of contraction, the resultant Vo_2-PVA relation was also linear with a correlation coefficient very close to unity ($r = 0.96$ on average).

We therefore obtained the following empirical equation to describe the Vo_2-PVA relation, both Vo_2 and PVA on a per-beat basis.

$$Vo_2 = a\text{PVA} + b$$

where a is the slope of the Vo_2-PVA relation and b is the Vo_2 intercept of this relation. Slope coefficient a has dimensions of ml O_2/(mmHg ml) and intercept b has the same dimensions as Vo_2, i.e., ml O_2/beat per 100 g left ventricle. On average, a(mean ± SE) was $(1.64 \pm 0.12) \times 10^{-5}$ ml O_2/(mmHg ml) and b was 0.019 ± 0.003 ml O_2/beat per 100 g [48].

The Vo_2-PVA relation is essentially the same whether or not both Vo_2 and PVA are normlaized relative to the left ventricular weight (LVW). When both

Vo_2 and PVA are raw values, $100 \times Vo_2/LVW$ and $100 \times PVA/LVW$ are their values normalized to 100 g left ventricle. When the Vo_2-PVA relation is given with raw values for Vo_2 and PVA, the relation is $100 \times Vo_2/LVW = a \times 100 \times PVA/LVW + 100 \times b/LVW$. Dividing all terms by LVW/100 yields $Vo_2 = a\text{PVA} + b$. Both equations, whether raw or normalized, have the same slope value of a. The Vo_2 intercept is b or $100 \times b/LVW$. However, to ease the comparison of b values between different hearts, we normalized both Vo_2 and PVA for 100 g left ventricle.

The square of the correlation coefficient (r^2) is the coefficient of determination, and indicates the fraction of the variance of one variable (e.g., Vo_2) attributable to the variance of the other variable (PVA). For example, $r^2 = 0.92$ for $r = 0.96$ between Vo_2 and PVA indicates that approximately 92% of the variance of Vo_2 can be accounted for by the variance of PVA and the remaining 8% of Vo_2 should be attributed to the variance of factors other than PVA. Therefore, PVA could explain as much as 92% of Vo_2 in dog left ventricles.

Hisano and Cooper [51] applied the concept of PVA, which was originally developed for a ventricular chamber, to a papillary muscle preparation. The linear muscle version of PVA was called "force-length area" and was abbreviated as FLA. They studied the Vo_2-FLA correlation and regression in both isometric and afterloaded shortening contractions in ferret papillary muscles. They found that the correlation between Vo_2 and FLA (0.96 on the average) was better than any other correlation between Vo_2 and peak force (0.90), force-time integral for entire contraction (0.88) or force-time integral through end systole (0.93). Moreover, the Vo_2-FLA relation was common to both isometric and shortening contractions. These results indicate that the linear, load-dependent Vo_2-PVA relationship holds reasonably well in myocardium in the same manner as in the ventricle. In other words, the load-independent linear Vo_2-PVA relationship is intrinsic to myocardium and does not need to assume the complex shape of the ventricular chamber and myocardial fiber orientation within the ventricular wall. Gibbs [52] also examined the heat (instead of Vo_2) versus PVA relation in rabbit papillary muscles and confirmed the feasibility of this relation in myocardium.

Oxygen Equivalence of External Work and Potential Energy

We confirmed the uniqueness of PVA as a correlate of Vo_2 by a statistical method as follows [53]. After external mechanical work (EW) and end-systolic elastic potential energy (PE) were obtained in ejecting and isovolumic contractions in each dog left ventricle, they were multiplied by a_1 and a_2, respectively, and their sum, $a_1\text{EW} + a_2\text{PE}$, were correlated with Vo_2 to determine the best fit values for a_1 and a_2 in individual dog hearts with both ejecting and isovolumic data pooled.

The results showed that on the average a_1 was $(1.67 \pm 0.43) \times 10^{-5}$ ml O_2/(mmHg ml) and a_2 was $(1.74 \pm 0.49) \times 10^{-5}$ ml O_2/(mmHg ml). They were virtually the same in each individual heart ($P < 0.05$, paired t test) [53].

Moreover, these multiple correlation coefficients were nearly the same as the simple correlation coefficient between Vo_2 and PVA in each heart. This result indicates that instead of these two coefficients a_1 and a_2, a single coefficient a could serve satisfactorily as a common coefficient of both EW and PE as well as the sum of them, namely PVA. Thus, Vo_2 per unit EW, or the oxygen cost of EW, is virtually the same as Vo_2 per unit PE, or the oxygen cost of PE. In other words, Vo_2 does not discriminate between EW and PE, and the sum of them determines Vo_2. The same study showed that correlations of Vo_2 with EW alone and PE alone were 0.63 and 0.83, respectively.

The load independence of the Vo_2-PVA relation was confirmed not only in the baseline contractile state but also in an enhanced contractile state as long as the contractile state was stable [54]. Therefore, the energetic equivalence of EW and PE holds regardless of contractile states.

Comparison with Force-Time Integral

Correlation coefficients of the Vo_2-PVA and Vo_2-force time integral (FTI) relations were compared in a given contractile state [55]. PVA always had higher correlation coefficients (0.97 on the average) with Vo_2 than FTI had (0.93 on average), although the difference was small, in both isovolumic and ejecting contractions pooled. The same situation holds in papillary muscles as described previously [51]. These results indicate that FTI as well as PVA can serve in practice as a predictor of Vo_2.

FTI has two forms: FTI during contraction phase until end systole (FTIs) and FTI during the entire cardiac cycle (FTIc). The correlation coefficient between Vo_2 and FTIs (0.93 on average) was always higher than that between Vo_2 and FTIc (0.84) in individual hearts. The correlation between PVA and FTI was also high (0.97 for FTIs and 0.85 with FTIc). We consider that the high correlation between Vo_2 and FTI may be due to the high correlation between PVA and FTI [55]. This contention is reinforced below.

Same Vo_2 for Different Values of FTI

Although FTI has been shown to correlate fairly well with Vo_2 [19] in isovolumic contractions, there is also evidence that FTI does not consistently correlate with Vo_2 in ejecting contractions [19, 51, 55]. The reason for the contradictory conclusion seems to be due to different experimental protocols among studies. When Vo_2, PVA and FTI were pooled from variously preloaded and afterloaded contractions, FTI appears to correlate reasonably well with Vo_2 even in our study [56].

However, when loading conditions were varied while keeping PVA constant, Vo_2 remained unchanged whereas FTI did change [56]. For example, when PVA was kept constant at 1340 mmHg ml in isovolumic and ejecting contractions, Vo_2 also remained constant at 0.053 ml O_2. However, FTI through end systole gradually decreased by 32% from 164 to 111 g sec when stroke volume was increased from 0 to 15.4 ml in a representative dog left ventricle. Peak force was simultaneously decreased by 46% from 2360 to 1280 g. This study conclusively negated FTI as a candidate for the ideal predictor or determinant of V_{O_2}.

Inclusion of FTI

Since the correlation between V_{O_2} and PVA is very high, it is unreasonable to expect any improvement of the V_{O_2} predictability of PVA even if FTI is added to the predictive equation: $V_{O_2} = a\text{PVA} + b$. We actually examined this as follows [55]. We considered a multiple regression equation: $V_{O_2} = a\text{PVA} + k\text{FTI} + b$, where a and k are regression coefficients to be determined by multiple regression analysis, and b is the V_{O_2} intercept at zero PVA and FTI. Using both isovolumic and ejecting contractions pooled together, the multiple correlation coefficients were determined in each individual dog left ventricle. The multiple correlation coefficient between V_{O_2} and PVA was very close to unity (0.97 on the average). However, the multiple correlation coefficient between V_{O_2} and PVA plus FTI (0.98 on the average) was only slightly greater than the simple correlation coefficient between V_{O_2} and PVA (0.97). The coefficient of determination was 0.94 (mean) between V_{O_2} and PVA alone, and it was not always significantly increased by the addition of FTI (0.95). The standard partial regression coefficient of FTI was close to 0 was opposed to the value of nearly 1 for the PVA coefficient in all individual hearts. These statistical results indicate that the addition of FTI and PVA does not improve the predictability of V_{O_2} by PVA.

One could argue that the contribution of PVA will also be small if one starts with the V_{O_2} prediction by FTI. However, the multiple regression analysis we performed included both PVA and FTI from the beginning and PVA always had a better fit with V_{O_2} than FTI had [55]. Therefore, even if one starts with $V_{O_2} = k\text{FTI} + b$, he will end up with $V_{O_2} = a\text{PVA} + k\text{FTI} + b$ and the conclusion will be the same as above.

Abnormal Pressure-Volume Trajectory

All these results reviewed above show that the V_{O_2}-PVA relation is unique in both isovolumic and ejecting contractions and that this relation is superior to the relations of V_{O_2} with other mechanical indexes. We further reinforced the load-independence of the V_{O_2}-PVA relation as follows.

Various abnormal contractions were imposed on the left ventricle thanks to the high maneuverability of the servo pump we developed [57]. The onset of ejection and filling were varied widely so that the pressure-volume loop deviated from the normal rectangular shape and looked abnormal. However, V_{O_2}-PVA data points of the abnormal contractions were superimposable on the control V_{O_2}-PVA relation line of isovolumic and normally ejecting contractions.

When the onset of ejection was varied to produce abnormal contractions, we found that PVA was also changed [57]. However, when the onset of filling alone was advanced, PVA as a whole was not changed but the fraction of EW over one cardiac cycle decreased [58]. The decrement in EW during filling was equal to the increment in PE during the filling. Despite the changes in the relative magnitudes of EW and PE within a constant PVA, the Vo_2-PVA data points fell on the control Vo_2-PVA relation line of isovolumic and normally ejecting contractions [58].

Recently, we prolonged the ejection phase so that ejection continued even after end systole [59]. This procedure increased EW during ejection as well as in one cardiac cycle, and on the other hand decreased PE within a constant PVA. PVA was given by the systolic pressure-volume trajectory and the trajectory was fixed independent of changes in the ejection period. This procedure increased the fraction of EW in PVA to a surprisingly high value of about 96%. However, the Vo_2-PVA data points of these vastly ejecting contractions fell on the control Vo_2-PVA relation line of isovolumic and normally ejecting contractions [59]. This result also corroborated the load independence of the Vo_2-PVA relationship.

Negative Work

Ordinary ejecting contractions, both physiological and abnormal as above, have pressure-volume loop trajectories on which a working pressure-volume point moves counterclockwise. These contractions perform mechanical work on the outside of the ventricle. However, when a pressure-volume point moves clockwise, the heart receives mechanical work from the outside of the ventricle. Such work is called "negative work" of the heart. We produced left ventricular contractions performing such negative work. Ventricular filling occurred during the contraction phase and ejection occurred during the relaxation phase [60]. Despite the unphysiological contractions, Vo_2-PVA data points of these contractions with negative work fell on or near the control Vo_2-PVA relation line of isovolumic and normally ejecting contractions [60].

Quick Release

We filled the left ventricle to various end-diastolic volumes and allowed ejection against nearly zero pressure so that PVA was virtually zero [61]. Vo_2-PVA data points of these contractions fell on or near the control Vo_2-PVA relation line of ordinary contractions, or more specifically, on or near the Vo_2 intercept of this relation line. This result indicates that PVA determines Vo_2 in excess of the Vo_2 intercept (or unloaded Vo_2) independent of preloaded end-diastolic volume in a given contractile state. As a result, we can more reliably call Vo_2 above unloaded Vo_2 "PVA-dependent Vo_2" and the Vo_2 intercept or the unloaded Vo_2 "PVA-independent Vo_2" [6].

The result in this quick release study negates the following two possibilities. One is that a greater end-diastolic volume might increase PVA-independent Vo_2 due to the length-dependent activation. This possibility was suggested by Cooper [12, 62] in papillary muscles. However, we could not find evidence to support this possibility in the blood-perfused dog left ventricle. The mechanism of the difference between Cooper's [12, 62] and our observations remains to be elucidated [61].

The other is that ejection and myocardial shortening may accelerate the rate of cross-bridge dissociation and increase the rates of cross-bridge cycle and ATP hydrolysis. This mechanism has been postulated in cross-bridge kinetics [20]. However, we could not find any evidence that Vo_2 was increased by myocardial shortening above the unloaded Vo_2. This result is particularly interesting in the light of Yanagida et al.'s [41] recent finding that a mechanically unloaded crossbridge can travel along a several times longer distance than what has been believed to be a single cross-bridge reach by hydrolysing an ATP molecule. Thus, the coupling ratio between cross-bridge cycles and hydrolyzed ATP molecules may not be tight and could be variable depending on the loading conditions and shortening speed. This interesting point remains to be elucidated.

Another type of quick release applied to ventricular contractions was quick release of pressure and volume load at various instants during the course of isovolumic contraction [63]. PVA was developed until quick release occurred. Such a PVA was called "PVA(t)" where t is the instant of the quick release. PVA(t) increased with t until end systole, but was increased no more after end systole in isovolumic contractions at a fixed volume. PVA (end systole) is theoretically equal to PVA if E_{max} remains unchanged by the quick release.

We found that the Vo_2-PVA(t) relation was linear. This result supported the energetic consequence of the time-varying elastance model [63]. However, the slope of the Vo_2-PVA(t) relation, 1.49×10^{-5} ml O_2/(mmHg ml) on average, was smaller than the slope of the conventional Vo_2-PVA relation of entirely isovolumic contractions, 1.92×10^{-5} ml O_2/(mmHg ml) on average [63]. E_{max} of the end-systolic quick released contraction was 9% greater than E_{max} of the entirely isovolumic contraction at the same end-diastolic volume. Therefore, PVA (end systole) was 9% greater than PVA of the entirely isovolumic contraction. However, Vo_2 of the end-systolic quick released contraction was 5%–9% smaller than Vo_2 of the entirely isovolumic contraction; 5% for lower ejection velocity and 9% for higher ejection velocity [63]. If E_{max} of the end-systolic quick released contraction were the same as that of the entirely isovolumic contraction at the end-diastolic same volume, PVA (end systole) would be the same as PVA of the isovolumic contraction, and the quick released Vo_2 would be much smaller than the isovolumic Vo_2.

What has caused the difference in Vo_2 between the entirely isovolumic and end-systolic quick released contractions at comparable PVA(t) and PVA? A major difference is the abortion of force (or pressure)-time integral during the relaxation phase after end systole. In this respect, our result is similar to the finding of Monroe [64]. He found in the left ventricle of the excised, cross-circulated dog heart that Vo_2 of end-systolic quick released contraction was approximately 10% smaller than Vo_2 of entirely isovolumic contraction at the same volume. His ventricle preparation was air-loaded; we therefore speculate that the speed of release was relatively high because of the low viscosity of gas, and the quicker release decreased the force-time integral after end systole to a greater extent.

However, Cooper [12, 65] observed in cat papillary muscles that peak systolic quick release decreased Vo_2 by as much as 36% in isometric contractions at the length developing maximum force. We never observed such a large drop in Vo_2 by quick release in blood-perfused dog left ventricles [63]. Whether the difference was due to the animal species or the conditions of papillary muscle experiments, such as perfusion or temperature, remains unknown.

In this respect, two recent studies from different groups are interesting. One is from Duwel and Westerhof [66] and the other is from Gibbs et al. [67]. Duwel and Westerhof [66] showed that the mechanical events, including quick release during relaxation, did not affect Vo_2, basically supporting Monroe's [64] and Yasumura et al.'s [63] findings. However, the magnitudes of change in Vo_2 were much smaller than the 6%–10% [63, 64]. Gibbs et al. [67] showed that the magnitude of the energy (instead of Vo_2) decrease by the peak systolic quick release varied between 10% and 25% depending on the speed of contraction of normal and hypertrophied hearts, and speculated that even a smaller difference will be obtained in vivo. The mechanisms underlying the controversial effects of quick release on Vo_2 must be elucidated.

Yasumura and Suga [68] evaluated the effect of force-time integral on the Vo_2 predictability of PVA of quick released contractions. Although the contribution of FTI to the Vo_2 predictability by PVA was not proven in normal ejecting contractions [55], it was found to be significant for quick release contractions [68].

Cooper [65] and Teplick et al. [69] showed in cat papillary muscles and dog left ventricles, respectively, that the incremental ratio of Vo_2 to force-time integral was the greatest immediately after the onset of contraction, and decreased gradually with time during the contraction and relaxation plases. We calculated the same ratio and also the incremental ratio of Vo_2 to PVA(t) using the same data [63]. We found that the incremental ratio of Vo_2 to FTI was the largest at the onset of contraction and was rapidly decreased thereafter, whereas the incremental ratio of Vo_2 to PVA(t) was constant throughout systole [63]. Therefore, our results for the same oxygen cost of PVA at any time during systole are compatible with those of Cooper [65] and Teplick et al. [69]. Any difference between our results [63] and the other results [65, 69] seems to be due to the nonlinear relation between simultaneous increments in PVA and FTI during systole [63]. Therefore, the concept of PVA does not contradict cardiac energetics.

Heart-Rate-Independence of the Vo_2-PVA Relation

Since PVA represents mechanical energy per beat, we must correlate it with Vo_2 per beat in the steady state, but not with Vo_2 per min as is done conventionally. As long as the heart rate is fixed, the Vo_2-PVA relation is essentially the same, whether both Vo_2 and PVA are expressed on a per-beat or per-min basis. The empirical equation of $Vo_2 = a\text{PVA} + b$ obtained on a per-beat basis can be modified to $\text{HR} \times Vo_2 = \text{HR}(a\text{PVA} + b)$, where HR is heart rate per min. The latter equation returns to the former by dividing it with HR. The slopes of these two relations are identical regardless of whether the relation is expressed on a per-beat or per-min basis [70].

We studied the effects of heart rate on the Vo_2-PVA relation in the dog left ventricle [70]. The Vo_2-PVA relations at a lower heart rate (124 beats/min on average) and a higher heart rate (193 beat/min) were closely superimposable on each other. This tachycardia was associated with an approximately 10% increase in E_{max}. As will be described below, an increase in E_{max} by an ordinary inotropic intervention has been found to elevate the Vo_2-PVA relation in proportion to the increase in E_{max}. Therefore, we speculated that the small increase in E_{max} with tachycardia may have slightly increased the Vo_2 for excitation-contraction coupling or activation per beat. Basal metabolic Vo_2 per min can reasonably be assumed to be constant regardless of heart rate. Therefore, basal metabolic Vo_2 per beat probably decreased with tachycardia according to the inverse relation: basal metabolic Vo_2 per beat = (basal metabolic Vo_2 per min)/(heart rate). The reciprocally changing Vo_2 components for the activation and the basal metabolism may have cancelled out each other. This seems to be the reason why the PVA-independent Vo_2 did not change with tachycardia above the baseline heart rate [70].

On the contrary, when E_{max} decreases with bradycardia below the baseline heart rate, the PVA-independent Vo_2 will not be constant; it may increase hyperbolically with bradycardia because of the same inverse relation between the basal metabolic Vo_2 per beat and heart rate.

However, Maughan et al. [71] found that E_{max} decreased rapidly with decreases in heart rate below 80 beats/min. If this decrease in E_{max} is accompanied with a proportional decrease in Vo_2 for activation, the sum of Vo_2 for activation and basal metabolic Vo_2 may not increase hyperbolically as we expected with decreases in heart rate.

Contractility-Dependence of the Vo_2-PVA Relation

After establishing the load-independence of the Vo_2-PVA relation, we studied how it was affected by various positive and negative inotropic agents and interventions. In the following studies, we paced each heart at a constant rate before and under any inotropic intervention so that any heart rate-dependence of the Vo_2-PVA relation would not contaminate the effects of inotropic interventions.

Calcium

Cytosolic calcium ions are bound to troponin C and this binding allows cross-bridges to cycle by hydrolyzing ATP and to generate mechanical energy from the free energy change of ATP hydrolysis [20]. This mechanism is considered to be common in both skeletal and cardiac muscles [23]. Increased concentration of extracellular calcium increases calcium influx through voltage-dependent calcium channels during the depolarization phase. Increased calcium influx increases intracellular concentration of calcium ions, which augments total released calcium ions from the sarcoplasmic reticulum and enhances the contractile force as a function of length, i.e., contractility [72].

When intracoronary arterial administration of calcium chloride (0.05–0.2 meq/min) or its intravenous administration into the support dog (0.03 meq/min per kg) increased E_{max} by 50%–100%, the Vo_2-PVA relation was sensitively elevated in a parallel manner with a 50%–100% increase in the PVA-independent Vo_2 [54]. The parallel was confirmed by analysis of covariance. Therefore, the empirical equation $Vo_2 = a\text{PVA} + b$ is affected by calcium in such a manner that coefficient a remains unchanged and constant b is increased. On average, a was $(1.86 \pm 0.32) \times 10^{-5}$ ml O_2/(mmHg ml) before calcium and $(1.94 \pm 0.48) \times 10^{-5}$ ml O_2/(mmHg ml) under calcium, which enhnaced E_{max} from 7.5 ± 2.1 mmHg/ml to 12.9 ± 34.9 mmHg/ml per 100 g. Simultaneously, b increased from 0.024 ± 0.009 ml O_2/beat to 0.036 ± 0.010 ml O_2/beat per 100 g [54].

Catecholamines

Catecholamines are β-adrenergic receptor agonists that enhance contractility in two ways. β-Receptor stimulation causes increases in cyclic AMP which phosphorylates voltage-dependent calcium channels in the sarcolemma and phospholamban on the sarcoplasmic reticulum. The phosphorylated calcium channels increase calcium influx from the outside during the depolarization phase. The phosphorylated phospholamban accelerates calcium uptake by the calcium pump ATPase on the sarcoplasmic reticulum from the cytosol and hence accelerates calcium release from the sarcoplasmic reticulum [73]. These are considered to be the major mechanisms of the positive inotropism of catecholamines. Cyclic AMP also phosphorylates troponin and decreases its calcium sensitivity, which in turn accelerates relaxation [72].

We administered epinephrine in the coronary circulation at a rate (2 μg/min) which increased E_{max} by 50%–100%. We found that the Vo_2-PVA relation was elevated in a parallel manner with a 50%–100% increase in the PVA-independent Vo_2, similar to the effect of calcium described above. On average, a was $(1.75 \pm 0.25) \times 10^{-5}$ ml O_2/(mmHg ml) before epinephrine and $(2.04 \pm 0.44) \times 10^{-5}$ ml O_2/(mmHg ml) under epinephrine when E_{max} was increased from 6.3 ± 1.4 mmHg/ml to 11.3 ± 1.6 mmHg/ml per 100 g, and b increased from 0.019 ± 0.006 ml O_2/beat to 0.003 ± 0.011 ml O_2/beat per 100 g simultaneously. Figure 4 shows a representative case.

We expected that the elevation of the Vo_2-PVA relation for a comparable increase in E_{max} was greater for epinephrine than calcium because of the oxygen wasting effect of catecholamines [74]. A greater oxygen wastage of epinephrine may be accounted for by the reduced sensitivity of the phosphorylated troponin C to calcium, the uncoupling of oxidative phosphorylation

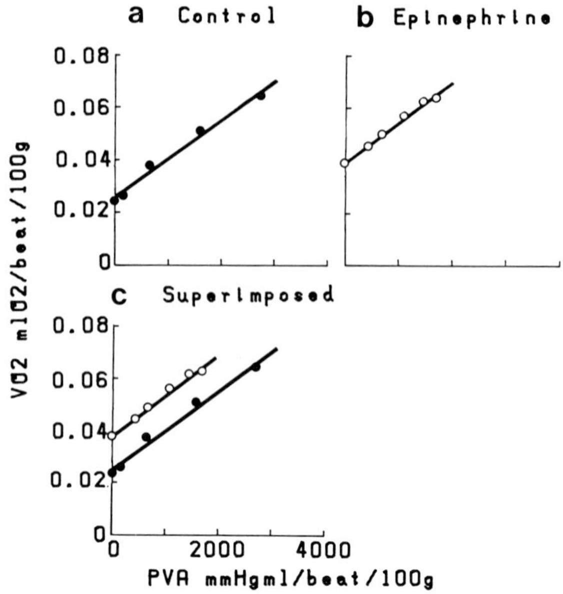

Fig. 4. Left ventricular oxygen consumption per beat (Vo_2) versus systolic pressure-volume area (*PVA*) relations in a control contractile state (Panel **a**) and an enhanced contractile state with epinephrine (Panel **b**). Panel **c** superimposes both data from Panels **a** and **b**. (From [143] with permission)

and the recruitment of lipid metabolism [74]. However, the increase in the elevation of the Vo_2-PVA relation by epinephrine was not significantly different from that by calcium [54].

Besides epinephrine, other β-adrenergic catecholamines, such as norepinephrine, dobutamine, isoproterenol and denopamine (a partial β_1-agonist), were used to examine the parallel upward elevation of the Vo_2-PVA relation. The parallel was common for all these agents [6, 75, 76]. Burkhoff et al. [77] confirmed the parallel Vo_2-PVA relation using dobutamine.

Phenylephrine, an α-adrenergic agonist with a weak β-agonist, given at a high dose (0.1–0.2 mg/min intracoronary arterially), increased E_{max} by 30% and elevated the Vo_2-PVA relation proportionally in a parallel manner [6]. However, the pure α-agonist methoxamine, even at a high bolus dose of 4 mg, increased neither E_{max} nor Vo_2 in dog hearts [6]. Dog hearts are known to be insensitive in contractility to α-agonists. Therefore, the effects of α-agonists on both E_{max} and the Vo_2-PVA relation remain to be studied in the hearts of species, such as rabbit, which are known to respond to α-adrenergic agonists.

Digitalis

Ouabain, a short-acting digitalis, enhances contractility by inhibiting the Na, K pump ATPase, the inhibition of which accumulates Na intracellularly and facilitates Na/Ca exchange, in turn increasing intracellular calcium. Therefore, the net effect of digitalis is similar to increased calcium administration [78].

When E_{max} was increased by ouabain (0.1 mg intra coronary arterially) by 60%, the Vo_2-PVA relation was elevated in a parallel manner with a 30% increase in PVA-independent Vo_2 [79]. When we compared the degree of the elevation per unit increase in E_{max} by ouabain and epinephrine in paired experiments in dog hearts, the degrees were comparable between these two cardiotonic agents despite their different pharmacological mechanisms [79]. This surprising result seems consistent with the similar oxygen wastage of catecholamines and digitalis per comparable increases in contractility in terms of V_{max} and maximum dp/dt [10].

Paired Pulse Stimulation

Paired pulse stimulation is a non-pharmacological positive inotropic intervention. The mechanism of its inotropism is considered to be the augmentation of the total released calcium for the post-extrasystolic potentiated contraction due to a prolonged diastole after the preceding premature contraction. When E_{max} was enhanced by 170% by the maximum post-extrasystolic potentiation, the Vo_2-PVA relation was markedly elevated in a parallel manner with an 82% increase in PVA-independent Vo_2 [80]. The magnitude of the elevation per unit increase in E_{max} was comparable to calcium and catecholamines.

The frequency of electrical activation and the succeeding excitation-contraction coupling is twice the frequency of the post-extrasystolic potentiated beat. We found that the PVA-independent Vo_2 per potentiated beat was slightly but significantly more than twice the PVA-independent Vo_2 of the control regular beat, where basal metabolic Vo_2 was subtracted beforehand from both PVA-independent Vo_2 values. However, E_{max} of the potentiated beat was less than twice E_{max} of the control beat.

We studied E_{max} and the Vo_2-PVA relation while changing the coupling interval of the premature beat to the previous potentiated beat in a steady-state bigeminy while keeping heart rate per min constant [81]. The sum of two E_{max} values of a premature beat and a potentiated beat was virtually the same as those of two control regular beats over a wide range of the coupling interval. Likewise, the relation of the sum of two Vo_2 values against the sum of two PVA values of the same pair of premature and potentiated beats was the same as those of the summed Vo_2 against the summed PVA of two control regular beats. This seems to imply that the sum of the total released calcium in a premature beat and that in a potentiated beat was the same as those in two regular beats.

As the coupling interval was further shortened, the premature beat was fused into the preceding potentiated beat. The E_{max} of the potentiated beat increased and the E_{max} of the premature beat decreased, and the summed E_{max} was not further increased. However, the summed Vo_2-summed PVA relation was further elevated and the summed PVA-independent Vo_2 was also increased. Therefore, the increase in the sum of two PVA-independent Vo_2 of a premature and a potentiated beat per unit increase in E_{max} was greater as the prematurity was increased. This might be accounted for by a saturation of contractile force despite an augmented total released calcium in the maximal and submaximal potentiated beats.

New Cardiotonic Agents

New cardiotonic agents are non-catecholamine, non-digitalis agents which have been developed recently. They are designed to increase cyclic AMP to augment calcium handling in the excitation-contraction coupling or to increase the calcium sensitivity or responsiveness of contractile proteins [24, 25].

We studied the effect of milrinone, which is known to inhibit phosphodiesterase and in turn increase the intracellular level of cyclic AMP. Milrinone simply elevated the Vo_2-PVA relation in proportion to E_{max} in the same way as catecholamines and calcium [82]. For an increase in E_{max}, milrinone and epinephrine elevated the Vo_2-PVA relation to a comparable extent.

We also studied the effects of some agents which are known to have a calcium sensitizing effect in addition to the phosphodiesterase inhibition. They include sulmazole [82], OPC-8212 [83], DPI 201-106 [82] and UDCG-115 [84]. We expected a smaller increase in Vo_2 for calcium handling and hence both a smaller increase in the PVA-independent Vo_2 and a smaller elevation of the Vo_2-PVA relation per unit increase in E_{max}. We compared the energetic effects of these cardiotonic agents with those of catecholamines and calcium. The results showed that none of the new cardiotonic agents tested had a smaller PVA-independent Vo_2 per unit increase in E_{max}.

We speculated about the reasons why the tested agents, which are said to be calcium sensitizers, did not save the oxygen cost for increasing E_{max}. All of these calcium sensitizers still serve as phosphodiesterase inhibitors and their calcium sensitizing effect may not be effective enough to save oxygen cost for calcium handling. The calcium sensitivity of contractile proteins and the amount of calcium needed to raise E_{max} are discussed in the following section.

Propranolol

Propranolol is a β-adrenergic receptor blocker and depresses ventricular contractility by decreasing the (AMP level and hence depressing phosphorylation of calcium channels and phospholamban. E_{max} is considered to be decreased by these mechanisms.

When E_{max} was decreased from the baseline level of 11.6 mmHg/ml to 5.6 mmHg/ml per 100 g, the Vo_2-PVA relation was lowered in a parallel manner with a decrease in PVA-independent Vo_2 from 0.027 ml O_2/beat to 0.019 ml O_2/beat per 100 g [75, 85]. The slope of the relation was 1.76 ml O_2/(mmHg ml) before propranolol and 1.64 ml O_2/(mmHg ml) after propranolol. This response is opposite to the response to a positive inotropic intervention.

Verapamil and Niphedipine

Verapamil is a calcium antagonist and depresses ventricular contractility by decreasing calcium influx via calcium channels. When E_{max} was decreased by 30%–60% from the baseline contractile state, the Vo_2-PVA relation was lowered in a parallel manner with a 20%–30% decrease in PVA-independent Vo_2 (unpublished). Niphedipine also lowered the Vo_2-PVA relation in a parallel manner [77]. These responses are opposite to the response to extracellular calcium administration, but similar to the response to propranolol.

Myocardial Cooling

Myocardial contractility is enhanced by cooling. This effect is known as cooling inotropy. When the excised, cross-circulated dog heart was cooled from 36°C to 29°C, E_{max} was increased by 50%. However, the Vo_2-PVA relation was not significantly elevated [86], unlike the other positive inotropic interventions we tested. The linearity of the Vo_2-PVA relation was preserved and the slope of this relation was not changed.

Oxygen Cost of PVA and Contractile Efficiency

All these experimental results have shown that the Vo_2-PVA relation obtained in a stable contractiler state is largely independent of loading conditions, although the relation is elevated or lowered (except for cooling) by changes in E_{max}. The slope of the Vo_2-PVA relation was not significantly altered by the tested inotropic interventions.

Thanks to the load-independent and contractility-dependent Vo_2-PVA relationship, Vo_2 can be divided into two major components as shown in Fig. 5. One is the PVA-independent Vo_2 below the Vo_2 intercept of the Vo_2-PVA relation, and the other is the PVA-dependent Vo_2 above this Vo_2 intercept (Panel A). The PVA-independent Vo_2 is considered to be constant at any PVA according to the experimental observation of the constancy of Vo_2 for different preloaded contractions mentioned above. Vo_2 above the level of the PVA-independent Vo_2 is called "PVA-dependent Vo_2" because this Vo_2 increases with PVA. The Vo_2-PVA relation can therefore be characterized by the sum of the PVA-independent Vo_2 and the PVA-dependent Vo_2. Since the experimental results have shown that the Vo_2-PVA relation is virtually linear over physiological ranges of PVA and Vo_2, the slope of this relation describes the increment of Vo_2 per unit increment in PVA, or in other words, the oxygen cost of PVA.

The slope of the Vo_2-PVA relation, namely the slope coefficient a in the empirical equation $Vo_2 = a\text{PVA} + b$, was 1.8×10^{-5} ml O_2/(mmHg ml) on average. This means that 1.8×10^{-5} ml O_2 is needed to increase PVA by 1 mmHg ml per beat, or 0.018, 0.036 and 0.054 ml O_2 per beat to increase PVA by 1000, 2000 and 3000 mmHg ml per beat, respectively, which are representa-

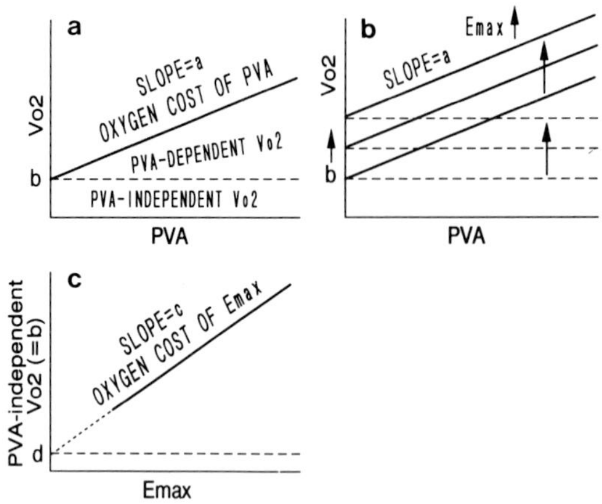

Fig. 5. Vo_2-PVA-E_{max} relations. In Panel **a**, the *thick diagonal line* schematically shows the Vo_2-PVA relation in a stable contractile state. Slope *a* of this relation represents the oxygen cost of PVA. Vo_2 intercept *b* of this relation divides Vo_2 into the PVA-independent Vo_2 which is equal to *b* and the PVA-dependent Vo_2 above *b*. In Panel **b**, the *thick diagonal lines* schematically show the Vo_2-PVA relations at three different contractile states (or E_{max} levels). Slope *a* remains unchanged despite the changes in Vo_2 intercept or PVA-independent Vo_2 *b*. In Panel **c**, the *thick diagonal line* schematically shows the relation between the PVA-independent Vo_2 (*b*) and corresponding E_{max}. Slope *c* of this relation represents the oxygen cost of E_{max}. PVA-independent Vo_2 intercept *d* represents the PVA-independent Vo_2 extrapolated to zero E_{max}

tive PVA values for the hearts of 12–15 kg dogs. When the heart rate is 100 beats/min, these Vo_2 values are 1.8, 3.6 and 5.4 ml O_2.

The reciprocal of the oxygen cost of PVA describes the fraction of PVA in the PVA-dependent Vo_2, or the efficiency of PVA from the PVA-dependent Vo_2. We call this efficiency "contractile efficiency." To express the contractile efficiency in percentages, both Vo_2 and PVA must be expressed in a common unit of energy. One ml O_2 is biochemically equivalent to approximately 20 J, or more precisely 19.5–20.5 J depending on the metabolic substrate used [87]. As a metabolic substrate burnt with O_2, glucose has the largest value of caloric energy (or enthalpy) per ml O_2 (20.84 J/ml O_2), free fatty acids have the smallest (19.36 J/ml O_2 for palmitate), and lactate has the middle value (20.33 J/ml O_2) [87]. One mmHg ml of PVA is physically equivalent to 1.333×10^{-4} J. The average value of the oxygen cost of PVA, 1.8×10^{-5} ml O_2/(mmHg ml), therefore corresponds to approximately 0.4 (dimensionless) or 40% of the contractile efficiency.

The experimental results show that the oxygen cost of PVA falls within 30%–50% around a mean value of 40% [6]. It was unchanged among different species, dogs [6], rabbits [88] and ferrets [51]; between different types of preparation, whole heart and papillary muscles; between different methods of energy measurements, Vo_2 [6] and heat production [2].

What are the sources of energy loss of as much as 60% of Vo_2? To answer this, we have to consider the efficiency of oxidative phosphorylation because contractile efficiency is the product of the chemochemical efficiency of the oxidative phosphorylation from Vo_2 to ATP production and the chemomechanical efficiency of the cross-bridge cycling from ATP hydrolysis to mechanical energy.

The efficiency of oxidative phosphorylation is related to the P:O ratio, namely, the atomic ratio of phosphate, to be used to produce ATP, to oxygen consumed in the mitochondria [87]. The ratio is nominally 3 for lactate, in that one mole of Vo_2 is consumed to generate 6 moles of ATP. It is approximately 3.2 for glucose, including glucolysis in which ATP is produced anaerobically. It is approximately 2.8 for a free fatty acid. Thus, the P:O ratio falls wihtin ±7% around 3.0.

The efficiency of oxidative phosphorylation falls in the range of 60%–70% based on the ratio of the enthalpies of the metabolic substrates oxidized and the ATP produced. The former enthalpy is approximately 20 J/ml O_2 or 448 kJ/mol O_2 and the latter enthalpy is 48 kJ/mol ATP or 288 kJ/6 moles ATP. Their ratio according to the 3:1 atomic P:O ratio yields 64%. The rest is converted into heat as energy loss.

From an oxidative phosphorylation efficiency of 64% and a contractile efficiency of 40%, we calculated that the chemomechanical efficiency of cross-bridge cycling is 63% (0.63 = 0.40/0.64), as shown in Fig. 6. Is this high or low

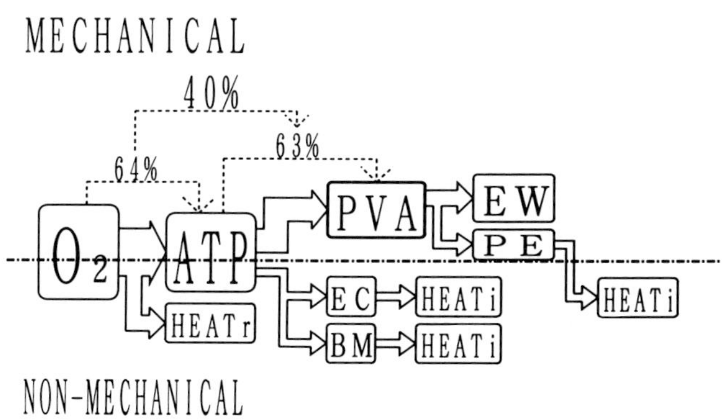

Fig. 6. Energy flow diagram from myocardial O_2 consumption to ATP, PVA, EW and heat. O_2, myocardial O_2 consumption; *ATP*, adenosine 5′-triphosphate; *PVA*, total mechanical energy generated by ventricular contraction measured by systolic pressure-volume area; *EW*, external mechanical work; *PE*, mechanical potential energy; *EC*, energy utilization of excitation-contraction coupling or calcium handling; *BM*, basal metabolic energy utilization; $Heat_i$, initial heat, which is related to ATP utilization; $Heat_r$ recovery heat, which is related to the energy loss in the oxidative phosphorylation to resynthesize ATP. The *percent values* indicate the efficiencies of the energy conversions across the steps marked by the dashed brackets and arrows. The *thick horizontal chained line* divides energies and their conversion steps into mechanical and non-mechanical parts. (Modified from [6] with permission)

relative to the estimated thermodynamic efficiency of 75%–95% in cross-bridge cycling [20]? At present, we cannot answer this question because the chemomechanical efficiency of cross-bridge cycling remains to be elucidated for myocardium.

When the contractile efficiency changes, there is a possibility that the efficiency of oxidative phosphorylation or the efficiency of cross-bridge cycling changes, or that both change. In our experiments, we cannot differentiate between which efficiency changes. Evidence exists that oxidative phosphorylation changes its efficiency when metabolic substrates shift between free fatty acids to lactate and glucose, when the fraction of anaerobic metabolism changes, and when uncoupling occurs in the P:O ratio in the mitochondria. Catecholamines, ischemia, acidosis, and other factors change this efficiency [74].

The verified equivalence between PE and heat [42] indicates that PE quantified the total mechanical potential energy stored in the cross-bridge elasticity and any series elasticity. If PE were equivalent to a fraction of total potential energy, heat would be greater than PE because heat is the sum of PE and any loss from it. It is therefore most likely that the thermodynamic efficiency is close to 0.64 rather than 0.75–0.95 which are the assumed values in the cross-bridge model of skeletal muscles [20]. Since the thermodynamic efficiency of cross-bridges has not been determined, our estimation of 0.64 may be a reasonable estimate of the true value. How this value is related to myosin isozymes and ATPase remains to be elucidated.

Oxygen Cost of E_{max}

When Vo_2-PVA relations are obtained at different levels of contractility or E_{max}, they are different in their elevations but their slopes are virtually the same, as schematically shown in Fig. 5B. The elevation increases with E_{max}. Burkhoff et al. [77] actually obtained these parallel Vo_2-PVA relations at several different E_{max} levels altered by positive (dobutamine) and negative (niphedipine, coronary occlusion) inotropic interventions. When the PVA-independent Vo_2 values or Vo_2 intercept values of the Vo_2-PVA relations at different E_{max} levels were plotted against E_{max} values, the relation was linear [77], as schematically shown in Fig. 5C. The relation was formulated as PVA-independent $Vo_2 = cE_{max} + d$, where c represents the slope of this relation and d the PVA-independent Vo_2 intercept or the PVA-independent Vo_2 extrapolated to zero E_{max}. Slope c describes the oxygen cost of E_{max} in that it indicates the increment in Vo_2 per unit increment in E_{max}. Burkhoff et al. [77] obtained 0.0036 ± 0.0011 ml O_2/(mmHg/ml) for c per beat 100 g left ventricle when E_{max} was changed with dobutamine, niphedipine and coronary low perfusion. They obtained 0.010 ± 0.004 ml O_2 for d per beat per 100 g. The correlation coefficient was 0.96 on average, validating the linearity of the relation over the tested E_{max} range of 2.8–9.6 mmHg/ml per 100 g.

We also calculated an average oxygen cost of E_{max} using pooled Vo_2-PVA data before and after a single dose of epinephrine or calcium administration in multiple dog hearts [89]. The data are the same as those obtained in our previous study [54]. The *c* and *d* values for epinephrine were 0.0024 ml O_2/(mmHg/ml) and 0.005 ml O_2 per beat per 100 g; those for calcium were 0.0014 ml O_2/(mmHg/ml) and 0.015 ml O_2 per beat per 100 g. Because of the inter-heart variation, the correlation coefficient for epinephrine or calcium was 0.64 or 0.57, respectively, and these *c* and *d* values were not significantly different between epinephrine and calcium. When both epinephrine and calcium data were pooled, *c* and *d* values were 0.0018 ml O_2/(mmHg/ml) and 0.010 ml O_2 per beat per 100 g. Our *c* value is about half of the value obtained by Burkhoff et al. [77] and our *d* value is the same as theirs. Our analysis could not find any significant correlation between E_{max} and slope *a* of the Vo_2-PVA relation before and after epinephrine and calcium [89].

The method used by Burkhoff et al. to determine the oxygen cost of E_{max} seems time-consuming because a stable level of E_{max} is required to sample at least two Vo_2-PVA data points to obtain a Vo_2-PVA relation line, and E_{max} has to be changed to several levels in each individual heart [77]. Our method to determine the oxygen cost of E_{max} [89] seems liable to be influenced by the inter-heart variation of this oxygen cost. To circumvent these problems, we devised a new method [90].

When the intracoronary infusion rate of calcium or epinephrine was gradually increased while end-diastolic and end-systolic volumes and hence stroke volume were kept unchanged, E_{max}, PVA and Vo_2 were increased gradually. The Vo_2-PVA data points linearly moved right upward with the increases in E_{max}, deviating upward from the control Vo_2-PVA line in the Vo_2-PVA diagram [90], as schematically shown in Fig. 7A.

From this relation, we determined the PVA-independent Vo_2 for each E_{max} by drawing a line through the data point in parallel to the control Vo_2-PVA relation, based on the already established parallels of the Vo_2-PVA relations for different E_{max} levels [90]. PVA-independent Vo_2 values were plotted against the corresponding E_{max} values, as schematically shown in Fig. 7B, and the relation was linear. This relation could be formulated by an empirical equation: PVA-independent $Vo_2 = cE_{max} + d$. Slope coefficient *c* indicates the oxygen cost of E_{max}. Constant *d* indicates the PVA-independent Vo_2 intercept of the relation. On average, *c* was 0.001 ml O_2/(mmHg/ml) and *d* was 0.017 ml O_2 per beat per 100 g.

Since the basal metabolic Vo_2 of a KCl-arrested heart was not increased by calcium and epinephrine administration [54], we considered that the increases in PVA-independent Vo_2 in proportion to E_{max} were primarily due to increases in the total released calcium and hence increases in the Vo_2 for the increased calcium handling in the excitation-contraction coupling. This consideration is based on the tight 2:1 stoichiometry between the amount of calcium ions sequestered and the amount of ATP molecules hydrolysed by the Ca pump ATPase of the sarcoplasmic reticulum [73].

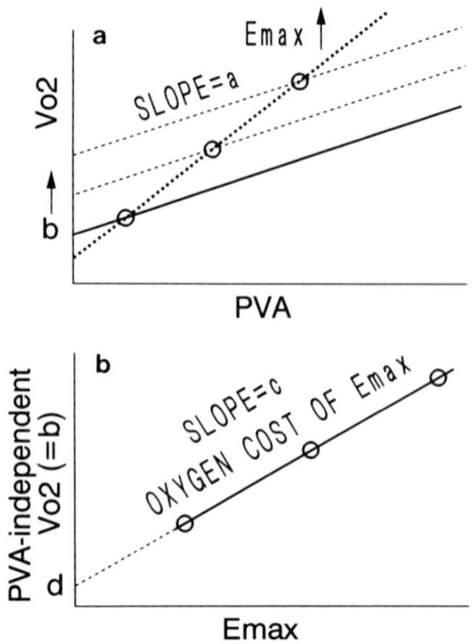

Fig. 7. Schematic illustration of the new method to obtain the oxygen cost of E_{max}. In Panel **a**, the *solid diagonal line* is the control Vo_2-PVA relation. The *solid circle* is a Vo_2-PVA data point in the control contractile state. The *open circles* are the Vo_2-PVA data points of contractions whose end-diastolic volume is kept constant and contractility (or E_{max}) is enhanced in two steps. The two *dotted lines* are drawn through these data points in parallel to the control Vo_2-PVA relation. The Vo_2 intercept of these *dotted lines* is considered to represent the PVA-independent Vo_2 (*b*) at the respective E_{max} levels. Panel **b** plots the PVA-independent Vo_2 (*b*) values against the respective E_{max} levels. Slope *c* of this relation represents the oxygen cost of E_{max}. PVA-independent Vo_2 intercept *d* of this relation represents the PVA-independent Vo_2 extrapolated to zero E_{max}

The PVA-dependent Vo_2 at zero E_{max}, namely *d*, represents the Vo_2 for minimal calcium handling when contractility is null in an electrically beating heart. Beating means that the membrane excitation still exists and Na, K pump ATPase is consuming Vo_2. Therefore, *d* consists of basal metabolic Vo_2 and Vo_2 for electrical activation, as discussed in the next section.

Oxygen Cost of Electrical Activation

The oxygen cost of electrical activation is due to energy utilization by the Na, K pump ATPase, which pumps out sodium ions during the membrane repolarization which has entered during the membrane depolarization. Klocke et al. [91] reported that the Vo_2 of electrical acvtivation was about 0.0004 ml O_2/100 g per activation, which is less than 1% of the total Vo_2. Since then, its contribution to the total Vo_2 has often been neglected.

However, Chapman [5] considered that it may not always be negligibly small. He referred to Langer's [92] data of sodium flux per activation of 66 nmol/g myocardium. Assuming a sodium pump stoichiometry of 3 Na^+ ions per ATP molecule and −48 kJ/mol for the enthalpy of ATP hydrolysis in vivo, the 66 nmol/g of Na^+ would generate initial heat of about 1 mJ/g myocardium or 1.8 mJ/g if the recovery heat is included. Chapman [5] considered that this is probably an upper limit. This energy cost corresponds to 0.01 ml O_2/100 g per activation. This is 25 times more than what Klocke et al. [91] obtained experimentally in dog hearts.

We estimated the oxygen cost of membrane excitation by a new method. The zero-E_{max} PVA-independent Vo_2, which is *d* in Fig. 5C, is considered to be the sum of basal metabolic Vo_2 and the Vo_2 for electrical activation because the PVA-independent Vo_2 at zero E_{max} can be assumed to have virtually no Vo_2 for calcium handling. Basal metabolic Vo_2 per min in KCl-arrested hearts is typically 1.4 ml O_2/100 g [93]. The zero-E_{max} PVA-independent Vo_2 per min at a heart rate of 150 beats/min is typically 2–3 ml O_2/100 g [94], which is 50%–100% greater than the basal metabolic Vo_2. Therefore, Vo_2 for electrical activation per minute at 150 beats/min is calculated to be 0.6–1.6 ml O_2/100 g, and that per beat is 0.004–0.011 ml O_2/100 g per activation. This value is comparable to the value calculated by Chapman [5] but is 10–28 fold greater than the value obtained by Klocke et al. [91].

Another oxygen cost to be considered in relation to the Na, K pump ATPase would be that for pumping Na^+ which has entered by the Na/Ca exchanger. This exchanger is known to remove intracellular Ca^{2+} when the Ca pump ATPase of the sarcoplasmic reticulum is not effectively functioning. To remove one Ca^{2+} to the outside of the sarcolemma, the exchanger allows three Na^+ to enter the cell. These Na^+ ions have to be pumped out by the Na, K pump ATPase. The net stoichiometry is one Ca^{2+} per one ATP. This coupling ratio is half the coupling ratio of the Ca pump ATPase. Therefore, if the sarcoplasmic reticulum Ca pump ATPase has a reduced capability of Ca^{2+} removal, Ca^{2+} removal is performed by the Ca/Na exchanger and the Na, K pump ATPase at an oxygen cost that is two times higher. This hypothesis remains to be tested experimentally.

Basal Metabolism

The basal metabolism of myocardium is the energy utilization of myocardial activitites other than the electrical activation and the mechanical contraction. It can be determined by different methods, and can be directly measured in resting myocardium. A myocardial preparation can rest when it is not stimulated and the resting energy utilization is the basal metabolism [95]. However, whole heart preparations do not relax due to the spontaneous sinus rhythm. They can be relaxed under high K^+ (10–20 mM) perfusion and basal metabolic Vo_2 can be measured directly [4, 93].

Basal metabolism can be indirectly obtained by extrapolating Vo_2 of unloaded contractions at various heart rates to zero heart rate. Basal metabolic Vo_2 is around 1.4 ml O_2/min per 100 g, but it is reported to vary depending on substrates, catecholamines, animal species, temperature, and other factors [2, 4].

We determined basal metabolic Vo_2 under KCl arrest. Administration of KCl into the coronary arterial circulation (14 meq) caused cardiac arrest without interfering with the support dog's condition for 20–30 min [54]. KCl flowing into the support dog seems to be diluted by about ten times and 20–30 min seemed to be necessary for KCl to depress the support dog's heart and systemic blood pressure. When the coronary venous return to the support dog was dialyzed to remove excess KCl, the experiment was able to continue longer without cardiac depression and hypotension [96].

We found that the basal metabolic Vo_2 was 1.24 ± 0.59 ml O_2 at 5 min under KCl arrest, decreased to 1.01 ± 0.53 ml O_2 within the next 5 min, and did not significantly decreased thereafter until 30 min under KCl arrest [96]. The KCl concentration in the coronary circulation was measured to be about 13 meq. However, thanks to the dialysis, the KCl concentration in the support dog's circulation increased slightly from 1.9 to 3.5 meq/1 over 60–90 min of KCl arrest.

The KCl-arrested basal metabolic Vo_2 did not significantly increase with increases in end-diastolic volume from V_0 (about 7 ml) to 50 ml [96]. It did not significantly increase with dobutamine (10–25 µg/min intracoronary arterially). This dose of dobutamine increased E_{max} by 50%–100%.

The basal metabolic Vo_2 of myocardium is considered to include ATP utilization for protein synthesis, maintenance of membrane polarization by the Na, K pump ATPase, and phosphorylation of various proteins. However, much remains to be elucidated as to the components of basal metabolic energy utilization. In particular, information is lacking as to how basal metabolic Vo_2 changes with loading, heart rate and inotropic conditions.

Related Topics

In addition to the considerable clarification of cardiac energetics by our new concepts and studies, some other related topics have been also studied. The results of these studies either corroborate the concept of PVA or expand the utility of PVA.

PVA and Cross-Bridges

The concept of PVA as a measure of the total mechanical energy of ventricular contraction derives from a time-varying elastance model. An unsolved question is the relation between the time-varying elastance model and the cross-bridge mode. We consider that these two models are too far apart to relate them directly using present knowledge on cross-bridge kinetics [39]. There are two opposing opinions. One opinion is that the time-varying elastance model simulates the fundamental pressure-volume relationship of the ventricle and hence must reasonably represent the overall, lumped contractile characteristics of cross-bridge kinetics [8, 97]. The other opinion is that cross-bridge kinetics does not theoretically predict such a simple, zero-order mechanical model as described by a time-varying elastance [98]. We believe that this gap must be closed from both sides to better understand PVA and its feasibility and limitation.

As a first step, from the magnitude of PVA and the estimated concentration of myosin heads in cardiac muscle, we can estimate the number of cycles of one cross-bridge per contraction in dog hearts. This calculation was based on Suga's personal discussion with Prof. Roger C. Woledge of the University College, London, on September 18, 1990 in London. Woledge suggested that if the calculated number of cycles of one cross-bridge were far more than a few cycles per twitch, the concept of PVA would be ridiculous.

The maximal value of PVA in dog left ventricles is about 4000 mmHg ml/100 g or 0.53 J/100 g = 5.3 mJ/g. The concentration of myosin heads is known to be about 0.15 μmol/g wet myocardium. PVA divided by this myosin head concentration yields 35.3 kJ/mole myosin head. Dividing this further by the free energy of ATP hydrolysis of −57 kJ/mole yields 0.62 (dimensionless). This value indicates the fraction of ATP free energy that is converted to mechanical energy per each cross-bridge cycle. The figure 0.62 is 62% in terms of the mechanical efficiency of a cross-bridge.

This 62% efficiency coincides with the efficiency value (63%) calculated from the contractile efficiency and the oxidative phosphorylation efficiency (Fig. 6). This coincidence implies that each cross-bridge cycles once on average in a twitch contraction. A smaller value than 0.62 would imply that each cross-bridge cycles more than once on average in one cardiac cycle. A greater value than 0.62 would imply that each cross-bridge cycles less than once on average in one cardiac cycle. For example, 0.31 instead of 0.62 implies that each cross-bridge cycles twice on average per contraction, and 1.24 implies that each cross-bridge cycles 0.5 times on average per contraction. The fact that the actual Vo_2-PVA data predict one cycling per cross-bridge per contraction supports PVA as a candidate for a measure of the total mechanical energy of ventricular contraction.

The relatively slow cycling rate of cross-bridges within one cardiac cycle is consistent with the results of quick release experiments [63, 64, 66]. When the average cycling rate of a cross-bridge is one cycle per contraction, the ATP consumption will not be affected whether the force during the relaxation falls naturally or quick-released. On the contrary, if the cross-bridge cycling rate is far greater than one cycle per contraction, the cross-bridges made during systole will be partially or entirely broken during relaxation and the force during relaxation requires new cross-bridges to be made. Therefore, if the force during relaxation is aborted by quick release, the new formation of cross-bridges is not necessary and the quick release will save ATP and Vo_2. Thus, the degree of Vo_2 saving by quick release at peak contraction will depend on the cross-bridge cycling rate. This mechanism may be the basis of the observation of the variable degree of energy saving by quick release [67].

In the present cross-bridge model as originally proposed by Huxley [43] or as modified by others [20], the energetics of each cross-bridge is assumed to be energized instantly by the free energy of ATP hydrolysis when it is made Fig. 8 and the mechanical potential energy is given to the cross-bridge elasticity [99]. This potential energy is then either used for mechanical work while shortening under load or, if unused, dissipated into heat when the cross-bridge is broken. It is generally considered that the amount of energy of mechanical contraction is proportional to the number of ATP molecules hydrolysed in the contractile machinery and also to the number of cross-bridge cycles made. In this respect, the mechanical model of muscle consisting of multiple cross-bridges has essentially a time-varying elastic nature [100].

Recently, Mast and Elzinga [42] found that the total mechanical energy assessed by the PVA matched the heat generated during relaxation in rabbit papillary muscles. This heat equivalence strongly supports the PVA concept and the equivalence between PVA and ATP consumption. The result negated the feasibility of the Hill model for cardiac muscle, supporting our contention [101].

This heat equivalence also supports our contention that the PVA concept is compatible with the Huxley crossbridge model. The free energy profile of a cross-bridge [20] shows that the thermodynamic efficiency (w/e) is smaller than the free energy change of ATP hydrolysis because of two factors. One is the energy loss when the cross-bridge is attached. The other is the energy loss when the cross-bridge is detached. These energy losses are dissipated as heat. The heat equivalence of PVA is consistent with the heat equivalence of the potential energy of a cross-bridge, as shown in Fig. 8.

PVA and the Fenn Effect

The Fenn effect is generally considered to be characteristic of muscles in general [97, 102, 103]. The discovery of this effect by Fenn led to the discarding of the viscoelastic model of muscle, called the cocked spring model or new elastic body, as a realistic model of skeletal muscle. However, the cardiac Fenn effect is different from the skeletal Fenn effect in that the isometric energy utilization is always greater than the energy utilized by a shortening contraction in cardiac muscles whereas the former is sometimes smaller than the latter in skeletal muscles [102]. In terms of Mommaerts' unifying concept of the Fenn effect, the Fenn effects of both muscles are essentially the same [103].

As Chapman and Gibbs [99] commented, the conventional cross-bridge model assumes cross-bridge kinetics similar to the classic cocked spring or new elastic body in the quantum level. Each cross-bridge does not show the Fenn effect within one cross-bridge cycle. The Fenn effect is manifested by the frequency of cross-bridge cycles, which increases with increases in the shortening speed by making and breaking more cross-bridges with adjacent actin sites over longer lengths. The frequency of cross-bridge cycling is minimal in isometric contraction. The total number of cross-bridge cycles within a contraction and hence the Fenn effect will therefore depend on two factors: one is

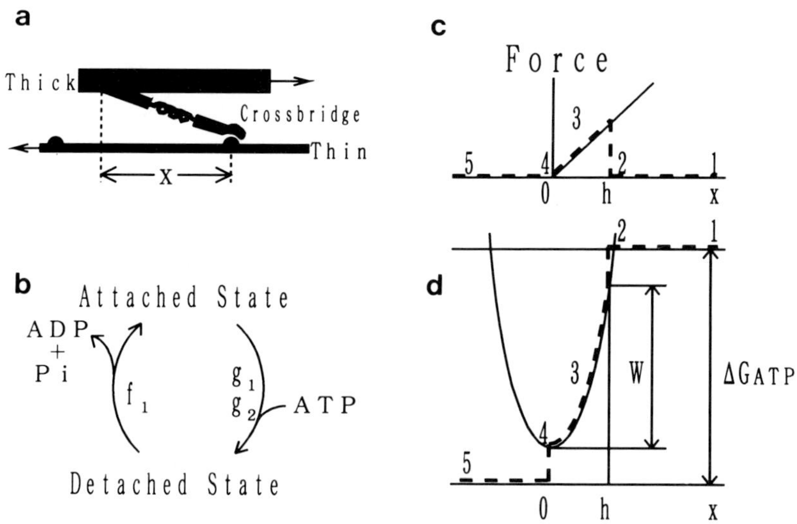

Fig. 8. Huxley's cross-bridge model, its kinetics and free energy changes. Panel **a** schematically shows Huxley's 1957 cross-bridge model. *Thick*, thick filament consisting of myosin; *Thin*, thin filament consisting of actin and other contractile proteins; x, distance between the neutral position of the cross-bridge and actin. Panel **b** shows the two states of the cross-bridge: the attached state and detached state. Cross-bridge attachment occurs at a rate constant of f_1 and detachment occurs at a rate constant of g_1 in the forward position ($x > 0$) and g_2 in the backward position ($x < 0$). One attachment and detachment cycle hydrolyzes one ATP. Panel **c** shows the force (*thick dashed curve*) generated by a cross-bridge as a function of x. The numbers (*1–5*) show different ranges of the cross-bridge position. In the *1–2* range, the cross-bridge is detached, generating no force. In the *3* range, the cross-bridge is attached, generating force. In the *4–5* range, the cross-bridge is detached, generating no force. Panel **d** shows the free energy profile (*thick dashed curve*) of the cross-bridge. ΔG_{ATP}, free energy change of ATP hydrolysis; *PE*, potential energy; *W*, mechanical work. The parabolic curve describes the mechanical potential energy curve of the cross-bridge. The numbers (*1–5*) correspond to those in Panel **c**

the length-dependence of cross-bridge cycles, and the other is the rates of cross-bridge making and breaking during shortening. Even if the latter is the same, differences in the former will cause the difference between the skeletal and cardiac types of the Fenn effect.

Figure 9 shows the Fenn effect of PVA per se and the Fenn effect of the Vo_2-PVA relation. These Fenn effect curves were theoretically obtained [6]. Gibbs [104] found experimentally that our PVA concept was compatible with the cardiac Fenn effect. We also found that the compatibility between the Vo_2-PVA relation and the Fenn effect held in any of control, enhanced or depressed contractile states [75]. Since PVA is based on the time-varying elastance model, this compatibility means that the energetic consequences of the time-varying elastance are reconcilable with the cardiac Fenn effect.

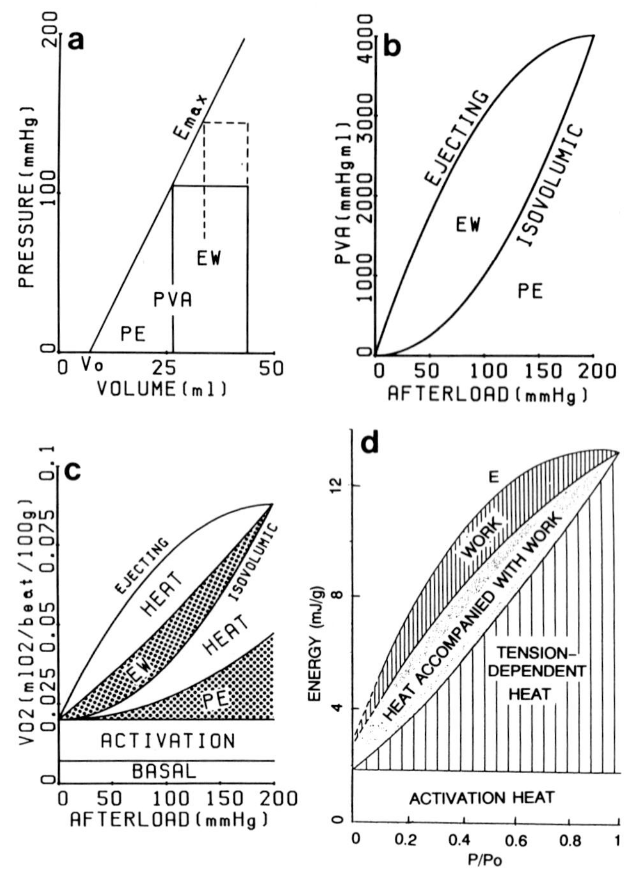

Fig. 9. Fenn effect of PVA, Vo_2 and heat. Panel **a** schematically shows a left ventricular pressure-volume diagram and PVA. E_{max}, E_{max} line or end-systolic pressure-volume relation; *EW*, external work; *PE*, potential energy. Panel **b** shows PVA as a function of afterload pressure (ejection pressure of afterloaded isobaric contraction). *EJECTING curve* shows the PVA-afterload pressure relation of ejecting contractions, in which PVA = EW + PE. *ISOVOLUMIC curve* shows the PVA-afterload pressure relation of isovolumic contractions, in which PVA = PE because their EW is zero. Panel **c** schematically indicates the Vo_2-afterload pressure relation. *EJECTING curve* shows the VO_2-afterload pressure relation of ejecting contractions, in which *HEAT* is the heat dissipated in association with *EW* (*upper dotted zone*). *ISOVOLUMIC curve* shows the Vo_2-afterload pressure relation of isovolumic contractions, in which *HEAT* is the heat dissipated in association with *PE* (*lower dotted zone*). *ACTIVATION* means the Vo_2 used for both the membrane electrical activation and the excitation-contraction coupling. *BASAL* means the basal metabolic Vo_2. Panel **d** shows the Fenn effect of the energy utilization of myocardium as a function of afterload (P/Po). The *E curve* is the energy utilization of afterloaded-isotonically shortening contractions. *WORK* (*upper hatched zone*) is the mechanical work. *TENSION-DEPENDENT HEAT* (*lower hatched zone*) means the energy utilization of isometric contractions. The *shaded zone* in the middle is the heat associated with *WORK*. *ACTIVATION HEAT* means the energy utilization of activation consisting of both electrical activation and excitation-contraction coupling. Basal metabolism is omitted. (Panels **a–c**; from [6] with permission. Panel **d**; from [2] with permission)

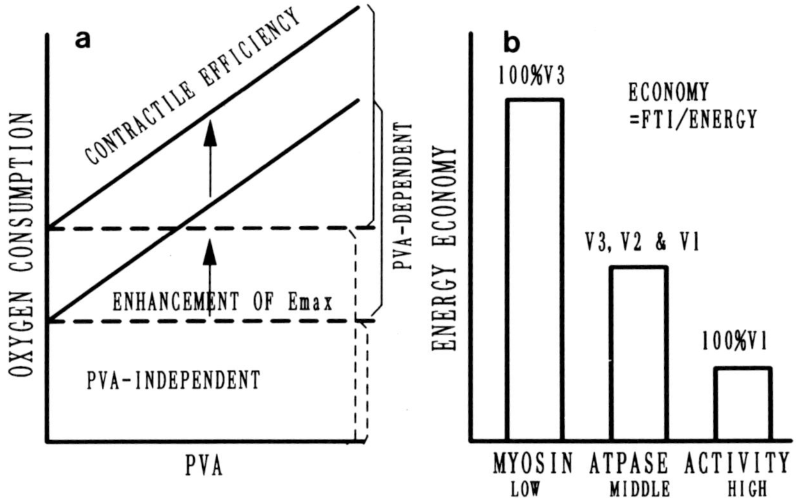

Fig. 10. Constant contractile efficiency versus variable energy economy. Panel **a** schematically shows that the slope of the Vo_2-PVA relation remains unchanged despite the change in the elevation by *enhancement of* E_{max}. *Contractile efficiency* is the reciprocal of the slope of the Vo_2-PVA relation. Panel **b** schematically shows the inverse relation between the energy economy and myosin ATPase activity. The economy is defined as the ratio of the force-time integral divided by the energy utilized. *100%* V_3 means that all or nearly all isomyosins are V_3-type. *100%* V_1 means that all or nearly all isomyosins are V_1-type. V_3, V_2 *&* V_1 means the three different types of isomyosins are mixed

Contractile Efficiency Versus Energy Economy

The contractile efficiency as well as the maximum mechanical efficiency has been shown to be largely independent of inotropic conditions [2, 105], whereas the economy has been shown to change considerably with inotropic interventions [106]. A massive shift of myosin isozyme from V_3 to V_1 by hyperthyroidism decreases heat economy to one half or one third [106] but only slightly decreases contractile efficiency in rabbit hearts [107]. However, increased cross-bridge cycling rate by hyperthyroidism without a myosin isozyme shift from V_3 in dog hearts did not decrease contractile efficiency [108]. Therefore, we consider that contractile efficiency is resistant to changes of myosin isozyme whereas the heat economy is affected by its changes. The mechanism underlying this dissociation must be elucidated for a better understanding of the concept of PVA.

Figure 10 compares the relative constancy of contractile efficiency and the variability of energy economy [105]. Contractile efficiency, as defined by the reciprocal of the slope of the Vo_2-PVA relation (Fig. 5A), is dimensionless because the denominator Vo_2 and the numerator PVA have dimensions of [energy]. However, the energy (or heat or thermal) economy of force which is defined by the force-time integral per energy (or heat) accompanied by the force generation and maintenance [106] has dimensions of 1/[speed]; the denominator has dimensions of [energy] whereas the numerator has dimensions of [force] × [time] [109]. Namely, 1/[speed] = [force] × [time]/[energy] = [force] × [time]/([force] × [length]). When the speed is normalized for a reference length, 1/[speed] is reduced to [time]. That is, 1/([speed]/[length]) = [time]. Recently, the force-time integral per cross-bridge was proposed as a quantum index of the energy economy of muscle contraction [110]. The dimensions of this index are [force] × [time]. Whichever the case, the energy economy of contraction has the dimensions of [time] in the numerator. This means that the time factor of contraction, such as the speed and duration of contraction, shortening velocity (V_{max}), the time-derivative of force or pressure development, myosin ATPase activity, myosin isozyme changes, and other factors may affect the value for the economy. This contrasts with the efficiency which has no time factor [105].

Recently, we considered the theoretical relation between the maximum mechanical work efficiency and the energy economy of muscle contraction in general. Although mechanical work efficiency is different from the contractile efficiency so far discussed, the former is a fraction of the latter and the maximum work efficiency is about two-thirds of the contractile efficiency [111, 112]. We started from the Hill characteristic equation of muscle [113].

Although the theoretical procedure is not described here, our analysis shows that the maximum mechanical efficiency is a logarithmic function of Po/a. Po is the isometric force, a is the shortening heat constant (note that this constant a is different from slope coefficient *a* of the Vo_2-PVA relation), and Po/a is a measure of the curvature of the hyperbolic force-velocity curve and serves as an index of the thermodynamic efficiency [20]. We tacitly assumed that cardiac muscles show a mechanoenergetic relation similar to Hill's characteristic equation. Our result indicates that the expectable range of maximum mechanical efficiency falls within 40%–60%. These values are high because recovery energetics is excluded. Assuming that the energy ratio of the initial process to the recovery process is 2:1 (which is essentially the same as the oxidative phosphorylation efficiency of 67%), the above efficiency range would be reduced to 27%–40%. Whichever efficiency is taken, its range is only 1.5-fold as opposed to the approximately 3-fold range of Po/a between cardiac muscles of V_1 and V_3 isomyosin predominance.

On the other hand, we showed that the heat economy of force could theoretically be formulated by a second-third power function of Po/a, although the theoretical procedure is not described here [113]. When Po/a changes three-fold, the thermal economy would change 27-fold in contrast to only a 1.5-fold change in the maximum efficiency.

Oxygen Cost of E_{max} and Calcium Kinetics

The energy utilization for calcium handling is erroneously considered to be relatively small, based on the observation that the free cytosolic Ca^{2+} concen-

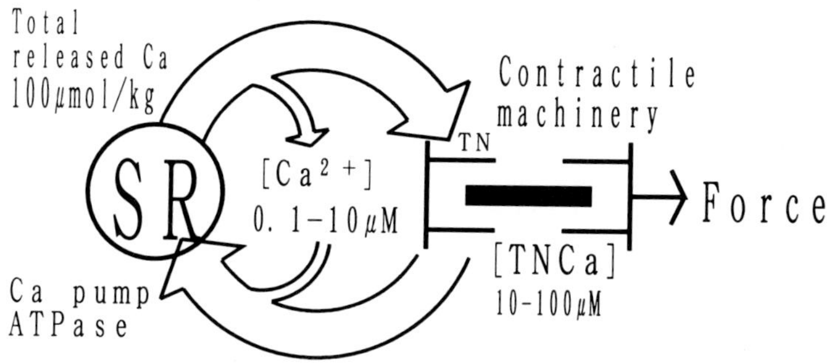

Fig. 11. Relation of the total released calcium from sarcoplasmic reticulum (*SR*), the cytosolic free calcium concentration ([Ca^{2+})], and the concentration of the calcium bound to troponin ([*TNCa*]). *TN*, troponin; *Force*, contractile force. Most of the total released calcium ions are bound to troponin and some remain as free calcium ions during contraction. Most of these calcium ions are sequestered by the Ca pump ATPase into the sarcoplasmic reticulum. The fraction of [Ca^{2+}] will vary with the calcium sensitivity of the contractile machinery. Therefore, the relation between [Ca^{2+}] and total released calcium is complex

tration needed to activate mechanical contraction is in the order of 0.5–2 μM [114]. However, the amount of Ca^{2+} ions to be related with energy utilization is the total Ca^{2+} removed by Ca^{2+} pump ATPase. The total Ca^{2+} removed is nearly equal to the total Ca^{2+} released from sarcoplasmic reticulum. The order of this Ca^{2+} is considered to be 50–200 μmol/kg wet myocardium [72, 73]. This amount is 25–400 times greater than the free Ca^{2+} measured as the Ca^{2+} transient [114]. Figure 11 depicts this relation. As shown above, a significant fraction of the PVA-independent Vo_2 is used for calcium handling. This is the basis of the oxygen cost of E_{max}.

The recognition of the difference between the Ca^{2+} transient and the total released Ca^{2+} is essential to a better understanding of cardiac energetics. To visualize this difference, we performed a computer simulation of the calcium kinetics [115]. The result clearly shows that the even if the total released Ca^{2+} is unchanged, the peak Ca^{2+} transient decreases inversely with the calcium sensitivity of the contractile machinery. This result indicates that one cannot assess the energy utilization of calcium handling from the Ca^{2+} transient unless a change in the calcium sensitivity of the contractile machinery is known.

Based on this simulation, other investigators' experimental observations [24, 25] that calcium sensitizers increased contractile force without increasing the Ca^{2+} transient must be interpreted carefully. For example, Allen and Lee [116] observed that EMD 53998, a new cardiotonic agent with a calcium sensitizing effect, increased contractile force but slightly decreased the peak Ca^{2+}. This should not be interpreted as an unchanged or slightly decreased calcium handling in the excitation-contraction coupling. We could interpret their result to indicate that the total released Ca^{2+} increased, based on the simultation. The

Ca^{2+} transient could decrease even if the total released calcium increase when calcium binding to the contractile proteins was augmented.

Another example would be the effect of acidosis. Acidotic myocardium shows an increased Ca^{2+} transient despite a decreased contractile force [117]. The increased Ca^{2+} transient may be interpreted as augmented calcium handling. However, acidosis decreases the calcium sensitivity of the contractile machinery. Therefore, the increased Ca^{2+} transient could occur even if the total released calcium was unchanged or even decreased. In fact, our unpublished study showed that the PVA-independent Vo_2 decreased by acidosis. Thus, the naive estimation of a change in the total released calcium from an observed change in the Ca^{2+} transient will lead to an erroneously opposite conclusion.

Optimal Contractility for Maximum Efficiency

Our studies have shown that the Vo_2-PVA relation is elevated in proportion to E_{max} due to the proportional increases in the PVA-independent Vo_2 [6, 90]. One may wonder if maximum work efficiency in the ventricule would decrease with increases in E_{max}. However, an increase in E_{max} increases maximum mechanical work [112]. As a net result, the maximum efficiency may not considerably be changed [2]. Digitalis is known to increase cardiac efficiency of a severely failing heart, but it decreases the efficiency of a normal heart [118]. This result has suggested the existence of an optimal contractility for a maximum mechanical efficiency of the heart [119].

Using the empirical Vo_2-PVA relation, we predicted how Vo_2 would change as a function of E_{max} in a heart which is required to pump a constant cardiac output against a constant arterial pressure and hence perform constant work [120]. Figure 12 shows representative results. As illustrated, Vo_2 for a constant work output has a minimum at a relatively low E_{max} within the working range. The optimal E_{max} increases with increases in the afterload pressure and hence the work output.

We attempted to obtain such an optimal E_{max} in dog left ventricles. However, we found that the end-diastolic pressure reached 25–30 mmHg before E_{max} was decreased to an optimal level [121]. We considered that such a result was obtained in non-failing hearts. We are curious to know whether optimal contractility can be easily obtained in the middle of the working E_{max} range when failing hearts are used, because Covell et al. [118] were successful in increasing cardiac mechanical efficiency only when the heart was severely failing.

Pathophysiology

Ischemia

Ventricular contractility changes with coronary perfusion. Decreases in mean coronary perfusion pressure from 80 mmHg to 50 mmHg and 33 mmHg pro-

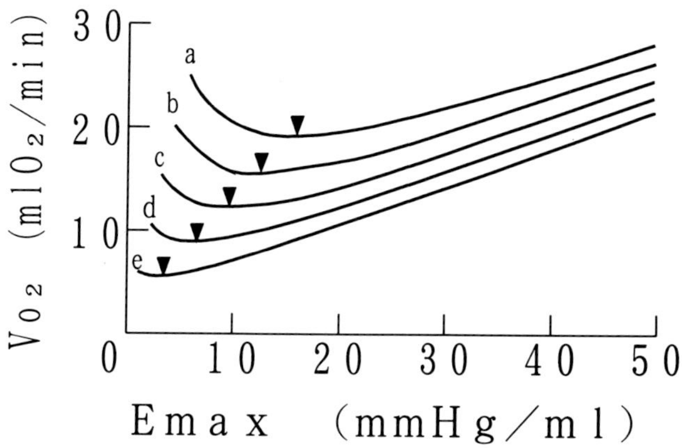

Fig. 12. Theoretical relation of cardiac oxygen consumption as a function of ventricular contractility (E_{max}). Cardiac output is constant at 1200 ml/min. Mean ejection pressure is variable between 50 mmHg for the lowest curve (*e*) and 250 mmHg for the highest curve (*a*) in steps of 50 mmHg for the three intermediate curves (*b* – *d*). Heart rate is constant at 150 beats/min. External mechanical work is constant for each curve: 60,000 mmHg ml/min for the lowest curve (*e*), 120,000 mmHg ml/min for the second lowest curve (*d*), 180,000 mmHg ml/min for the middle curve (*c*), 240,000 mmHg ml/min for the second highest curve (*b*), and 300,000 mmHg ml/min for the top curve (*a*). The *arrow heads* indicate the Vo_2 nadirs of the individual curves. E_{max} values at the *arrow heads* can be called optimal contractility in the sense that Vo_2 at the *arrow head* is minimal under the conditions of constant cardiac output, constant mean arterial pressure, constant heart rate and hence constant external work. These optimal contractilities fall within a physiological range of E_{max}. (Modified from [120] with permission)

portionally decreased E_{max} [85]. The Vo_2-PVA relation was lowered in a parallel manner at 50 mmHg. However, at 33 mmHg, the Vo_2-PVA relation was tilted to increase its slope. E_{max} of contractions decreased gradually with increases in PVA at this severely reduced coronary perfusion pressure. We found that the coronary arteriovenous oxygen content difference markedly increased with increases in PVA at this coronary perfusion pressure. Therefore, we speculated that the gradual decreases in coronary reserve decreased E_{max} with increases in PVA. These results were not associated with lactate production, but lactate uptake by the coronary circulation gradually decreased with decreases in coronary perfusion pressure and increases in PVA. Although net lactate production was not observed even at the largest PVA at 33 mmHg except for one heart, we speculated that the endocardial layers may have been suffering ischemia.

The KCl-arrested Vo_2 also decreased with decreases in coronary perfusion pressure. This indicated that, unlike other negative inotropic interventions, coronary underperfusion decreases not only the Vo_2 for calcium handling but also basal metabolic Vo_2. There is a possibility that the smaller slope of the Vo_2-PVA relation at the coronary perfusion pressure of 33 mmHg was partly due to the gradual decrease in basal metabolic Vo_2 with increases in PVA.

Goto et al. [122] increased coronary perfusion pressure and flow separately and studied their individual effects on E_{max} and the Vo_2-PVA relation. Adenosine injected into the coronary circulation of excised, cross-circulated rabbit hearts increases coronary flow. Coronary perfusion pressure was maintained unchanged so that only the flow of coronary perfusion was changed, although the coronary transmural flow pattern may have been altered. Adenosine increased E_{max} and elevated the Vo_2-PVA relation in proportion to E_{max}.

Stunned Myocardium

We produced myocardial stunning in dog hearts by producing a 15-min normothermic global ischemia followed by reperfusion for up to 2h [123]. Immediately after reperfusion, coronary perfusion flow was markedly increased, and E_{max} was considerably lower than control. However, the Vo_2-PVA relation was only slightly lowered, in disproportion to the decrease in E_{max}. At 1 or 2h under reperfusion, E_{max} gradually recovered halfway, but the Vo_2-PVA relation recovered to the control level. Thus, PVA-independent Vo_2 increased in disproportion to E_{max}.

When calcium was given to increase E_{max} to the control level in postischemic reperfused hearts, the Vo_2-PVA relation was elevated far above the control level. The full contractile return implies that the heart is stunned, because a full return means that the depressed contractility was not due to an energy deficiency.

We found that the oxygen cost of E_{max} determined with increased intracoronary Ca^{2+} administration was nearly doubled in the stunned state as compared to the pre-ischemic control. For a given E_{max}, the PVA-independent Vo_2 was therefore nearly two times greater after stunning. This could account for the nearly unchanged PVA-independent Vo_2 of stunned hearts despite the decreased E_{max}. So far, stunning is the only known intervention that significantly increased the oxygen cost of E_{max}.

We speculated on the mechanisms of the increased oxygen cost of E_{max} as follows. The increased oxygen cost of E_{max} means that more Vo_2 is needed for calcium handling to keep E_{max} constant. This situation will occur when the calcium sensitivity of the contractile machinery is decreased, or when the sarcoplasmic reticulum becomes leaky and futile calcium cycling is increased, or both. An increased Ca^{2+} transient despite a decreased contractile force in stunned myocardium [124] indicates a decrease in the calcium sensitivity of the contractile machinery. The sarcoplasmic reticulum is shown to be leaky during ischemia but to recover after reperfusion [125]. This finding supports the importance of a decrease in the calcium sensitivity of the contractile proteins as a cause of the increased oxygen cost of E_{max} in stunned myocardium.

Hyperthyroidism

The thyroid state is known to affect the gene expression of contractile proteins and result in a myosin isozyme shift between V_1 (or α type), V_2 (or αβ type) in the middle and V_3 (or β type) [126, 127]. In small mammals like rats, V_1 myosin isozyme is normally dominant and hypothyroidism shifts it to V_2 and further to V_3. In mid-size mammals like rabbits, myosin isozyme is a mixture of V_1, V_2 and V_3, and hyperthyroidism shifts them exclusively to V_1 and hypothyroidism exclusively to V_3 [106]. However, in large mammals like dogs and man, V_3 isomyosin is normally dominant, and shifts to V_2 and V_1 hardly ever occur [127].

Goto et al. [107] compared the Vo_2-PVA relations of euthyroid and hyperthyroid rabbit hearts. The hyperthyroid Vo_2-PVA relation was higher and steeper than the euthyroid control. This response consisted of an increased PVA-independent Vo_2 and an increased oxygen cost of PVA. They correlated these changes to an increased calcium pump ATPase activity and massive myosin shift from V_2 and V_3 to V_1 and a decrease in thermal economy of cross-bridges.

Suga et al. [108] made dogs hyperthyoid by the same method as used to make hyperthyroid rabbits, i.e., by daily intramuscular administration of L-thyroxine (0.3–1 mg/kg) for 3–5 weeks. Hyperthyroid dogs were characterized by tachycardia which was not blocked by propranolol even after being excised and cross-circulated. It was also characterized by a 20%–70% increased force transient responses in glycerinated myocardium, which is considered to reflect an increased cross-bridge cycling rate. However, unlike in rabbits, neither E_{max} nor the Vo_2-PVA relation were different from the control of euthyroid hearts. Myosin isozyme was exclusively V_3 in both euthyroid and hyperthyroid dog hearts. We therefore consider that the myosin isozyme shift to V_1 without an increased cross-bridge cycling rate is a prerequisite for a steeper Vo_2-PVA relation.

Arrhythmia

We studied the effect of steady-state bigeminy on the Vo_2-PVA relation [81]. We have already described the results of the bigeminy when the coupling ratio between the potentiated beat and the following premature beat is considerably shortened. Except for such a short coupling, the sum of E_{max} values of a potentiated beat and a premature beat is nearly two times that of the E_{max} of a regular beat. The same holds for both Vo_2 and PVA. Therefore, the relation between Vo_2 and PVA of two consecutive beats (one potentiated and one premature beat) is virtually the same as that of two regular beats.

We also studied the relation between Vo_2 and PVA, both of which were summed for total beats per minute, when the absolute arrhythmia was produced by electrically maintained atrial fibrillation [128]. The Vo_2-PVA relation on a per-min basis was nearly the same for both regular beats and arrhythmias.

Both results suggest that the PVA-independent Vo_2 and the Vo_2 for calcium handling in the excitation-contraction coupling of all beats per min remains unchanged whether the beats are regular or irregular unless the coupling becomes very short.

Fibrillation

We also studied the Vo_2 of fibrillating hearts. A fibrillating left ventricle has an almost stationary pressure-volume point in the pressure-volume diagram. However, the Vo_2 per min under fibrillation is variably greater than that under regular beating. Even when the fibrillating ventricle produces a stationary pressure, we consider that different ventricular wall regions are contracting asynchronously. Under such asynchronous contractions, each region must be contracting isobarically, not isovolumically, generating a finite regional PVA [129]. At this point, the total PVA of a fibrillating ventricle can be obtained as the sum of the regional PVAs of all individual regions. We found theoretically that it can be obtained as the PVA between the end-systolic and end-diastolic pressure-volume relation curves obtained under regularly beating conditions and under an isobaric line through the working pressure-volume point. The assumption used was that the diastolic and systolic properties of individual regions remain unchanged by fibrillation. We call such a PVA of a fibrillating ventricle the "equivalent PVA."

We plotted Vo_2 per min against the equivalent PVA and compared this relation with the Vo_2 per min plotted against PVA of a regular beat. The Vo_2 per min-PVA relation at a given heart rate was extrapolated to different heart rates assuming that both basal metabolic Vo_2 per min and the Vo_2 for calcium handling per beat were unchanged by fibrillation. We found that the fibrillation Vo_2 per min-equivalent PVA relation was superimposable on a regular-beat Vo_2 per min-PVA relation at a specific heart rate. This heart rate was considered to be the average number of isobaric contractions of an individual wall region of a fibrillating ventricle, and this heart rate was called the "equivalent heart rate" [130]. It was 224 ± 34 beat/min. This frequency is about one third of the dominant frequency (about 10 Hz) of a fibrillation electrocardiogram. However, the electrocardiographic frequency could simply be a composite frequency of the slower mechanical contractions of individual regions [130].

Asynchronous Contraction

Burkhoff et al. [131] studied the effects of atrial and ventricular electrical pacing on E_{max} and the Vo_2-PVA relation. As the pacing site was moved from the atrium to the ventricle and from the left ventricle to the right ventricular free wall, E_{max} was considerably decreased. However, the Vo_2-PVA relation was virtually unchanged. They accounted for this observation by assuming that the entire ventricle is consuming the same PVA-independent Vo_2 regardless of the degree of synchrony but some ventricular regions are not contributing to E_{max}, PVA and Vo_2.

We came across a natural case in which the excised, cross-circulated dog heart showed a spontaneous irreversible intraventricular block. The duration of the QRS wave of a left ventricular electrocardiogram was widened by 50% suddenly and irreversibly, and E_{max} was nearly halved. We suspected that an intraventricular block occurred. However, the Vo_2-PVA relation after the block passed through the control Vo_2-PVA data point before the block, indicating no change in the PVA-independent Vo_2. This observation is consistent with Burkhoff et al.'s observation mentioned above.

To account for this observation, we made a simulation study in which the ventricle consisted of two compartments which share the same ventricular pressure but divide the total ventricular volume [132]. The two compartments were made to contract with a variable time interval to simulate a variable degree of asynchronicity. Isovolumic contractions at a constant total ventricular volume were produced with different intervals of contraction of the two compartments. E_{max} and PVA of the two compartments as well as the entire ventricle were obtained. Both E_{max} and PVA of the entire ventricle decreased with increasing degree of asynchronicity although the E_{max} of individual compartments remained unchanged. The PVA of the entire ventricle is the sum of the PVAs of the two compartments. The unchanged E_{max} of the individual compartments despite the changed asynchronicity resulted in no change in the PVA-independent Vo_2 of the individual compartments and of the entire ventricle. Therefore, the outcome of the simulation suggests that the Vo_2-PVA relation would not change its elevation regardless of the degree of asynchronicity, and that the Vo_2-PVA data point would fall along the same Vo_2-PVA relation as the asynchronicity increases. In this simulation, it was not necessary to consider any ventricular compartment which required the same PVA-independent Vo_2 regardless of the asynchronicity but did not contribute to E_{max} and PVA as Burkhoff et al. [131] assumed.

Hypertrophy

Nakamura et al. [133] studied the effects of left ventricular pressure-overloaded hypertrophy on E_{max} and the Vo_2-PVA relation. The pressure overload was produced by the aortic banding in puppies maintained between one half to one year. They found that when normalized for left ventricular weight, both E_{max} and the Vo_2-PVA relation were superimposable for both normal and hypertrophied hearts. This may be a reasonable result, considering that the predominance of V_3 isomyosin does not change with hypertrophy in dog hearts unlike the pressure-overloaded hypertrophy in rabbit hearts.

Remaining Problems

Although the PVA concept has been shown to be useful in cardiac mechanoenergetics, many aspects of the PVA concept still have to be further elucidated as touched upon above. The two aspects that follow must also be recognized as problems.

Load-Dependence of E_{max}

As long as the end-systolic pressure-volume is linear or virtually so, both E_{max} and PVA are easily determined conceptually and practically. This is usually the case over a wide middle range of E_{max} [134]. However, the end-systolic pressure-volume relation is convex downward in a very low E_{max} range and convex upward in a very high E_{max} range. When the nonlinear end-systolic pressure-volume relation is obtained in a stable contractile state, this contractile state cannot be represented by a single E_{max} value. There are a few different methods to quantify the contractility. One is to obtain a single E_{max} as the slope coefficient of the regression line through experimentally obtained end-systolic pressure-volume data points. Another is to obtain E_{max} as the slope of the line connecting V_0 and the end-systolic pressure-volume point of each individual contraction and calculate the mean of the E_{max} values. A third is to fit a mathematical function, e.g., $y = ax^2 + bx + c$, or $y = a(1 - e^{-b(V-Vo)})$, and to use the a and b values instead of E_{max} [134, 135] (Note that these a, b and c are different from those in the Vo_2-PVA-E_{max} relation).

PVA does not need a linear end-systolic pressure-volume relation. It can be either upward or downward convex as long as the contractile state is stable. PVA can be determined under the curvilinear end-systolic pressure-volume relation by definition [80, 136]. When such PVAs under a nonlinear end-systolic pressure-volume relation were plotted against Vo_2, the Vo_2-PVA relation was found to be virtually linear and a change in E_{max} shifted the relation in a parallel manner [80, 88, 136].

However, the end-systolic pressure-volume relation can level off and even descend with increases in volume due to mechanical overload. The overload would compromise coronary circulation and cause subendocardial ischemia. In such a case, we found that the Vo_2-PVA relation was tilted downward. We attributed this change to gradual decreases in both basal metabolic Vo_2 and Vo_2 for excitation-contraction coupling [85].

This does not necessarily mean that the Vo_2-PVA relation with a smaller slope than control is due to gradual decreases in the contractile state with PVA. We have to determine the mechanisms underlying the nonlinearity of the end-systolic pressure-volume relation. We probably have to know the contributions of various factors which influence contractile force as a function of preload and afterload. They include the length- and load-dependent activation, calcium sensitivity, cross-bridge association and dissociation rate constants [44, 137].

Load-dependence of Vo_2-PVA Relation

We have established the linearity of the Vo_2-PVA relation under a variety of pre- and afterloading conditions in a stable contractile state. Yasumura and Suga [138] analyzed the effects of shortening activation [139, 140] and shortening deactivation [141] on the Vo_2-PVA relation. Ejecting contractions with relatively small ejection fractions develop end-systolic pressures and E_{max} values greater than those of the isovolumic contractions at the corresponding end-systolic volumes. However, their Vo_2-PVA data points were virtually on the isovolumic Vo_2-PVA relation. The Vo_2-PVA data points of shortening deactivated contractions were also on the isovolumic Vo_2-PVA relation. From these results, Yasumura and Suga [138] speculated that the PVA-independent Vo_2 was not affected by shortening activation and deactivation.

However, recently, it was showed that when considerable shortening activation occurred, the Vo_2-PVA data point was situated below the isovolumic Vo_2-PVA relation Burkhoff 1990, personal communication. The degree of this lower deviation was proportional to the degree of the shortening activation. This result indicated that the enhanced E_{max} of the shortening-activated contraction was not associated with an increased PVA-independent Vo_2 and probably not accompanied by increased calcium handling. The mechanism underlying this intriguing phenomenon remains to be elucidated.

Conclusion and Perspective

We have summarized our theoretical considerations and experimental findings on ventricular energetics. They have provided us with an important new concept that Vo_2 can be described logically, more than phenomenologically, by a combination of total mechanical energy (PVA), oxygen cost of PVA, contractile efficiency and oxygen cost of contractility (E_{max}). These key concepts have theoretical and empirical advantages over conventional determinants of Vo_2. Despite some problems yet to be solved, the new concepts have already started to help us look into various characteristic changes in mechanoenergetics of normal and failing hearts under the influence of a variety of mechanical loading conditions, heart rates and inotropic interventions. We are challenged not only to solve the remaining problems, but also to apply the new concepts to hearts under different pathophysiological conditions.

In the context of the cardiology of chronic failing hearts, the new concepts will also be powerful tools in the evaluation of therapeutic effects of mechanical or pharmacological interventions such as pre- and afterload reduction and cardiotonic agents. In particular, the new concepts seem to be useful to evaluate the oxygen saving effect of calcium sensitizers as cardiotonic agents.

Acknowledgments. This work was partly supported by a Grant-in-Aid from the Ministry of Education, Science and Culture (B61480102), a grant for Cardiovascular Diseases from the Ministry of Health and Welfare of Japan (1A-1), and a grant from the Nissan Science Foundation.

We cordially thank our colleagues for their energetic and productive research activity, whose names appear in the authors of our papers in the reference list. Without these colleagues, our energetics studies would not have advanced with such a high efficiency.

We thank Dr. Tad W. Taylor, a Japan Science and Technology Agency fellow (1990–) joining our research group from the Yale University School of Medicine, for his valuable advice in the final draft of the manuscript.

References

1. Drake-Holland AJ, Noble MIM (1983) Cardiac Metabolism. Wiley, New York
2. Gibbs CL (1978) Cardiac energetics. Physiol Rev 58:174–254
3. Gibbs CL, Chapman JB (1979) Cardiac energetics. In: Bern RM, Sperelakis N, Geiger SR (eds) The Cardiovascular System I. American Physiol Soc, Bethesda, pp 775–804 (Handbook of physiology)
4. Gibbs CL (1982) Modification of the physiological determinants of cardiac energy expenditure by pharmacological agents. Pharmac Ther 18:133–157
5. Chapman JB (1983) Heat production. In: Drake-Holland AJ, Noble MIM (eds) Cardiac Metabolism. Wiley, New York, pp 239–256
6. Suga H (1990) Ventricular energetics. Physiol Rev 70:247–277
7. Jacob R, Just HJ, Holubarsch CH (1987) Cardiac Energetics. Basic Mechanisms and Clinical Implications. Steinkopff, Darmstadt
8. Suga H (1990) Cardiac mechanics and energetics—from E_{max} to PVA. Front Med Biol Eng 2:3–22
9. Evans CL, Matsuoka Y (1915) The effect of various mechanical conditions on the gaseous metabolism and efficiency of the mammalian heart. J Physiol (London) 49:378–405
10. Braunwald E (1971) Control of myocardial oxygen consumption. Physiologic and clinical considerations. Am J Cardiol 27:416–432
11. Gibbs CL, Chapman JB (1979) Cardiac heat production. Annu Rev Physiol 41:507–519
12. Cooper G IV (1990) Load and length regulation of cardiac energetics. Annu Rev Physiol 52:505–522
13. Baller D, Bretschneider HJ, Hellige G (1981) A critical look at currently used indirect indices of myocardial oxygen consumption. Basic Res Cardiol 76:163–181
14. Rooke GA, Feigl EO (1982) Work as a correlate of canine left ventricular oxygen consumption, and the problem of catecholamine oxygen wasting. Circ Res 50: 273–286
15. Schipke JD, Burkhoff D, Kass DA, Alexander J, Schaefer J, Sagawa K (1990) Hemodynamic dependence of myocardial oxygen consumption indexes. Am J Physiol 258:H1281–1291
16. Futaki S, Goto Y, Ohgoshi Y, Yaku H, Kawaguchi O, Takaoka H, Suga H (1990) Comparison between Bretschneider's total myocardial energy demand (E_t) and our total mechanical energy (PVA) as a predictor of cardiac oxygen consumption in dogs. Jpn J Physiol 40:809–825
17. Suga H (1979) Total mechanical energy of a ventricular model and cardiac oxygen consumption. Am J Physiol 236:H498–H505
18. Sarnoff SJ, Braunwald E, Welch GH, Case RB, Steinsby WN, Marcruz R (1958) Hemodynamic determinants of oxygen consumption of the heart with special reference to the tension time index. Am J Physiol 192:148–156
19. Weber KT, Janicki JS (1977) Myocardial oxygen consumption: the role of wall force and shortening. Am J Physiol 233:H421–H430
20. Woledge RC, Curtin NA, Homsher E (1985) Energetic aspects of muscle contraction. Academic, London
21. Fenn WO (1923) A quantitative comparison between the energy liberated and the work performed by the isolated sartorius muscle of the frog. J Physiol (London) 58:175–203
22. Suga H, Goto Y, Nozawa T, Yasumura Y, Futaki S, Tanaka N (1987) Force-time integral decreases with ejection despite constant oxygen consumption

and pressure-volume area in dog left ventricle. Circ Res 60:797–803
23. Braunwald E, Ross J Jr, Sonnenblick EH (1976) Mechanisms of contraction of the normal and failing heart, 2nd edn. Little, Brown, Boston
24. Endoh M, Yanagisawa T, Taira N, Blinks JR (1986) Effects of new inotropic agents on cyclic nucleotide metabolism and calcium transients in canine ventricular muscle. Circulation 73(suppl III):117–133
25. Rüegg JC (1988) Calcium in Muscle Activation. Springer, Berlin, pp 36–37
26. Suga H, Hisano R, Hirata S, Hayashi T, Yamada O, Nonomiya I (1983) Heart rate-independent energetics and systolic pressure-volume area in dog heart. Am J Physiol 244:H206–H214
27. Yasumura Y, Nozawa T, Futaki S, Tanaka N, Goto Y, Suga H (1987) Dissociation of pressure-rate product from myocardial oxygen consumption in dog. Jpn J Physiol 37:657–670
28. Britman NA, Levine H (1964) Contractile element work: a major determinant of myocardial oxygen consumption. J Clin Invest 43:1397–1408
29. Coleman HN, Sonnenblick EH, Braunwald E (1969) Myocardial oxygen consumption associated with external work: the Fenn effect. Am J Physiol 217:291–296
30. Suga H (1979) Total internal mechanical work of ventricle assessed from quick release pressure-volume curve. Jpn J Physiol 29:227–237
31. Suga H (1979) External mechanical work from relaxing ventricle. Am J Physiol 236:H494–H497
32. Graham TP, Covell JW, Sonnenblick EH (1968) Control of myocardial oxygen consumption: relative influence of contractile state and tension development. J Clin Invest 47:375–385
33. Suga H (1969) Time course of left ventricular pressure-volume relationship under various end-diastolic volumes. Jpn Heart J 10:509–515
34. Suga H (1971) Theoretical analysis of a left ventricular pumping model based on the systolic time-varying pressure/volume ratio. IEEE Trans Biomed Eng BME-18:47–55
35. Suga H, Sagawa K, Shoukas AA (1973) Load independence of the instantaneous pressure-volume ratio of the canine left ventricle and effects of epinephrine and heart rate on the ratio. Circ Res 32:314–322
36. Suga H, Sagawa K (1974) Instantaneous pressure-volume relationships and their ratio in the excised, supported canine left ventricle. Circ Res 35:117–126
37. Sunagawa K, Sagawa K (1982) Models of ventricular contraction based on time-varying elastance. CRC Critical Rev Biomed Eng 7:193–228
38. Sagawa K, Maughan L, Suga H, Sunagawa K (1988) Cardiac contraction and the pressure-volume relationship. Oxford University Press, New York
39. Yasumura Y, Suga H (1988) Cross-bridge model compatible with the linear relation between left ventricular oxygen consumption and pressure-volume area. Jpn Heart J 29:335–347
40. Taylor TW, Goto Y, Futaki S, Kawaguchi O, Hata K, Takasago T, Saeki A, Suga H (1991) Computer simulation of cardiac energetics using a cardiac muscle cross-bridge analysis (abstract). In: World Congress on Medical Physics and Biological Engineering, July 7–12 1991, Tokyo
41. Yanagida T, Arata T, Oosawa F (1985) Sliding distance of actin filament induced by a myosin cross-bridge during one ATP hydrolysis cycle. Nature 316:366–369
42. Mast F, Elzinga G (1990) Heat released during relaxation equals force-length area in isometric contractions of rabbit papillary muscle. Circ Res 67:893–901

43. Huxley AF (1957) Muscle structure and theories of contraction. Prog Biophys Biophys Chem 7:255–318
44. Panerai RB (1980) A model of cardiac muscle mechanics and energetics. J Biomech 13:929–940
45. Monroe RG, French GN (1961) Left ventricular pressure-volume relationships and myocardial oxygen consumption in the isolated heart. Circ Res 9:362–374
46. Khalafbeigui F, Suga H, Sagawa K (1979) Left ventricular systolic pressure-volume area correlates with oxygen consumption. Am J Physiol 237:H566–H569
47. Suga H, Sagawa K (1977) End-diastolic and end-systolic ventricular volume clamper for isolated canine heart. Am J Physiol 233:H718–H722
48. Suga H, Hayashi T, Shirahata M (1981) Ventricular systolic pressure-volume area as predictor of cardiac oxygen consumption. Am J Physiol 240:H39–H44
49. Shepherd AP, Burgar CG (1977) A solid-state arteriovenous oxygen difference analyzer for flowing whole blood. Am J Physiol 232:H437–H440
50. Suga H, Futaki S, Ohgoshi Y, Yaku H, Goto Y (1989) Arteriovenous oximeter for O_2 content difference, O_2 saturations, and hemoglobin content. Am J Physiol 257:H1712–H1716
51. Hisano R, Cooper G IV (1987) Correlation of force-length area with oxygen consumption in ferret papillary muscle. Circ Res 61:318–328
52. Gibbs CL (1987) Cardiac energetics and the Fenn effect. Basic Res Cardiol 81(suppl2):61–68, or in: Jacob R, Just Hj, Holubarsch Ch (eds) Cardiac Energetics. Steinkopff, Darmstadt, pp 61–68
53. Suga H, Hayashi T, Shirahata M, Suehiro S, Hisano R (1981) Regression of cardiac oxygen consumption on ventricular pressure-volume area in dog. Am J Physiol 240:H320–H325
54. Suga H, Hisano R, Goto Y, Yamada O, Igarashi Y (1983) Effect of positive inotropic agents on the relation between oxygen consumption and systolic pressure-volume area in canine left ventricle. Circ Res 53:306–318
55. Suga H, Nozawa T, Yasumura Y, Futaki S, Ohgoshi Y, Yaku H, Goto Y (1990) Force-time integral does not improve predictability of cardiac O_2 consumption from pressure-volume area (PVA) in dog left ventricle. Heart Vessels 5:152–158
56. Suga H, Goto Y, Nozawa T, Yasumura Y, Futaki S, Tanaka N (1987) Force-time integral decreases with ejection despite constant oxygen consumption and pressure-volume area in dog left ventricle. Circ Res 60:797–803
57. Suga H, Yamada O, Goto Y, Igarashi Y (1984) Oxygen consumption and pressure-volume area of abnormal contractions in canine left ventricle. Am J Physiol 246:H154–H160
58. Suga H, Goto Y, Yamada O, Igarashi Y (1984) Independence of myocardial oxygen consumption from pressure-volume trajectory during diastole in canine left ventricle. Circ Res 55:734–739
59. Hata K, Goto Y, Futaki S, Kawaguchi O, Takasago T, Saeki A, Taylor TW, Suga H (to be published) (1991) External work during relaxation period does not affect myocardial oxygen consumption (abstract). In: World Congress on Medical Physics and Biomedical Engineering, July 7–12 1991, Kyoto
60. Suga H, Goto Y, Yasumura Y, Nozawa T, Futaki S, Tanaka N, Uenishi M (1988) Oxygen-saving effect of negative work in dog left ventricle. Am J Physiol 254: H34–H44
61. Yasumura Y, Nozawa T, Futaki S, Tanaka N, Suga H (1989) Minor preload dependence of O_2 consumption of unloaded contraction in dog heart. Am J Physiol 256:H1289–H1294

62. Cooper G IV (1981) Influence of length changes on myocardial metabolism in the cat papillary muscle. Circ Res 49:423–433
63. Yasumura Y, Nozawa T, Futaki S, Tanaka N, Suga H (1989) Time-invariant oxygen cost of mechanical energy in dog left ventricle: consistency and inconsistency of time-varying elastance model with myocardial energetics. Circ Res 64:763–778
64. Monroe RG (1964) Myocardial oxygen consumption during ventricular contraction and relaxation. Circ Res 14:294–300
65. Cooper G IV (1979) Myocardial energetics during isometric twitch contractions of cat papillary muscle. Am J Physiol 236:H244–H253
66. Duwel CMB, Westerhof N (1988) Feline left ventricular oxygen consumption is not affected by volume expansion, ejection or redevelopment of pressure during relaxation. Pflugers Arch 412:409–416
67. Gibbs CL, Wendt IR, Kotsanas G, Young IR (1990) The energy cost of relaxation in control and hypertrophic rabbit papillary muscles. Heart Vessels 5:198–205
68. Yasumura Y, Suga H (1989) Addition of internal mechanical energy loss to PVA improves prediction of Vo_2 in canine heart (abstract). Circulation 80(suppl II): II-154
69. Teplick R, Haas GS, Trautman E, Geffin G, Dagget WM (1986) Time dependence of the oxygen cost of force development during systole in the canine left ventricle. Circ Res 59:27–38
70. Suga H, Hisano R, Hirata S, Hayashi T, Yamada O, Ninomiya I (1983) Heart rate-independent energetics and systolic pressure-volume area in dog heart. Am J Physiol 244:H206–H214
71. Maughan WL, Sunagawa K, Burkhoff D, Graves WL, Hunter WC, Sagawa K (1985) Effect of heart rate on the canine end-systolic pressure-volume relationship. Circulation 72:654–659
72. Solaro RJ, Pan B-S (1989) Control and modulation of contractile activity of cardiac myofilaments. In: Sperelakis N (ed) Physiology and pathophysiology of the heart, 2nd edn. Kluwer Academic, Boston, pp 291–303
73. Tada M, Shigekawa M, Kadoma M, Nimura Y (1989) Uptake of calcium by sarcoplasmic reticulum and its regulation and functional consequences. In: Sperelakis N (ed) Physiology and pathophysiology of the heart, 2nd edn. Kluwer Academic, Boston, pp 267–290
74. Opie LH (1984) The Heart. Physiology, Metabolism, Pharmacology and Therapy. Grune and Stratton, London
75. Nozawa T, Yasumura Y, Futaki S, Tanaka N, Uenishi M, Suga H (1989) The linear relation between oxygen consumption and pressure-volume area in left ventricle can be reconciled with the Fenn effect. Circ Res 65:1380–1389
76. Futaki S, Goto Y, Ohgoshi Y, Yaku H, Kawaguchi O, Suga H (to be published) (1991) Denopamine (β_1-selective adrenergic receptor agonist) and isoproterenol (non-selective β-adrenergic receptor agonist) equally increase heart rate and myocardial oxygen consumption in dog heart. Jpn Circ J
77. Burkhoff D, Yue DT, Oikawa RY, Franz MR, Schaefer J, Sagawa K (1987) Influence of ventricular contractility on non-work-related myocardial oxygen consumption. Heart Vessels 3:66–72
78. Akera T, Brody TM (1982) Myocardial membranes: regulation and function of the sodium pump. Ann Rev Physiol 44:375–388
79. Wu D, Yasumura Y, Nozawa T, Tanaka N, Futaki S, Ohgoshi Y, Yaku H, Suga H (1989) Effect of ouabain on the relation between left ventricular oxygen con-

sumption and systolic pressure-volume area (PVA) in dog heart. Heart Vessels 5:17–24

80. Suga H, Futaki S, Tanaka N, Yasumura Y, Nozawa T, Wu D, Ohgoshi Y, Yaku H (1988) Paired-pulse pacing increases cardiac O_2 consumption for activation without changing efficiency of contractile machinery in canine left ventricle. Heart Vessels 4:79–87
81. Nozawa T, Yasumura Y, Futaki S, Tanaka N, Suga H (1990) Effects of bigeminies and paired-pulse stimulation on oxygen consumption in dog left ventricle. Circ Res 67:142–153
82. Futaki S, Nozawa T, Yasumura Y, Tanaka N, Suga H (1988) Effects of new inotropic agents on myocardial oxygen consumption vs. pressure-volume area relation (abstract). Jpn Circ J 52:723–724
83. Futaki S, Nozawa T, Yasumura Y, Tanake N, Suga H (1988) New cardiotonic agents, OPC-8212, elevates the myocardial oxygen consumption versus pressure-volume area (PVA) relation in a similar manner to catecholamines and calcium in canine hearts. Heart Vessels 4:153–161
84. Suga H, Goto Y, Hata K (1990) Cardiac energy supply-demand balance (abstract in Japanese). 1990 Interim Report of Grants for Cardiovascular Diseases (Heisei 2-nendo Junkankibyo-kenkyu-itakuhi niyoru Kenkyu-chukan-houkoku-yoshi), National Cardiovasvular Center, pp 78–79
85. Suga H, Goto Y, Yasumura Y, Nozawa T, Futaki S, Tanaka N, Uenishi M (1988) O_2 consumption of dog heart under decreased coronary perfusion and propranolol. Am J Physiol 254:H292–H303
86. Suga H, Goto Y, Igarashi Y, Yasumura Y, Nozawa T, Futaki S, Tanaka N (1988) Cardiac cooling increases E_{max} without affecting relation between O_2 consumption and systolic pressure-volume area in dog left ventricle. Circ Res 63:61–71
87. Elzinga G (1983) Cardiac oxygen consumption and the production of heat and work. In: Drake-Holland AJ, Noble MIM (eds) Cardiac Metabolism Wiley, UK, pp 173–194
88. Goto Y, Slinker BK, LeWinter MM (1990) Similar normalized E_{max} and O_2 consumption-pressure-volume area relation in rabbit and dog. Am J Physiol 255: H366–H374
89. Suga H, Igarashi Y, Yamada O, Goto Y (1985) Mechanical efficiency of the left ventricle as a function of preload, afterload and contractility. Heart Vessels 1: 3–8
90. Ohgoshi Y, Goto Y, Futaki S, Yaku H, Kawaguchi O, Suga H (1990) New method to determine oxygen cost for contractility. Jpn J Physiol 40:127–138
91. Klocke FJ, Braunwald E, Ross J (1966) Oxygen cost of electrical activation of the heart. Circ Res 18:357–365
92. Langer GA (1967) Sodium exchange in dog ventricular muscle. Relation to frequency of contraction and its possible role in the control of myocardial contractility. J Gen Physiol 50:1221–1239
93. Gibbs CL, Papadoyannis DE, Drake AJ, Noble MIM (1980) Oxygen consumption of the nonworking and potassium chloride-arrested dog heart. Circ Res 47: 408–417
94. Ohgoshi Y, Goto Y, Futaki S, Kawaguchi O, Yaku H, Takaoka H, Hata K, Takasago T, Suga H (to be published) (1991) Epinephrine and calcium have similar oxygen cost of contractility. Am J Physiol
95. Loiselle DS, Gibbs CL (1983) Factors affecting the metabolism of resting rabbit papillary muscle. Pflugers Arch 396:285–291

96. Nozawa T, Yasumura Y, Futaki S, Tanaka N, Suga H (1988) No significant increase in O_2 consumption of KC1-arrested dog heart with filling and dobutamine. Am J Physiol 255:H807–H812
97. Suga H (1990) Energetics of the time-varying elastance model, a visco-elastic model, matches Mommaerts' unifying concept of the Fenn effect of muscle. Jpn Heart J 31:341–353
98. Elzinga G, Westerhof N (1981) "Pressure-volume" relations in isolated cat trabecula. Circ Res 49:388–394
99. Chapman JB, Gibbs CL (1972) An energetic model of muscle contrction. Biophys J 12:227–236
100. Gibbs CL, Chapman JB (1985) Cardiac mechanics and energetics: chemomechanical transduction in cardiac muscle. Am J Physiol 249:H199–H206
101. Suga H (1980) Relaxing ventricle performs more external work than quickly released elastic energy. Europ Heart J 1(supp1A):131–137
102. Rall JA (1982) Sense and nonsense about the Fenn effect. Am J Physiol 242: H1–H6
103. Mommaerts WFHM (1970) What is the Fenn effect? Naturwissenschaften 57: 326–330
104. Gibbs CL (1987) Cardiac energetics and the Fenn effect. In: Jacob R, Just H, Holubarsch C (eds) Cardiac energetics. Basic mechanisms and clinical implication, Steinkopff, Darmstadt, pp 61–68
105. Suga H (to be published) (1990) Ventricular perspective on efficiency (abstract). In: Myocardial Optimixation and Efficiency. The 5th Symposium "Myocardial Optimization and Efficiency," the International Institute for Theoretical Cardiology, Graz, Austria. Walter de Gruyer , Berlin
106. Alpert NR, Mulieri LA (1986) Determinants of energy utilization in the activated myocardium. Fed Proc 45:2597–2600
107. Goto Y, Slinker BK, LeWinter MM (1990) Decreased contractile efficiency and increased nonmechanical energy cost in hyperthyroid rabbit heart. Relation between O_2 consumption and systolic pressure-volume area or force-time integral. Circ Res 66:999–1011
108. Suga H, Tanaka N, Ohgoshi Y, Saeki Y, Nakanishi T, Futaki S, Yaku H, Goto Y (to be published) (1991) Hyperthyroid dog left ventricle has the same oxygen consumption versus pressure-volume area (PVA) relation as euthyroid. Heart Vessels
109. Suga H, Futaki S, Ohgoshi Y, Yaku H, goto Y (1989) Load- and contractility-independent stoichiometry of energy conversion from excess oxygen consumption to total mechanical energy in canine left ventricle. Muscle Energetics. Alan R. Liss, pp 543–554
110. Alpert NR, Mulieri LA, Blanchard E, Litten RZ, Holubarsch C (1989) A myothermal analysis of absolute myosin cross-bridge cycling rates in rat hearts. Muscle Energetics. Alan R. Liss, pp 503–517
111. Sunagawa K, Maughan WL, Burkhoff D, Sagawa K (1983) Left ventricular interaction with arterial load studied in isolated canine ventricle. Am J Physiol 245: H773–H780
112. Yasumura Y, Tanaka N, Nozawa T, Futaki S, Suga H (1988) Dobutamine and calcium do not waste oxygen for mechanical efficiency in canine left ventricle (abstract). Circulation 78(supplII):II–68
113. Suga H (to be published) (1991) Constant efficiency versus variable economy of cardiac contraction. Jpn Heart J

114. Allen DG, Kurihara S (1980) Calcium transients in mammalian ventricular muscle. Eur Heart J 1(supplA):5–15
115. Suga H, Goto Y, Futaki S, Kawaguchi O, Yaku H, Hata K, Takasago T (to be published) (1991) Calcium kinetics and energetics in myocardium. Simulation study. Jpn Heart J
116. Allen DG, Lee JA (1989) EMD 53998 increases tension with little effect on the amplitude of calcium transients in isolated ferret ventricular muscle. J Physiol 416:43P
117. Allen DG, Orchard CH (1983) Intracellular calcium concentration during hypoxia and metabolic inhibition in mammalian ventricular muscle. J Physiol 339:107–122
118. Covell JW, Braunwald E, Ross J, Sonnenblick E (1966) Studies on digitalis. XVI. Effects on myocardial oxygen consumption. J Clin Invest 45:1535–1542
119. Suga H (1979) Minimal oxygen consumption and optimal contractility of the heart: theoretical approach to principle of physiological control of contractility. Bull Math Biol 41:139–150
120. Tanaka N, Yasumura Y, Nozawa T, Futaki S, Uenishi M, Hiramori K, Suga H (1988) Optimal contractility and minimal oxygen consumption for constant external work of heart. Am J Physiol 254:R933–R943
121. Tanaka N, Nozawa T, Yasumura Y, Futaki S, Hiramori K, Suga H (1990) Contractility to minimize oxygen consumption for constant work in dog left ventricle. Heart Vessels 6:9–20
122. Goto Y, Slinker BK, LeWinter MM (1991) Effect of coronary hyperemia on E_{max} and oxygen consumption in blood-perfused rabbit heart. Energetic consequences of Gregg's phenomenon. Circ Res 68:482–492
123. Ohgoshi Y, Goto Y, Futaki S, Yaku H, Kawaguchi O, Suga H (to be published) (1991) Increased oxygen cost of contractility in stunned myocardium of dog. Circ Res
124. Kusuoka H, Porterfield JK, Weisman HF, Weisfeldt ML, Marban E (1987) Pathophysiology and pathogenesis of stunned myocardium. Depressed Ca^{2+} activation of contraction as a consequence of reperfusion-induced cellular calcium overload in ferret hearts. J Clin Invest 79:950–961
125. Krause SM, Jacobus WE, Becker LC (1989) Alterations in cardiac sarcoplasmic reticulum calcium transport in the postischemic "stunned" myocardium. Circ Res 65:526–530
126. Yazaki Y, Raben MS (1975) Effect of the thyroid state on the enzymatic characteristics of cardiac myosin. Circ Res 36:208–215
127. Swynghedauw B (1986) Developmental and functional adaptation of contractile proteins in cardiac and skeletal muscles. Physiol Rev 66:710–771
128. Kawaguchi O, Goto Y, Suga H (to be published) (1991) Cardiac oxygen consumption under atrial fibrillation. Am J Physiol
129. Yaku H, Goto Y, Futaki S, Ohgoshi Y, Kawaguchi O, Suga H (to be published) (1990) Multicompartment model for mechanics and energetics of fibrillating ventricle. Am J Physiol 260
130. Yaku H, Goto Y, Futaki S, Ohgoshi Y, Kawaguchi O, Suga H (to be published) (1990) Equivalent pressure-volume area accounts for O_2 consumption of fibrillating heart. Am J Physiol
131. Burkhoff D, Oikawa RY, Sagawa K (1986) Influence of pacing site on canine left ventricular contraction. Am J Physiol 251:H428–H435
132. Suga H, Goto Y, Yaku H, Futaki S, Ohgoshi Y, Kawaguchi O (to be published) (1991) Simulation of mechanoenergetics of asynchronously contracting ventricle. Am J Physiol 259:R1075–R1082

133. Nakamura T, Kimura T, Motomiya M, Suzuki N, Arai S (1987) Myocardial oxygen consumption and mechanical efficiency in the pressure-overloaded hypertrophied canine left ventricle (abstract). Automedica 9:188
134. Burkhoff D, Sugiura S, Yue DT, Sagawa K (1987) Contractility dependent curvilinearity of end-systolic pressure-volume relations. Am J Physiol 252: H1218–H1227
135. Suga H, Yamada O, Goto Y, Igarashi Y (1986) Peak isovolumic pressure-volume relation of puppy left ventricle. Am J Physiol 250:H167–H172
136. Suga H, Yamada O, Goto Y, Igarashi Y, Yasumura Y, Nozawa T (1987) Left ventricular O_2 consumption and pressure-volume area in puppies. Am J Physiol 253:H770–H776
137. Jewell BR (1977) A reexamination of the influence of muscle length on myocardial performance. Circ Res 40:221–230
138. Yasumura Y, Nozawa T, Futaki S, Tanaka N, Suga H (1988) Ejecting activation and its energetics (abstract). Circulation 78(SupplII):II–225
139. Igarashi Y, Goto Y, Yamada O, Ishii T, Suga H (1987) Transient vs. steady end-systolic pressure-volume relation in dog left ventricle. Am J Physiol 252: H998–H1004
140. Sugiura S, Hunter WC, Sagawa K (1989) Long-term versus intrabeat history of ejection as determinants of canine ventricular end-systolic pressure. Circ Res 64:255–264
141. Suga H, Kitabatake A, Sagawa K (1979) End-systolic pressure determines stroke volume from fixed end-diastolic volume in isolated canine left ventricle under constant contractile state. Circ Res 44:238–249
142. Suga H, Goto Y, Igarashi Y, Yamada O (1987) The pressure-volume area as a predictor of cardiac oxygen consumption. CRC Press, Florida. pp 69–83

5

Left Ventricular Regional Mechanics and Energetics Assessed in the Wall Tension-Regional Area Diagram

Yoichi Goto[1], Hiroyuki Suga[2]

Summary. Assessment of regional contractile function of the left ventricle is important especially in clinical settings in diagnosis and treatment of patients with coronary artery disease. Unfortunately, however, many of the conventional indexes of regional function are influenced by not only myocardial contractility but also ventricular loading conditions. In addition, they cannot be used as a measure of regional myocardial oxygen consumption. Recently, we have proposed and validated a new approach assessing regional mechanics and energetics in the wall tension-regional area (T-A) diagram, by the analogy of the end-systolic pressure-volume relation and pressure-volume area (PVA) in the whole ventricle. In the T-A diagram, the area within a T-A loop during one cardiac cycle represents regional external work (in dimensions of energy [Joule]) performed by the region in both normal and ischemic hearts. The end-systolic T-A relation (ESTAR) can be approximated by a straight line. The slope of the ESTAR increases or decreases during positive or negative inotropic interventions reflecting regional myocardial contractility, except for regional ischemia during which the area-axis intercept of the ESTAR increases concomitantly with a decrease in the slope value. We defined "tension-area" area (TAA) as a specific area circumscribed by the ESTAR, the end-diastolic T-A relation, and the systolic T-A trajectory. TAA correlates highly linearly with regional myocardial oxygen consumption in a load-independent manner, indicating that TAA is a reliable measure of regional myocardial oxygen consumption. In conclusion, the ESTAR and TAA defined in the T-A diagram may be useful tools for assessing both mechanics and energetics of a ventricular region.

Key words: End systole — Myocardial contractility — Myocardial contraction — Myocardial oxygen consumption — Regional work — Tension-area relation

[1] Department of Cardiovascular Dynamics, National Cardiovascular Center Research Institute, Osaka, 565 Japan
[2] The Second Department of Physiology, Okayama University Medical School, Okayama, 700 Japan

Introduction

Assessment of regional contractile function of the left ventricle is important, especially in clinical settings in diagnosis and treatment of patients with coronary artery disease, because in the heart with coronary artery disease, myocardial contractile function is nonuniformly impaired. Assessment of regional function is also important in patients with cardiomyopathy, because hearts with hypertrophic [1] or dilated cardiomyopathy [2] have been reported to demonstrate regional abnormalities in contraction. Global indexes of left ventricular function (for example, ejection fraction) cannot detect such regional abnormalities of myocardial contractile function [3]. To assess regional myocardial contractile function, many indexes have been proposed, and these are listed in Table 1. Unfortunately, many of the indexes are influenced by not only myocardial contractility but also ventricular loading conditions. In addition, they cannot be used as a measure of regional myocardial oxygen consumption.

In the field of left ventricular global mechanics and energetics, the end-systolic pressure-volume relation (ESPVR) has been used to assess the global left ventricular contractile state [4, 5], and the systolic pressure-volume area (PVA) has been shown to be a reliable predictor of left ventricular oxygen consumption [6] as described in the previous chapter. By the analogy of the ESPVR and PVA in the global ventricle, we have recently proposed and validated a new approach assessing regional mechanics and energetics in the wall tension-regional area (T-A) diagram [7, 8]. In this chapter, we present an overview of conventional indexes of regional contractile function and describe our new method to assess regional contractile function, relating it to regional energetics using the T-A diagram.

Indexes of Left Ventricular Contractile Function: An Overview

Segment Shortening or Wall Thickening

At present, the most widely used indexes of regional contractile function are those quantifying the amount of muscle shortening during systole, such as segment shortening or wall thickening. This category of indexes includes segment shortening measured with ultrasonic dimension gauges [9–12] or radiopaque markers implanted in the ventricular wall [13], chord shortening [14–16] or fractional area shortening [14, 17–19] assessed by endocardial displacement using left ventriculography or two-dimensional echocardiography, and wall thickening assessed with ultrasonic dimension gauges [20–22] or in left ventricular tomographic images obtained by echo [23, 24], computed tomography [25, 26], or magnetic resonance [1, 27]. When regional myocardium is subjected to ischemia, the amount of segment shortening or wall thickening decreases, reflecting impairment of regional myocardial contractility.

However, the amount of shortening or thickening is also affected by changes in left ventricular afterload [28] or preload [29]. This load dependence is the

Table 1. Indexes of regional contractile function

1. Indexes of extent of myocardial shortening
segment shortening
chord shortening
fractional area shortening
wall thickening
2. Indexes of regional work
pressure-length loop
pressure-thickness loop
wall tension-area loop
wall stress-ln(1/thickness) loop
preload-recruitable stroke work index
3. Indexes at end systole
end-systolic pressure-length relation
end-systolic pressure-thickness relation
end-systolic tension-area relation
end-systolic stress-ln(1/thickness) relation

major limitation of indexes of this category. In addition, our recent study [12] has shown that segment shortening in the anterior and posterior wall regions of the left ventricle decreases more than that in the lateral wall within 5 s after sudden pulmonary artery constriction (Fig. 1). Because it takes more than 7 s for reflex increases in sympathetic nerve activity to take place [22], this finding suggests that local factors such as regional radius of curvature, myocardial fiber orientation, and tethering between fiber layers also affect the amount of shortening or thickening [30–32]. Therefore, results obtained with these indexes must be interpreted cautiously.

Indexes of Regional Work

Indexes of left ventricular regional work assess pump performance of a ventricular region during one cardiac cycle. By the analogy of left ventricular stroke work quantified by pressure-volume loop area, Forrester et al. [33] and Tyberg et al. [34] proposed pressure-segment length loop area as an index of regional work (Fig. 2). The pressure-length loop analysis provides precise information about behavior of a segment of the ventricular wall, and has been used by many investigators [16, 35, 36]. However, because myocardial fibers are variously oriented within the left ventricle [37], extents and time courses of segment shortening are influenced by the direction of the measured segment [7, 30, 31]. More importantly, as shown in Fig. 2, the dimensions of the pressure-length loop area (mmHg·cm) differ from those of work or energy (Joule). Another option of an index of regional work, the area within a pressure-wall thickness loop [38], may not be affected by myocardial fiber orientation. However, it may be affected by changes in blood volume within the ventricular wall [39, 40], and again, the dimensions of the pressure-thickness loop area (mmHg·cm) also differ from those of energy.

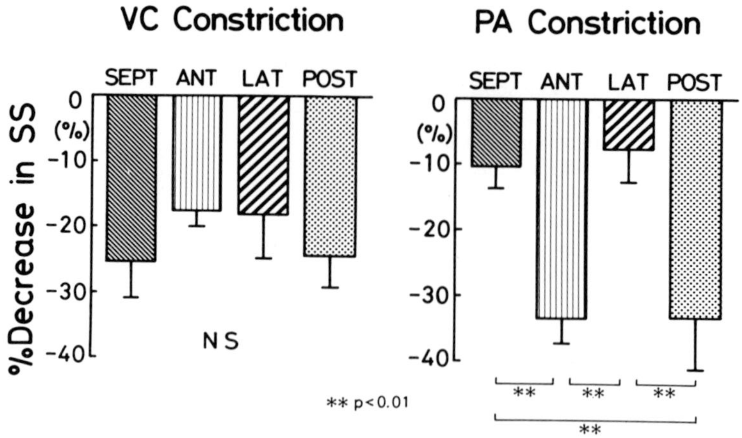

Fig. 1. Comparisons of decreases in systolic shortening (*SS*) of septal (*SEPT*), anterior (*ANT*), lateral (*LAT*), and posterior (*POST*) segments expressed as percentage of control shortening during venae caval (*VC*) and pulmonary artery (*PA*) constrictions with the intact paricardium. The decreases in *SS* are similar during *VC* constriction, whereas decreases in *SS* of the anterior and posterior segments are significantly greater than those of the septal and lateral segments during *PA* constriction. Mean ± SEM is indicated. (From [12] with permission)

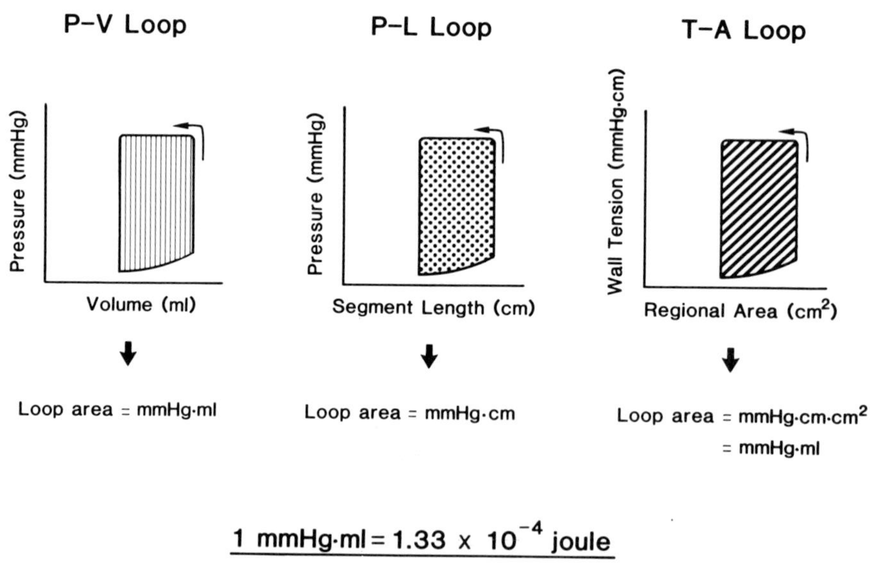

Fig. 2. Comparison of the pressure-volume (*P-V*), pressure-length (*P-L*), and wall tension-regional area (*T-A*) loops. The dimensions of the *P-V* and *T-A* loop area are equal to those of energy, whereas those of the *P-L* loop area are not. (From [53] with permission)

Recent studies from our [7, 8, 41] and other laboratories [42] have shown that regional work can be reliably measured by the area within a T-A loop with physically correct dimensions of energy as described below. Further, Nakano et al. [43] have proposed the wall stress-"logarithm of the reciprocal of wall thickness" [ln(1/thickness)] loop as a new method to quantify regional work normalized for a unit myocardial mass. These two methods provide physically rigorous, accurate measures of regional work.

Like indexes of myocardial shortening, indexes of regional work are also influenced by preload and afterload. Increased preload (e.g., increased end-diastolic segment length) increases regional work [34, 35, 41, 42], which is considered a manifestation of the Frank-Starling mechanism in a ventricular region. On the other hand, decreased afterload increases regional work [44]. Thus, indexes of regional work are not necessarily a measure of regional myocardial contractility although they quantify regional pump performance.

Recently, Glower et al. [35] proposed a preload-recruitable stroke work index in both the global ventricle and a local ventricular region. They have shown that the relation between global or regional preload (i.e., left ventricular volume or regional end-diastolic segment length) and global or regional stroke work, respectively, is linear and the slope reflects the myocardial contractile state independent of physiologic afterload in the conscious dog heart. Yun et al. [45] extended this concept to the relation between end-diastolic wall thickness and pressure-thickness loop area. These concepts seem to contradict the previous findings in excised hearts or in anesthetized animals that cardiac external work is a function of both preload and afterload [46]. Further study will be needed to elucidate whether the preload recruitable stroke work index is truly an afterload-independent index of myocardial contractility.

End-Systolic Measures of Regional Function

This category of indexes includes the end-systolic relations between left ventricular pressure and segment length [10, 47–49] or wall thickness [21, 22, 50, 51], between wall tension and regional area [52, 53], and between wall stress and logarithm of reciprocal of wall thickness [54]. In contrast to indexes of segment shortening and regional work, these end-systolic measures of regional function reflect myocardial contractility, for the most part independent of preload and afterload.

The linearity and load-independence of these relations originate from the characteristics of the end-systolic pressure-volume relations [4]. If we assume a linear end-systolic pressure-volume relation in a spherical ventricle, all the above end-systolic relations should be nonlinear with downward convexity [50, 53]. However, the actual end-systolic relations are well fitted to straight lines in physiologic contractile states [10, 48, 50, 51, 53], probably owing to the complex ventricular geometry and fiber orientation [55].

With enhanced or depressed global myocardial contractility, the slope of these linear end-systolic relations increases or decreases without changes in the X-axis intercept [22, 48, 51, 53]. However, during regional ischemia or infusion

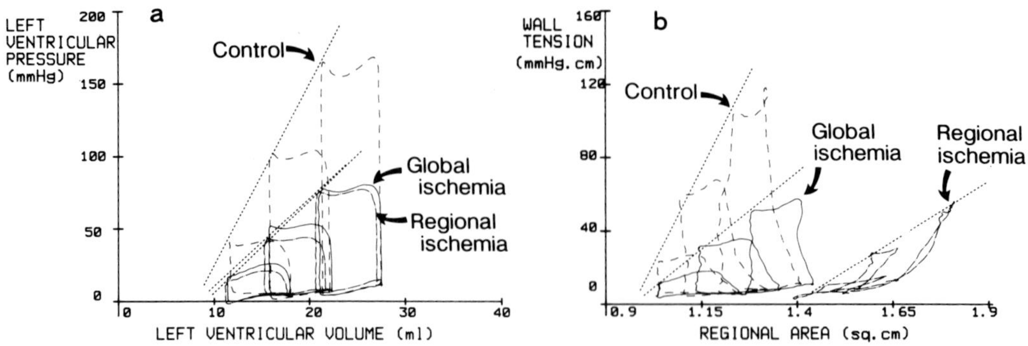

Fig. 3. Left ventricular pressure-volume loops (**a**) and wall tension-regional area (*T-A*) loops (**b**) during the control period, global ischemia, and regional ischemia. *Dashed lines* indicate the end-systolic pressure-volume or T-A relation. Regional ischemia resulted in not only a decrease in the slope of the end-systolic T-A relation but also a marked increase in the area axis intercept. (From [53] with permission)

of negative inotropic drugs into a selected coronary artery (i.e., regional depression of myocardial contractility), not only a decrease in the slope but also a shift in the X-axis intercept (increase in unloaded segment length or decrease in unloaded wall thickness) occurs initially (Fig. 3) [22, 53]. As regional myocardial contractility is progressively deteriorated, further shifts of the X-axis intercept occurs with no change or even paradoxical increases in the slope value [47, 48]. This mimics the rightward shift of the end-systolic pressure-volume relation no the whole ventricle during regional ischemia [56]. Therefore, in the case of regional depression of myocardial contractility, both slope and X-axis intercept values of the end-systolic relations have to be determined. In this context, many recent studies [22, 49, 50, 52, 57] have chosen to simply evaluate right or leftward shifts of the end-systolic relation per se relative to the control relation at the same pressure or tension range, rather than to compare the slope and intercepts of the two regression lines. Therefore, a rightward shift of the pressure-length relation or a leftward shift of the pressure-thickness relation is considered to indicate depressed regional myocardial contractility.

A limitation of the end-systolic pressure-length and pressure-wall thickness relations is that these relations cannot detect changes in regional wall stress resulting from changes in ventricular volume or regional radius of curvature. In our recent study [12] mentioned above, the end-systolic pressure-length relation in the left ventricular posterior wall region shifted right downward within 5 s after pulmonary artery constriction, but did not shift in the anterior and lateral wall regions (Fig. 4). This finding suggests that local factors other than myocardial contractility, such as regional radius of curvature and fiber orientation, affect the end-systolic pressure-length relation. Therefore, under conditions in which ventricular geometry changes greatly, these relations should be interpreted cautiously.

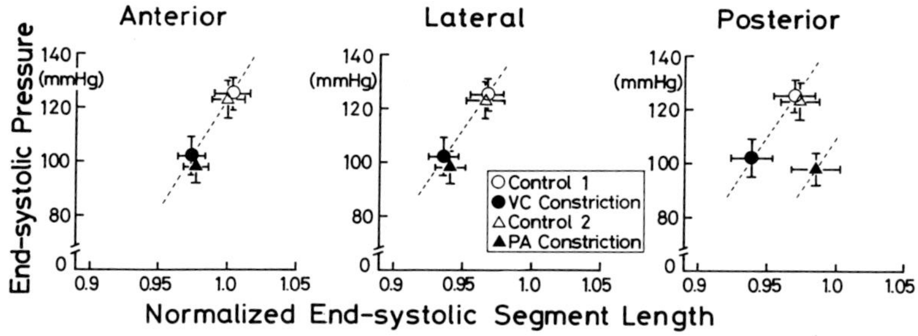

Fig. 4. Normalized end-systolic pressure-segment length relations in anterior, lateral, and posterior wall segments during two control periods and venae caval (*VC*) and pulmonary artery (*PA*) constrictions with the pericardium intact. The end-systolic pressure-length relation in the posterior wall segment, but not in the anterior and lateral wall segments, shifted right downward within 5 s after *PA* constriction

In contrast to the end-systolic pressure-length and pressure-thickness relations, the end-systolic stress-ln(1/thickness) relation represents the end-systolic myocardial elastance normalized for unit myocardial mass, and hence, is not influenced by ventricular size [54]. However, the use of mean wall stress cannot eliminate the influence of changes in regional radius of curvature on the relation. This also holds true in the case of the end-systolic T-A relation. Unfortunately, there is presently no means for directly measuring regional ventricular wall stress. However, an indirect method has been proposed by Janz [58] to compute local myocardial stress, which allows changes in geometric factors and wall thickness to be taken into account in assessment of regional myocardial function [59].

Assessment of Left Ventricular Regional Work from the Tension-area Loop

Theoretical Background

As mentioned above, the dimensions of the area within a pressure-length loop, a conventional regional work index, are not physically correct (Fig. 2). To determine regional work with physically correct dimensions, three theoretical methods can be considered [8], as shown in Fig. 5. The first method (Fig. 5a) assesses regional work from the product of unidirectional force acting on a linear segment in the ventricular surface plane and the amount of shortening of this segment. Regional work of the segment obtained by this method is equal to the area within a force-length loop during one cardiac cycle. However, because this method quantifies regional work in only one direction in a selected ventricular surface area, unidirectional regional work obtained by this method has to be summed in all directions to quantify total regional work of the area.

The second method (Fig. 5b) assesses regional work from the product of wall tension acting on the circumference of a plane in the ventricular surface

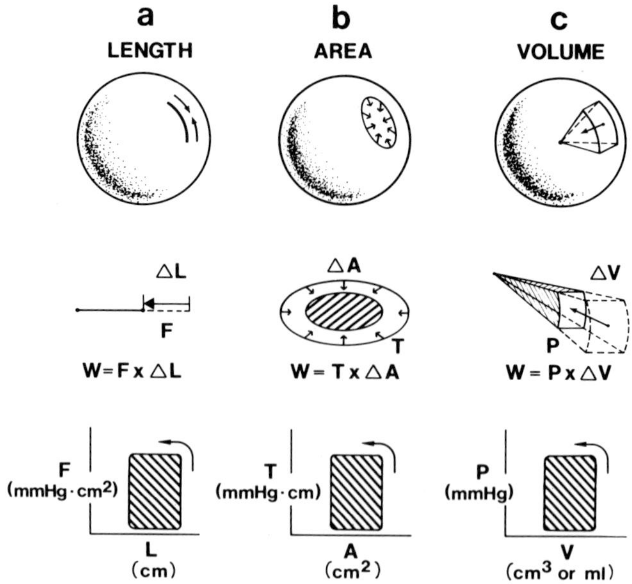

Fig. 5. Three theoretical methods of assessing regional work (*W*) of ventricular wall. **a**, force (*F*)-length (*L*) loop method; **b**, wall tension (*T*)-regional area (*A*) loop method; **c**, pressure (*P*)-"regional chamber volume (*V*)" loop method. (From [8] with permission)

and the amount of area shrinkage of the region circumscribed by the circumference. This has been proposed by Sugawara et al. [42] and us [7, 8] as:

$$RW = -\int_{t_1}^{t_2} T(dA/dt)dt$$

where RW is regional work, t_1 is onset of systole, t_2 is end of diastole, T is wall tension, and dA/dt is rate of change in regional area. Wall tension (force per unit circumferential length) used in this method differs from wall stress (force per unit cross-sectional area). Because the left ventricle is a thick-walled structure, and stresses and strains within the thick-walled shells have three orthogonal vectors and are not uniformly distributed [60–63], regional work cannot simply be obtained from these stresses and strains. However, our theoretical study has shown that lumping circumferential stress and strain into the endocardial layer allows correct assessment of regional work on the basis of the law of conservation of energy [64]. By using wall tension, we need not take the distribution of wall stress within the ventricular wall into account when we assess regional work over the entire thickness of the wall. Regional work obtained by this method is equal to the area within a T-A loop during one cardiac cycle.

The third method (Fig. 5c) assesses regional work from the product of ventricular pressure and the amount of ventricular surface displacement (i.e., a change in "regional chamber volume"), based on the assumption that all the

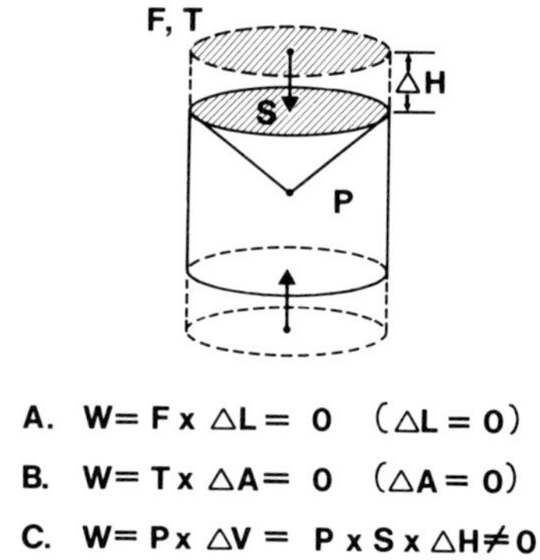

Fig. 6. A thin-walled cylindrical model of the ventricle that serves to examine validity of the three methods assessing regional work. *W*, work; *F*, force; *L*, length; *T*, tension; *A*, regional area; *P*, pressure; *V*, "regional chamber volume." (From [8] with permission)

points on the ventricular wall move toward a unique reference point in the ventricular lumen. According to this method, regional work performed by the regional chamber is equal to the area within a pressure-regional chamber volume loop.

Although all three methods give regional work with the same dimensions as energy, method C has a serious weakness under a certain condition of nonuniform ventricular contraction. Figure 6 shows a model of such a nonuniformly contracting ventricle. In this specific thin-walled cylindrical model of the left ventricle, the lateral wall contracts or shortens only in the longitudinal and not in the circumferential direction, while the upper and lower bases do not actively contract. During lateral wall contraction, the noncontracting bases are pulled passively toward the midpoint of the cylinder with a positive displacement and a constant area. When regional work of the upper base is assessed using the three methods mentioned above, it should be assessed to be zero by either method because the upper base does not actively contract. Methods A and B yield regional work of zero regardless of the value for force or wall tension during lateral wall contraction, because there is no change in length or regional area in the base plane. However, method C gives regional work of a positive value because all values for intraventricular pressure, base plane area, and the amount of base plane displacement are positive. As a result, method C yields incorrect results as if the noncontractile region actively performed positive external work under certain conditions. Thus, this model demonstrates that method C counts passive regional work given from the surrounding myocardium as active work performed by the observed noncontractile region, i.e., it cannot differentiate passive from active regional work in a nonuniformly contracting ventricle. This limitation of method C is attributable to the fact that this method does not directly measure muscle shortening per se but assesses resultant wall displacement. Therefore, method C requires an assumption that all the points on the ventricular wall move toward a unique reference point in the ventricular lumen, and hence, ventricular wall displacement is equivalent to active muscle shortening. However, in the case of nonuniform ventricular contraction, there could be a passive movement of the ventricular wall toward the reference point.

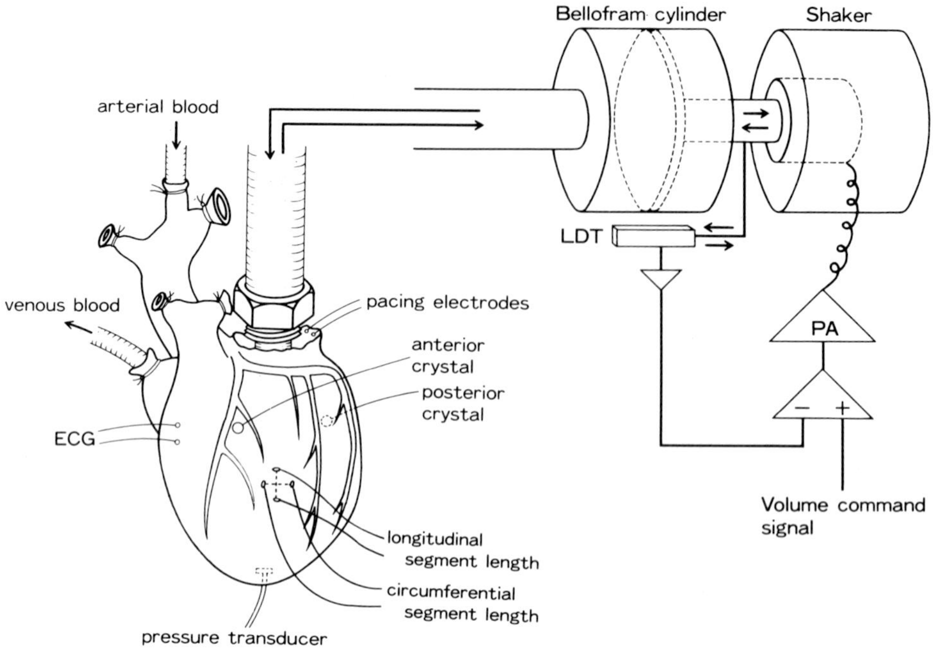

Fig. 7. Schematic drawing of excised, cross-circulated heart preparation connected to a volume servo pump. *ECG*, electrocardiogram; *LDT*, linear displacement transducer; *PA*, power amplifier

With regards to method A, although this method theoretically provides a correct assessment of regional work under such a specific condition mentioned above, it is practically difficult at present to integrate unidirectional regional work in all directions of the region on the ventricular surface plane. In contrast, method B, the T-A loop method, is practically feasible when regional area is measured by ultrasonic dimension gauges, and thus at present, is the most reasonable way to assess regional work with physically correct dimensions.

Validation in Normal and Globally Affected Hearts

To validate the T-A loop method for the assessment of regional work in normal and globally affected hearts, the following experiments were performed in excised, cross-circulated dog hearts [7]:

Materials and Methods. The surgical preparation has been described previously by us [7, 8]. In each experiment, two mongrel dogs were used. The heart donor dog was thoracotomized and the heart was excised after cross-circulation with the support dog was started (Fig. 7). After the left atrium was opened, a thin rubber balloon with a miniature pressure gauge was fitted in the left ventricle, and its mouth was secured at the mitral annulus. The balloon was connected to the same volume servo pump system used in research by Suga et al. [65]. With

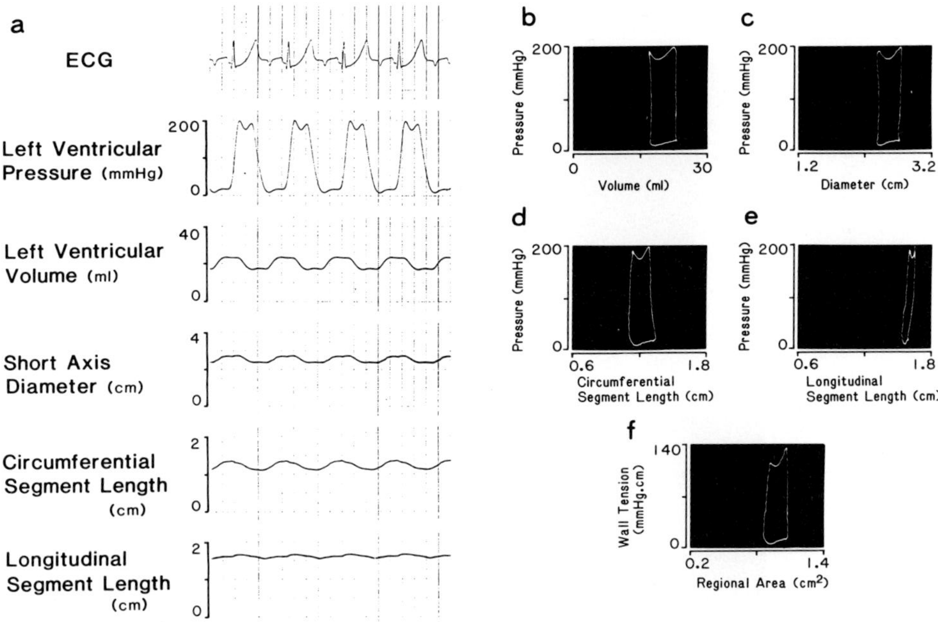

Fig. 8. **a**: examples of original tracings of electrocardiogram (*ECG*), left ventricular pressure, volume, and dimensions. **b-f**: pressure-volume (**b**), pressure-diameter (**c**), pressure-circumferential segment length (**d**), pressure-longitudinal segment length (**e**), and wall tension-regional area (**f**) loops constructed from data in **a**. Note that the time course and extent of shortening of the circumferential and longitudinal segments considerably differ from each other. (From [7] with permission)

this volume servo pump, we were able to precisely control left ventricular volume and accurately measure both instantaneous pressure and volume.

Left ventricular short axis (anterior-posterior) diameter and a pair of orthogonal segment lengths were measured with ultrasonic crystals (Fig. 7). The segment length crystals were placed in the subendocardium of the left ventricular anterior wall.

After surgical preparation, left ventricular loading conditions were altered by changing stroke volume or end-diastolic volume at each of the following contractile states: baseline, enhanced contractile state with dobutamine infusion, and depressed contractile state by lowering coronary perfusion pressure to 30–50 mmHg (global ischemia). During steady-state contractions under each loading condition, data were sampled to determine left ventricular stroke work from a pressure-volume loop and regional work from a T-A loop (Fig. 8). Wall tension (T, in mmHg·cm) was calculated according to the force equilibrium relation of a thick-walled sphere, assuming that the left ventricular contractile force is supported solely by the endocardial layer [64]. Namely, $T = \frac{1}{4}DP$, where D is left ventricular short axis diameter (cm) and P is left ventricular pressure (mmHg). Regional area (A, in cm^2) of the diamond-shaped region

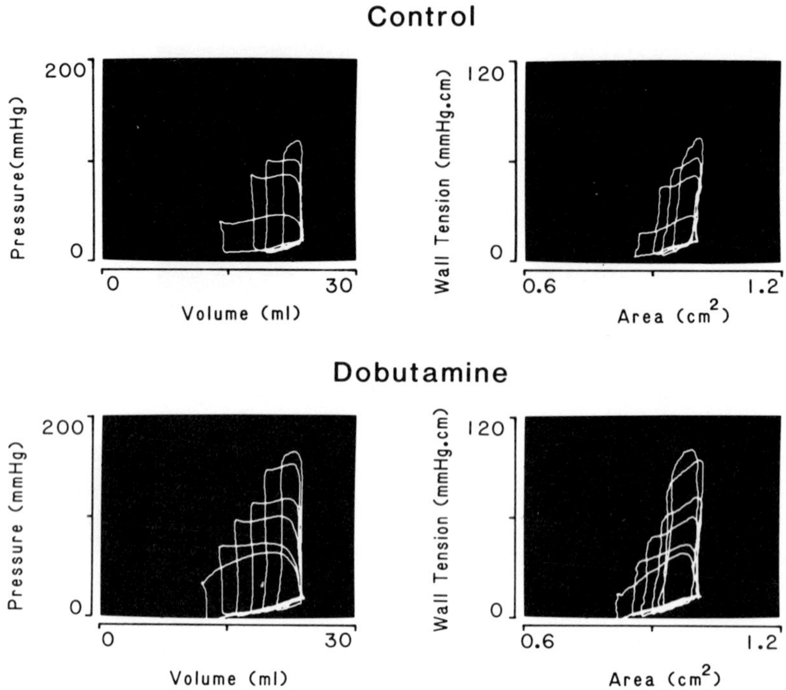

Fig. 9. Examples of pressure-volume loops (*left*) and wall tension-regional area loops (*right*) obtained during the control period (*upper*) and dobutamine infusion (*lower*)

surrounded by the four crystals was calculated as $A = \frac{1}{2}L_1L_2$ where L_1 and L_2 are circumferential and longitudinal segment lengths (cm). Regional work (mmHg·ml or dyne·cm) was then assessed from the integral of wall tension with respect to regional area, i.e., area within a T-A loop.

To compare measured regional work with predicted values, predicted regional work was calculated as the product of left ventricular stroke work obtained from the pressure-volume loop and the end-diastolic ratio of regional area to left ventricular endocardial surface area. Left ventricular endocardial surface area was calculated from the left ventricular volume and the short axis radius in an ellipsoid model.

Results. Figure 9 shows left ventricular pressure-volume loops (left) and T-A loops (right) in the baseline (control) and enhanced contractile states with dobutamine in a representative heart. Ventricular loading conditions were altered by changing stroke volume while end-diastolic volume was held constant. In each contractile state, increases in stroke volume caused proportional increases in regional area excursion, resulting in similar changes in shape between pressure-volume loops and T-A loops. At the same end-diastolic and stroke volumes, dobutamine infusion produced larger pressure-volume and T-A loop areas, i.e., greater external work for both the left ventricle and the

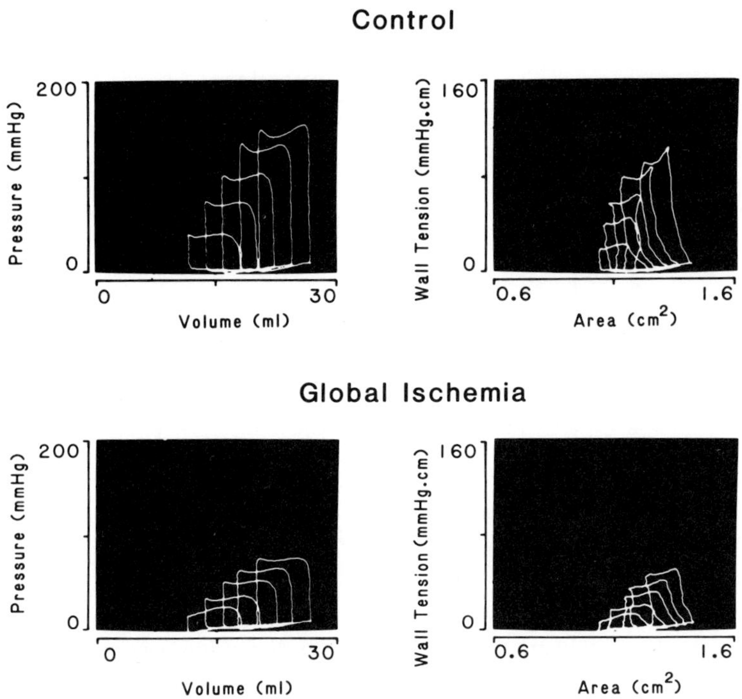

Fig. 10. Examples of pressure-volume loops (*left*) and wall tension-regional area loops (*right*) obtained during the control period (*upper*) and global ischemic (*lower*). (From [7] with permission)

observed region. Figure 10 shows left ventricular pressure-volume loops and T-A loops in the baseline and depressed contractile states with global ischemia in another representative heart. In this heart, end-diastolic volume was varied while stroke volume was kept constant. In each contractile state and loading condition, the shape of pressure-volume and T-A loops are quite similar. Global ischemia resulted in decreases in both left ventricular and regional work. These findings indicate that in normal and globally affected hearts, the whole ventricle and a ventricular region behave quite similarly regardless of changes in loading and inotropic conditions.

Figure 11 plots measured regional work from T-A loops against predicted regional work under various loading and inotropic conditions in a representative heart. Measured regional work closely agreed with predicted regional work over a wide range of regional work values regardless of changes in stroke volume, end-diastolic volume or contractile state. Similar close agreements between measured and predicted regional work were observed in six other hearts. In a total of 192 cardiac contractions under various experimental conditions in the seven left ventricles, the correlation between measured and predicted regional work yielded a linear regression equation as $y = 0.91x - 0.67$ ($r = 0.93$). From these findings, it was concluded that the T-A loop

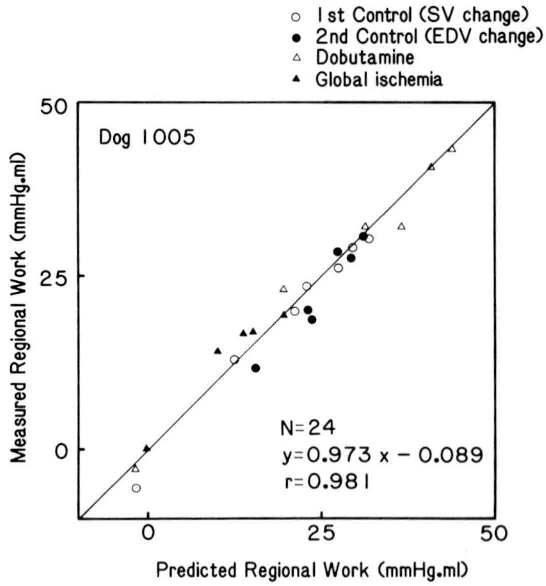

Fig. 11. Correlation between measured and predicted regional work in a representative heart. Measured values were obtained from a wall tension-regional area loop, and predicted values were calculated from left ventricular stroke work and percent regional area for the same contraction. *SV*, stroke volume; *EDV*, end-diastolic volume. *Solid line* indicates the identity line. (From [7] with permission)

method reliably quantifies left ventricular regional work in both normal and globally affected hearts.

Validation in Regionally Ischemic Heart

To validate the T-A loop method in a regionally ischemic heart, the following experiments were performed in 11 excised, cross-circulated dog hearts [52].

Materials and Methods. The surgical preparation of the isolated heart was the same as described above except for the placement of ultrasonic crystals and a coronary artery snare. In this protocol, two pairs of orthogonal segment lengths, one in the left ventricular anterior wall region and the other in the posterior wall region, were measured with pairs of ultrasonic crystals placed in the subendocardium. The anterior and posterior wall crystals were placed completely within the perfusion area of the left anterior descending and circumflex coronary arteries, respectively. A snare was placed on the left anterior descending (9 experiments) or circumflex (2 experiments) coronary artery for subsequent occlusion.

The left ventricular pressure-volume relation and T-A relations in the anterior and posterior wall regions were measured at various end-diastolic and stroke volumes during steady-state contractions before and during regional ischemia. Regional ischemia was produced by occluding either the left anterior descending or circumflex coronary artery with the snare. After each experiment, the ischemic zone size was determined by infusing barium sulfate suspension into the left main coronary artery. The non-opacified region in the X-ray photographs of slices of the heart were digitized as ischemic zone.

To validate the T-A loop method in the regionally ischemic heart, we compared globally integrated regional work with left ventricular stroke work obtained from the pressure-volume loop before and after coronary artery occlusion. Globally integrated regional work was calculated as the sum of the regional work for both ischemic and nonischemic zones. Regional work of each zone was calculated as regional work per unit area multiplied by the size of the ischemic or nonischemic zone.

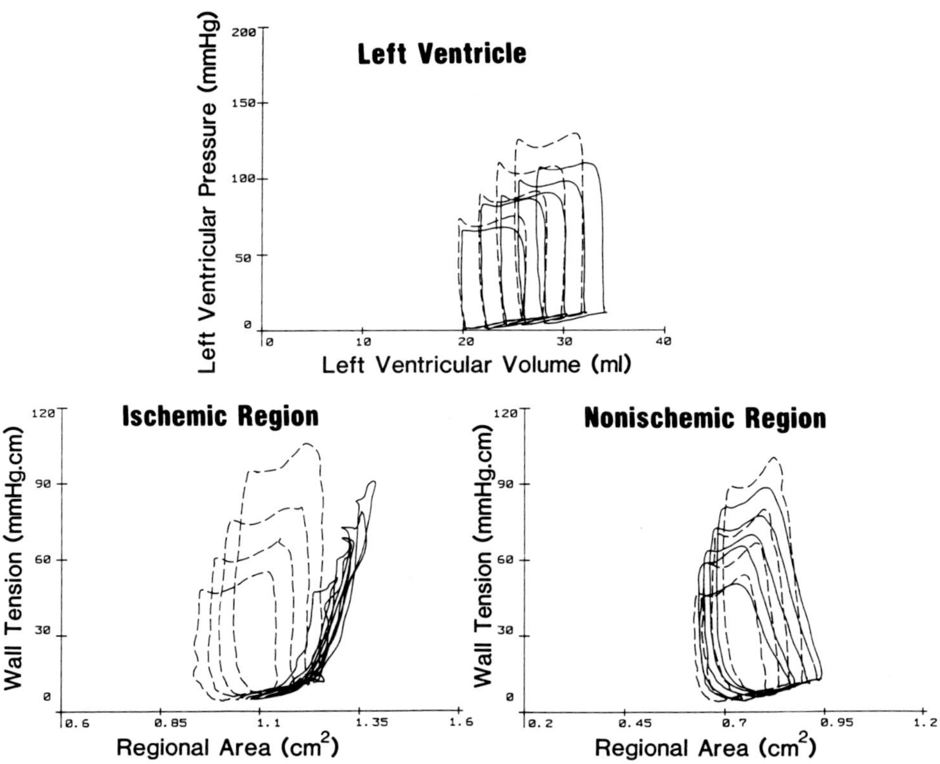

Fig. 12. Representative example of left ventricular pressure-volume loops and wall tension-regional area (T-A) loops in ischemic and nonischemic regions during the control period (*dashed line*) and regional ischemia (*solid line*). After coronary artery occlusion, the T-A loops in the ischemic region were markedly deformed and shifted to the right, whereas the T-A loops in the nonischemic region preserved the near rectangular shape. Note that the end-systolic T-A relation connecting the left upper corners of the loops in the nonischemic region was unchanged after coronary artery occlusion

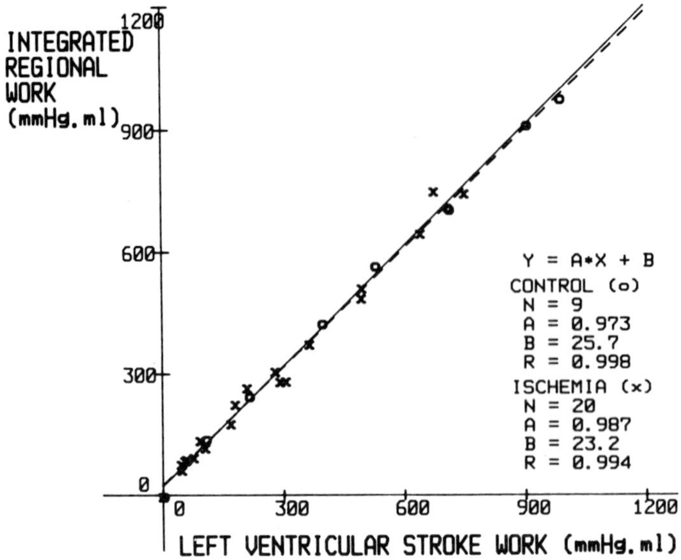

Fig. 13. Correlation between globally integrated regional work and left ventricular stroke work during the control period (*open cricle* and *dashed line*) and after coronary artery occlusion (*cross* and *solid line*). Globally integrated regional work obtained from the T-A loops closely agreed with left ventricular stroke work both before and after coronary occlusion. (From [8] with permission)

Results. Figure 12 shows left ventricular pressure-volume loops and T-A loops in the ischemic and nonischemic regions obtained before and after coronary artery occlusion in a representative heart. During the control period, all pressure-volume and T-A loops showed a similar rectangular shape. In addition, left ventricular stroke work and regional work indicated by the respective loop areas increased proportionally as end-diastolic ventricular volume and end-diastolic regional area increased. After coronary artery occlusion, left ventricular systolic pressure and stroke work moderately decreased at given end-diastolic and stroke volumes. The T-A loops in the ischemic region were markedly deformed and shifted to the right, resulting in marked decreases in regional work of the ischemic region. In contrast, the T-A loops in the nonischemic region preserved the near rectangular shape and hence, positive regional work. It should be noted that there is a significant area shrinkage during the isovolumic contraction period in the nonischemic region, corresponding to the area expansion during the same period in the ischemic region, while the end-systolic T-A relation connecting the left upper corners of the loops in the nonischemic region was virtually unaltered. This suggests that increased area shrinkage (hyperkinesis) in a nonischemic region during acute ischemia occurs at the same level of myocardial contractile state of the region (see the section Mechanism of Hyperkinesis in a Nonischemic Region).

In a total of 11 hearts, coronary artery occlusion resulted in decreases in both E_{max} from 10.0 ± 3.5 mmHg/ml to 5.1 ± 2.1 mmHg/ml and left ventricular stroke work by 49 ± 17% at matched end-diastolic and stroke volumes. Regional work of the ischemic region markedly decreased by 96 ± 23% on average, whereas regional work of the nonischemic region only moderately decreased by 42 ± 20% mainly because of a 45 ± 23% decrease in end-systolic wall tension. Figure 13 shows the correlation between globally integrated regional work and left ventricular stroke work before and after coronary artery occlusion in a representative heart. Despite marked deformations of the ischemic T-A loops and extreme reductions in ischemic regional work, globally integrated regional work closely agreed with left ventricular stroke work both before and after coronary artery occlusion. The two linear regression lines before and after regional ischemia were almost superimposable. The other ten hearts showed similar results. The linear regression equations for pooled data in the 11 hearts were $y = 1.00x - 70.0$ ($r = 0.92$) for 119 data points during the control period, and $y = 0.93x - 44.0$ ($r = 0.93$) for 141 data points after coronary artery occlusion. Neither a slope difference nor an elevation difference was indicated by analysis of covariance between two linear regression lines for pooled data obtained before and after coronary artery occlusion. Based on these results, it was concluded that left ventricular regional work can be reliably assessed by the T-A loop method even in a heart subjected to regional ischemia.

End-systolic Tension-area Relation (ESTAR)

Theoretical Background

The time-varying elastance model has been applied to the left ventricle to describe the systolic behavior of the ventricle under various loading conditions [4, 5]. The time-varying elastance E(t) is defined by the following equation:

$$E(t) = P(t)/[V(t) - V_0] \qquad (1)$$

where P(t) and V(t) are instantaneous ventricular pressure and volume, t is the time after the onset of contraction, and V_0 is an unloaded ventricular volume at which the ventricle does not generate positive pressure during systole [4]. Previous experimental results have shown that the maximal or end-systolic value of the elastance, which has been called E_{max}, represents the contractile state of the left ventricle independent of ventricular loading conditions under most circumstances [4, 5, 66]. Therefore, the linear end-systolic pressure-volume relation is expressed as:

$$P_{es} = E_{max}\,(V_{es} - V_0) \qquad (2)$$

where P_{es} and V_{es} are end-systolic left ventricular pressure and volume, and E_{max} and V_0 are the slope and the volume-axis intercept of the relation [4, 66].

If we assume a spherical ventricle, instantaneous wall tension T(t) and regional area A(t) are obtained as:

$$T(t) = r(t) \cdot P(t)/2 \qquad (3)$$

$$A(t) = k \cdot [4\pi r(t)^2] \tag{4}$$

where r(t) is the instantaneous radius of the spherical ventricle and k is the area ratio of an observed region to the whole ventricular endocardial surface. According to Eq. (1), we obtain the instantaneous relation between wall tension and regional area as:

$$T(t) = E(t) \cdot [A(t)^2 - A_0^{3/2} \cdot A(t)^{1/2}]/(24 \cdot \pi \cdot k) \tag{5}$$

where A_0 is an unloaded regional area at which peak systolic tension is zero. Thus, the instantaneous T-A relation can be defined as a function of ventricular elastance E(t). When E(t) reaches its end-systolic value E_{max}, the T-A relation is expressed as:

$$T_{es} = E_{max} \cdot (A_{es}^{\ 2} - A_0^{3/2} \cdot A_{es}^{\ 1/2})/(24 \cdot \pi \cdot k) \tag{6}$$

where T_{es} and A_{es} are end-systolic wall tension and regional area. This equation indicates a nonlinear function with downward convexity. Thus, according to the theoretical consideration, when the end-systolic pressure-volume relation is linear, the end-systolic T-A relation (ESTAR) is nonlinear with convexity toward the regional area axis.

Although the instantaneous slope of this ESTAR increases with increased regional area, Eq. (6) also indicates that the ESTAR reflects end-systolic elastance or myocardial contractile state. Therefore, the slope of the ESTAR can be used as an index of myocardial contractility of the region. However, a major limitation of the ESTAR as a contractility index is that it cannot be used for comparisons of myocardial contractility between different regions or different hearts, because regional area is not normalized. Thus, the ESTAR can be used only for comparisons of myocardial contractility in the same ventricular region. In this context, Nakano et al. [54] have reported that the exponential constant of the end-systolic relation between wall stress and the natural logarithm of the reciprocal of wall thickness represents the end-systolic myocardial stiffness normalized for a unit myocardial mass, and hence can be used for comparisons of myocardial contractility between different regions or between different hearts.

Linearity of the ESTAR

Figure 14 shows left ventricular pressure-volume loops (Panel A) and T-A loops in the anterior wall region (Panel B) which were measured simultaneously at a stable contractile state in one heart. The line connecting the left upper corners (end-systolic point) of the pressure-volume loops forms a highly linear end-systolic pressure-volume relation. In Panel B, the line connecting the left upper corners of the T-A loops, i.e., the ESTAR, is also well fitted by a straight line. Therefore, the ESTAR can be expressed as:

$$T_{es} = rE_{max}(A_{es} - A_0) \tag{7}$$

where rE_{max} is the slope of the ESTAR or regional E_{max} and A_0 is the area axis intercept of the linear ESTAR. The linearity of the ESTAR has also been

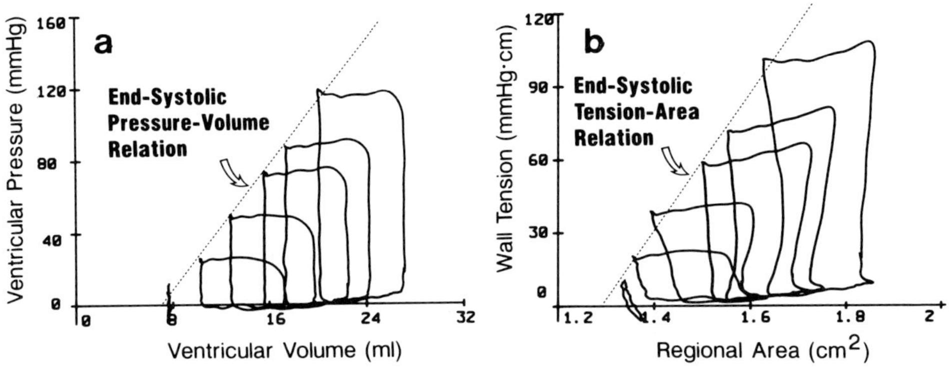

Fig. 14. Pressure-volume loops (**a**) and wall tension-regional area loops (**b**) which were measured simultaneously in one heart. *Dashed lines* indicated linear end-systolic pressure-volume and tension-area relations, respectively

demonstrated in Figs. 3, 9, 10, 12, and 15. In our recent study [67], the linearity of the ESTAR was demonstrated by a high median correlation coefficient of 0.983 among 15 ESTARs obtained in the baseline contractile state. Unlike theoretical predictions, these actually measured ESTARs are not necessarily convex downward. Sometimes the ESTAR even shows upward convexity as in Fig. 10 (upper right panel). This discrepancy between the theoretically predicted nonlinear ESTAR and the actually measured linear ESTAR may be attributable to the complex ventricular structure and geometry [32, 37, 55].

ESTAR as an Index of Regional Myocardial Contractility

To examine the ability of the ESTAR to sensitively reflect changes in regional myocardial contractility, the end-systolic pressure-volume relation and the ESTAR of the anterior wall region were simultaneously assessed before and during infusion of dobutamine into either the left anterior descending or circumflex coronary artery [67]. Results in a representative heart are shown in Fig. 15. When the myocardial contractility of the anterior wall was selectively

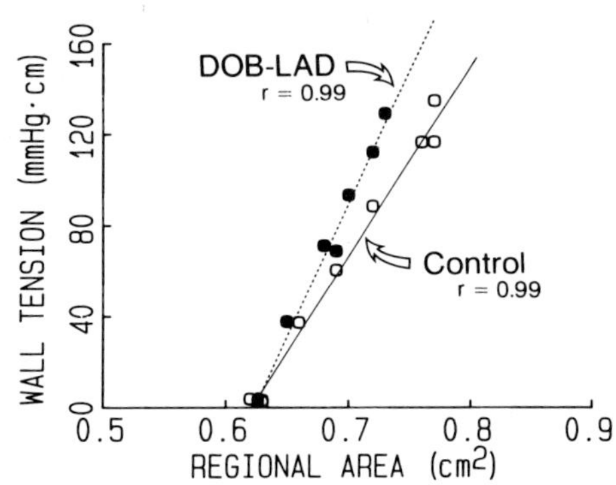

Fig. 15. The end-systolic wall tension-regional area relation in the anterior wall region before and during dobutamine infusion into the left anterior descending coronary artery. The relation was well fitted to a straight line in each state, and the slope increased with regional enhancement of myocardial contractility

enhanced with dobutamine, left ventricular global E_{max} modestly increased by 21 ± 23% from the baseline value of 8.2 ± 2.8 mmHg/ml, whereas regional E_{max} of the anterior wall region markedly increased by 117 ± 81% from the baseline value of 448 ± 258 mmHg/cm. In contrast, when myocardial contractility of the posterior wall was selectively enhanced with dobutamine, regional E_{max} of the anterior wall did not change, despite the similar (20 ± 15%) increase in left ventricular global E_{max}. These results indicate that the ESTAR sensitively and reliably reflects changes in myocardial contractility of the observed region independent of myocardial contractility of the opposite region.

In another study [68], effects of global and regional ischemia on the ESTAR were assessed in ten excised, cross-circulated dog hearts. In the same heart preparation as in Fig. 7, a snare was placed on the left anterior descending coronary artery and two pairs of ultrasonic crystals were placed in the subendocardium within the perfused area of the same coronary artery. Measurements for left ventricular pressure-volume relations and anterior wall T-A relations were made under the following four experimental conditions: the first control period, global ischemia produced by lowering coronary perfusion pressure from 93 ± 19 mmHg to 39 ± 5 mmHg, the second control period, and regional ischemia produced by occluding the left anterior coronary artery with the snare.

Results in a representative heart have already been shown in Fig. 3. Under each experimental condition, the ESTAR fitted reasonably well to a straight line as indicated by a median correlation coefficient of 0.960 during the first control period, 0.978 during global ischemia, 0.967 during the second control period, and 0.975 during regional ischemia. Figure 16 summarizes data for the ESTAR under four experimental conditions. During global ischemia, regional E_{max} (the slope of the ESTAR) markedly decreased by 53 ± 21% whereas A_0 (the area axis intercept) did not change. During regional ischemia, regional E_{max} significantly decreased by 46 ± 33%, the magnitude of which was similar to that during global ischemia. However, in contrast to the results during global ischemia, A_0 significantly increased by 22 ± 13% during regional ischemia. These results indicate that the ESTAR reflects depressed myocardial contractility during both global and regional ischemia. However, this study also demonstrated that during regional ischemia, both the slope and the area axis intercept of the ESTAR should be taken into account to assess regional changes in myocardial contractility.

Mechanism of Hyperkinesis in a Nonischemic Region

Hyperkinesis (increased systolic wall motion) has been observed in a nonischemic region of an acutely ischemic heart in experimental animals and in patients. The mechanism of this hyperkinesis has been ascribed to increased sympathetic activity [69], to the Frank-Starling mechanism [9], or to a combination of the Frank-Starling mechanism and mechanical unloading due to intraventricular regional interaction [11]. To elucidate the primary mechanism

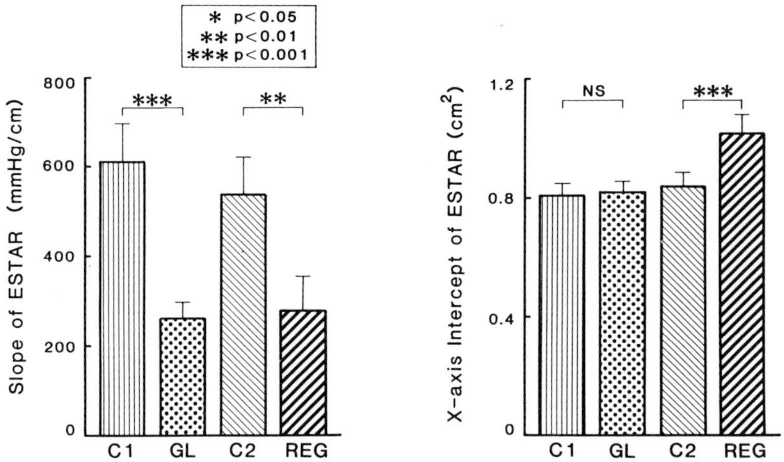

Fig. 16. Effects of global and regional ischemia on the slope (*left*) and the area axis intercept (*right*) of the end-systolic wall tension-regional area relation. Global ischemia (*GL*) decreases the slope without affecting the area axis intercept. In contrast, regional ischemia (*REG*) results in a significant increase in the area axis intercept for a similar decrease in the slope. *C1*, first control; *C2*, second control

of hyperkinesis in a nonischemic region, the T-A relations were assessed in both ischemic and nonischemic regions before and after occlusion of either the left anterior descending or circumflex coronary artery in the same isolated heart preparation as in Fig. 7 [52]. In this study, to determine whether hyperkinesis occurs without utilization of the Frank-Starling mechanism, regional ischemia was produced while left ventricular end-diastolic and stroke volumes were kept constant.

Figure 17 shows pressure-volume loops (A) and T-A loops in the ischemic (B) and nonischemic (C) regions in a representative heart. Figure 18 summarizes data for stroke volume and systolic area shrinkage in 12 experiments. After measurements during the control period (Fig. 17), regional ischemia was produced at constant left ventricular end-diastolic and stroke volumes. In the ischemic region (Fig. 17B), end-diastolic regional area increased despite the same end-diastolic wall tension, suggesting creep or passive stretch of the ischemic myocardium. The direction of rotation of the T-A loop was reversed, resulting in a negative regional work. On average, systolic area shrinkage decreased markedly by 109 ± 30% (Fig. 18). On the other hand, end-diastolic regional area in the nonischemic area decreased slightly during regional ischemia (Fig. 17C). With this decreased regional preload, the T-A loop in the nonischemic region showed a noticeable area shrinkage during the isovolumic contraction period, corresponding reciprocally to changes in the ischemic region. As a result, systolic area shrinkage increased by 33 ± 41% (Fig. 18) despite the apparent lack of utilization of the Frank-Starling mechanism. When left ventricular end-diastolic volume was increased (Fig. 17) to simulate a

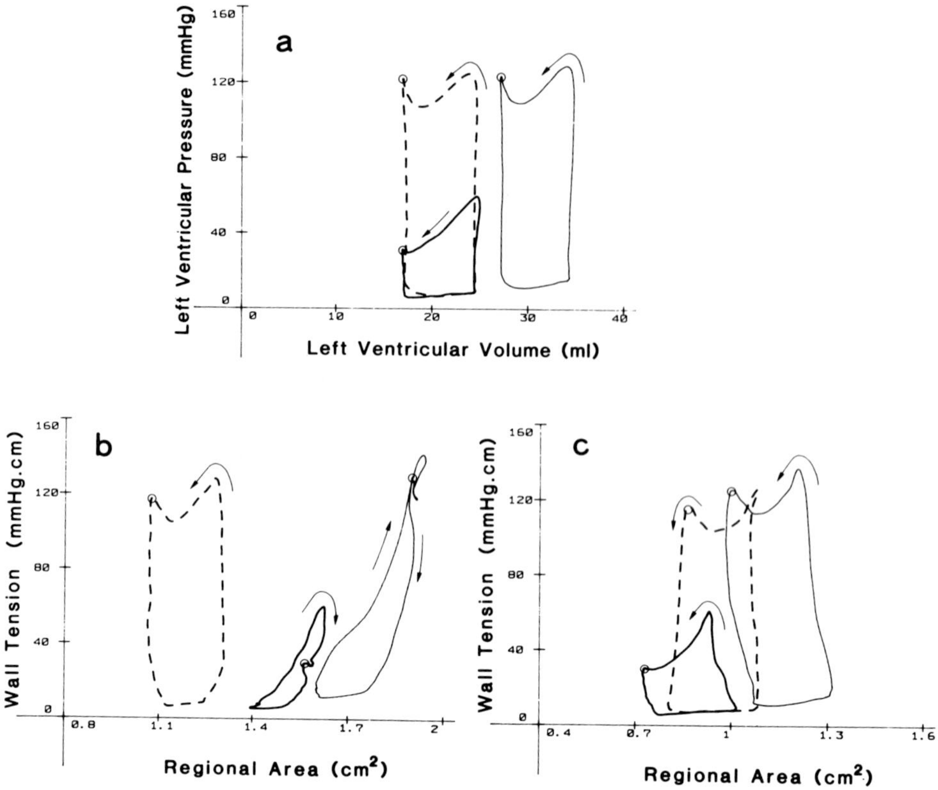

Fig. 17. A representative example of left ventricular pressure-volume loops (**a**) and wall tension-regional area loops in ischemic (**b**) and nonischemic (**c**) regions during the control period (*dashed line*), regional ischemia at constant left ventricular end-diastolic and stroke volumes (*thick solid line*), and regional ischemia with increased end-diastolic volume (*thin solid line*). Increased systolic area shrinkage in the nonischemic region, not associated with an increased regional preload, corresponds to the systolic bulging in the ischemic region, indicating intraventricular regional interaction. (From [52] with permission)

clinical condition in which left ventricular stroke work is compensated for by increased ventricular preload, systolic area shrinkage in the nonischemic region increased further at the expense of a further decrease in area shrinkage in the ischemic region despite the constant stroke volume (Fig. 18).

To examine whether enhanced regional myocardial contractility in the nonischemic region is responsible for hyperkinesis, the ESTAR was assessed in the ischemic and nonischemic regions during the control period and during regional ischemia (Fig. 19). Compared to the marked rightward shift of the ESTAR in the ischemic region, the ESTAR in the nonischemic region was almost unchanged during regional ischemia. This unaltered ESTAR in the nonischemic region during regional ischemia has also been demonstrated in Fig. 12. These findings indicate that myocardial contractility in the nonischemic

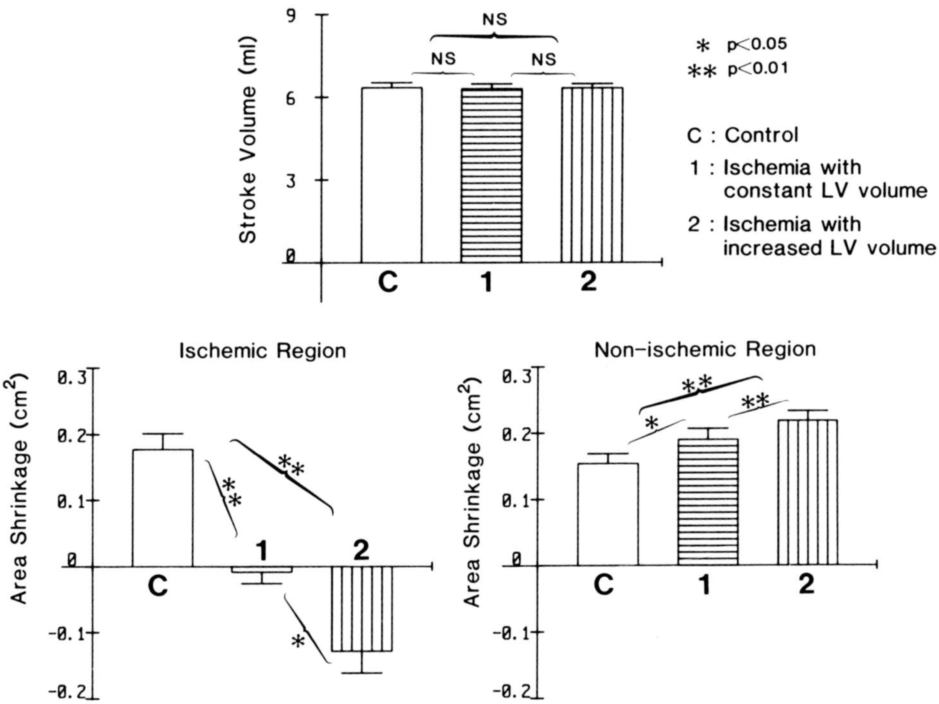

Fig. 18. Comparisons of stroke volume (*top*) and systolic area shrinkage in the ischemic (*bottom left*) and nonischemic (*bottom right*) regions during the control period and regional ischemia. Means ± SEM are indicated. (From [52] with permission)

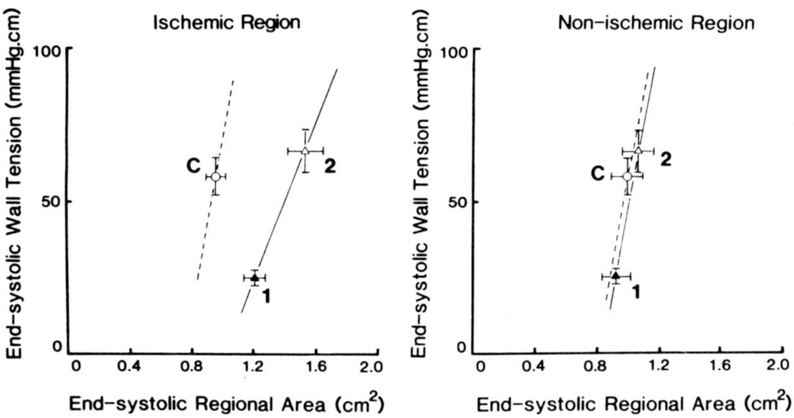

Fig. 19. The end-systolic wall tension-regional area relation in the ischemic (*left*) and nonischemic (*right*) regions during the control period (*open circle* and *dashed line*) and regional ischemia (*triangles* and *solid line*). The end-systolic tension-area relation in the ischemic region shifted markedly to the right after coronary occlusion, whereas the relation in the nonischemic region was almost unchanged. Means ± SEM are indicated. (From [52] with permission)

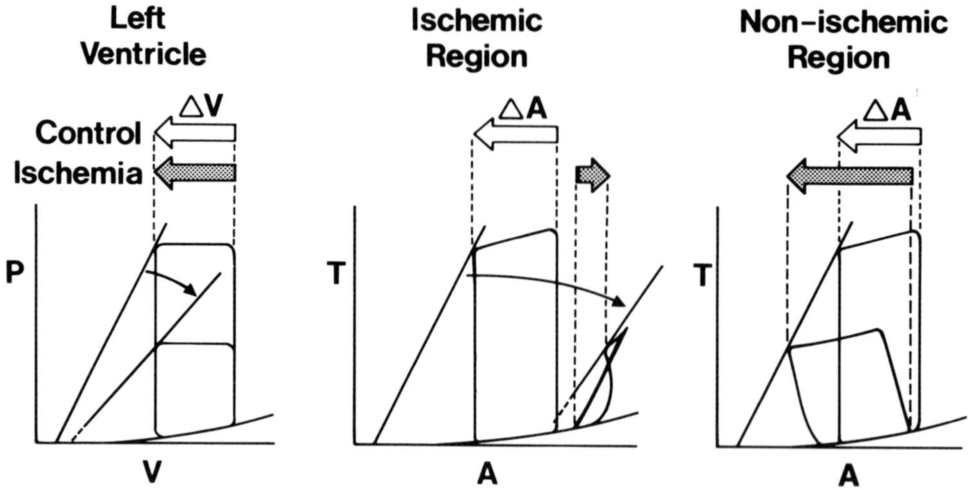

Fig. 20. Schematic illustration for explanation of the mechanism of hyperkinesis without utilization of the Frank-Starling mechanism. Left ventricular pressure-volume (*P-V*) loops (*left*) and wall tension-regional area (*T-A*) loops in the ischemic (*middle*) and nonischemic (*right*) regions during control and regional ischemic periods are shown. End-diastolic and stroke volumes are constant under both conditions. *Open* and *shaded arrows* indicate stroke volume (ΔV) and the amount of systolic area shrinkage (ΔA) during the control (*open arrows*) and regional ischemia (*shaded arrows*) periods. The *lines* passing through the *left upper corners* of the loops indicate end-systolic P-V or T-A relations. During regional ischemia, ΔA in the ischemic region becomes negative (systolic bulging) with a marked rightward shift of the end-systolic T-A relation, whereas ΔA in the nonischemic region increases (hyperkinesis) without any increase in preload or enhancement of myocardial contractility of the region. (From [52] with permission)

region is unchanged, and hence, it is unlikely that hyperkinesis of the nonischemic region is caused by an enhanced regional myocardial contractility.

Another interesting finding in this study was that regional work of the nonischemic region significantly decreased during regional ischemia at constant end-diastolic and stroke volumes, despite the presence of hyperkinesis. This mimics an unloaded whole ventricle in which a decrease in afterload results in an increase in ventricular stoke volume (or shortening) and a concomitant reduction in stroke work [46]. Thus, hyperkinesis is not a "compensatory" mechanism for the decreased contractile performance of the ischemic region, but a natural consequence of mechanical unloading of the nonischemic region.

Our hypothetical explanation of the mechanism of hyperkinesis without utilization of the Frank-Starling mechanism is illustrated in Fig. 20. During regional ischemia at constant end-diastolic and stroke volumes, the ESTAR in the ischemic region markedly shifts to the right due to depressed myocardial contractility. During the isovolumic contraction period, the ischemic region is no longer able to support the wall tension that is generated by the nonischemic myocardium, resulting in systolic bulging. In contrast, myocardial contractility in the nonischemic region is virtually unchanged, and hence the ESTAR is unaltered. Because systolic wall tension of the left ventricle which acts as afterload on the nonischemic region decreases, the nonischemic region can shorten to a greater extent even at a constant contractility and slightly lower preload.

Thus, this study [52] demonstrated that regional afterload reduction due to an intraventricular mechanical interaction between ischemic and nonischemic regions rather than the Frank-Starling mechanism may be the primary mechanism of hyperkinesis in the nonischemic region.

Tension-area Area (TAA) as an Index of Regional Myocardial Oxygen Consumption

Conventional Indexes of Regional Myocardial Oxygen Consumption

Most variables previously reported as an index of myocardial oxygen consumption (VO_2), such as pressure-rate product [70], force-time integral [71], tension-time index [72], peak wall tension [73], and pressure-work index [74], are global rather than regional mechanical variables and therefore reflect whole ventricular VO_2 rather than regional VO_2. On the other hand, most variables of regional myocardial contractile function such as segment shortening [75, 76], wall thickening [77], and regional work index [78], have not been systematically analyzed to determine whether they reliably reflect regional VO_2 under various loading conditions. With regards to this, Gayheart et al. [76] have recently reported a significant correlation between segment shortening and regional Vo_2. However, the correlation was modest ($r = 0.7$) and they did not analyze variables other than segment shortening. Thus, there has been no reliable measure of regional VO_2.

In contrast, recent studies [6, 65, 79] have shown that left ventricular systolic pressure-volume area (PVA) defined in the pressure-volume diagram (Fig. 21)

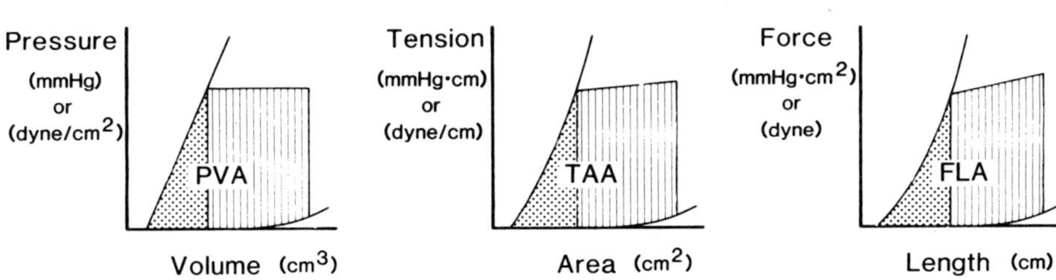

Fig. 21. Schematic illustrations of pressure-volume area (*PVA*) in the P-V diagram, wall tension-regional area area (*TAA*) in the T-A diagram, and force-length area (*FLA*) in the F-L diagram. The *hatched* and *dotted areas* in each diagram indicate external work and potential energy portions, respectively. All three areas have the same dimensions equivalent to energy

is a reliable predictor of left ventricular VO_2 regardless of loading conditions as described in the previous chapter. Further, we have demonstrated that the T-A loop area represents regional work with physically correct dimensions of energy and that the ESTAR reliably reflects regional myocardial contractility. Thus, it is quite conceivable that the T-A diagram is mechanically and energetically equivalent to the left ventricular pressure-volume diagram, i.e., the T-A diagram may be a regional version of the whole ventricular pressure-volume diagram.

Therefore, by the analogy of PVA in the left ventricular pressure-volume diagram, T-A area (TAA) [80] was defined in the T-A diagram as a specific area surrounded by the ESTAR, the end-diastolic T-A relation, and the systolic T-A trajectory as shown in Fig. 21. The dimensions of TAA are the same as those of PVA ($mmHg \cdot ml \cdot beat^{-1} \cdot 100\,g^{-1}$) and equivalent to energy (Joule). Because PVA theoretically represents total mechanical energy generated by the whole ventricle and linearly correlates with whole ventricular VO_2 [6], it seems reasonable to expect that TAA represents total mechanical energy generated by the observed region during contraction and that TAA linearly correlates with regional VO_2 of the region.

According to the theoretical consideration shown in Fig. 5, another equivalent of PVA, the force-length area (FLA), can be derived in the force-length diagram (Fig. 21). Because of its unidirectional nature, FLA may be suitable for mechanoenergetic analysis in a linear muscle preparation. In fact, the load-independent, linear relation between VO_2 and FLA has already been reported in papillary muscle preparations by Hisano and Cooper [81]. In contrast, TAA may be suitable for mechanoenergetic analysis in a region of the left ventricle because it can assess multidirectional contractile function [82, 83] of the region.

Correlation between Regional Oxygen Consumption and TAA

In the same isolated heart perparation as shown in Fig. 7, the left anterior descending coronary artery and the anterior interventricular vein were cannulated to measure region VO_2 in the anterior wall region [80]. The T-A relation of the anterior wall region was measured with ultrasonic crystals placed within the perfused area of the left anterior descending coronary artery. The correlation between TAA and regional VO_2 was assessed under various loading conditions by changing left ventricular end-diastolic and stroke volumes in a stable contractile state. In this study, a linear fit to the ESTAR was used to calculate TAA as shown in Fig. 14.

Figure 22 depicts correlations between various variables and regional VO_2 in a representative heart, in which both isovolumic and ejecting contractions were produced. The correlation between TAA and regional VO_2 (Fig. 22A) was highly linear and was not affected by the mode of contraction. In a total of ten experiments, the correlation coefficient between regional VO_2 and TAA (median $r = 0.96$) was slightly higher ($0.05 < P < 0.2$) than that for force-time integral ($r = 0.95$), tension-time integral ($r = 0.94$), or peak dP/dt ($r = 0.93$), and significantly higher ($P < 0.05$) than that for peak wall tension ($r = 0.89$),

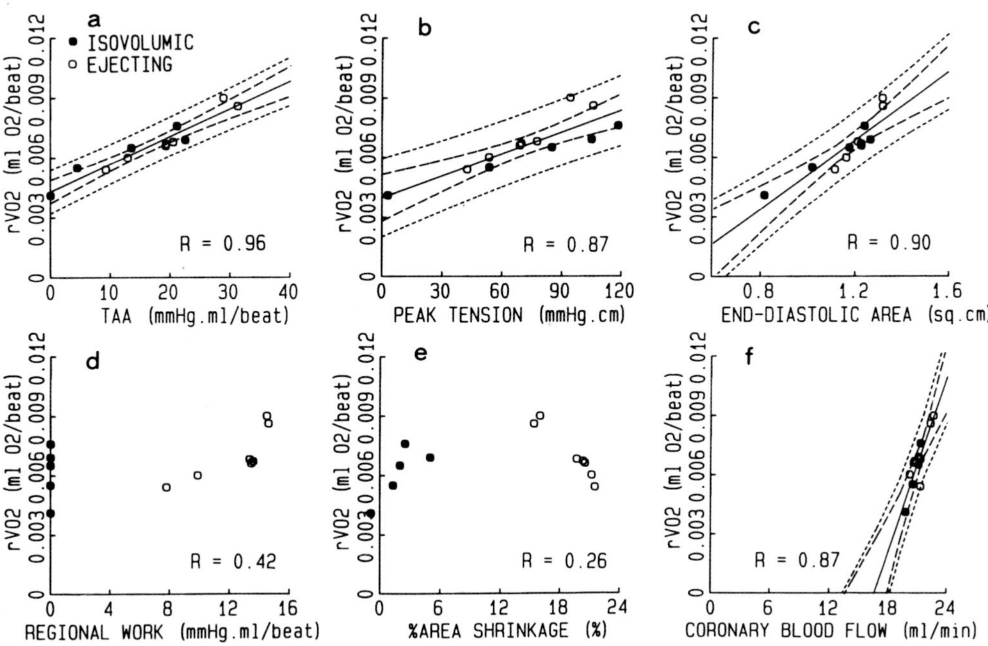

Fig. 22. Correlations between regional myocardial oxygen consumption (*rVO*$_2$) and various mechanical variables obtained in a representative heart in which both isovolumic and ejecting contractions were produced. The correlation for tension-area area (*TAA*) was linear, independent of modes of contraction, and accompanied by the highest correlation coefficient among the variables

end-diastolic regional area (r = 0.90), coronary blood flow (r = 0.86), end-systolic pressure (r = 0.83), regional work (r = 0.74), or percent area shrinkage (r = 0.41) by two-way analysis of variance.

An interesting observation in this study was that the reciprocal of the TAA-regional VO_2 relation (38 ± 8%), which we call "regional contractile efficiency," was very close to the previously reported value of the left ventricular contractile efficiency (35%–45%) [6, 84, 85] which is the reciprocal of the PVA-VO_2 relation. This contractile efficiency indicates the efficiency of energy conversion from oxygen used exclusively for mechanical contraction to total mechanical energy generated by a contraction. The close agreement between regional and global contractile efficiencies also supports the validity of TAA as a measure of regional mechanical energy expenditure. Thus, it was concluded that TAA is a reliable predictor of regional VO_2, which reflects regional mechanical energy expenditure regardless of the mode of contraction.

In a recent study [67], the relation between regional VO_2 and TAA was assessed during regional enhancement of myocardial contractility by selective infusion of dobutamine into the left anterior descending coronary artery. The purpose of this study was to examine whether the regional VO_2-TAA relation reflects regional changes in myocardial contractility. During infusion of

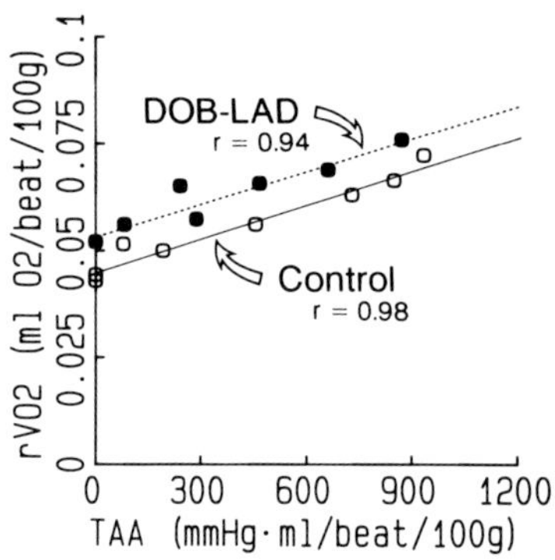

Fig. 23. The relationship between regional myocardial oxygen consumption (*r*VO_2) and tension-area area (*TAA*) in the anterior wall region during control period and dobutamine (*DOB*) infusion into the left anterior descending coronary artery (*LAD*) in the same heart as in Fig. 15. During regional enhancement of myocardial contractility with dobutamine, the linear relation between *r*VO_2 and *TAA* shifted upward in a parallel manner

dobutamine into the left anterior descending coronary artery, the regional E_{max} increased, as already shown in Fig. 15, indicating regional enhancement of myocardial contractility. Figure 23 shows the regional VO_2-TAA relation obtained in the same heart as in Fig. 15. The regional VO_2-TAA relation was highly linear during both the control period and dobutamine infusion. With dobutamine, it shifted upward in a parallel manner. This parallel upward shift with dobutamine is similar to the findings for the VO_2-PVA relation obtained in the whole left ventricle [79]. Thus, the regional VO_2-TAA relation sensitively reflects regional changes in myocardial contractility in the same manner as that for the whole ventricular VO_2-PVA relation.

Conclusion and Perspective

There are three methods to assess regional myocardial contractile function: segment shortening (or wall thickening), regional work, and end-systolic measures. At present, end-systolic measures appear the most reliable measure of regional myocardial contractility, because they are for the most part independent of loading conditions, unlike segment shortening and regional work. In this article, we have mainly described the T-A relation; the T-A loop method allows us to quantify regional work of the left ventricle with physically correct dimensions. In addition, the ESTAR is linear and can be used as an index of regional myocardial contractility. By analyzing the T-A relations during regional ischemia, we have demonstrated that the primary mechanism of hyperkinesis in a nonischemic region may be regional afterload reduction due to intraventricular regional interaction between ischemic and nonischemic regions.

The major limitation of the ESTAR as an index of regional myocardial contractility is that it is not normalized for unit myocardial mass so that it cannot be used to compare myocardial contractility between different regions or different hearts. For this purposes, the end-systolic myocardial stiffness constant proposed by Nakano et al. [54] may be more suitable because it is normalized for a unit myocardial mass. However, because regional ischemia causes not only a decreased slope of the ESTAR (regional E_{max}) but also an increased area axis intercept (A_0), assessment of systolic myocardial stiffness alone could potentially result in an underestimation of the decreased contractile function during regional ischemia. Further study is necessary to determine a load and size-independent measure of regional myocardial contractility, especially in the case of regional ischemia.

With regards to regional myocardial energetics, TAA defined in the T-A diagram linearly correlates with regional VO_2 in a load-independent manner, representing regional myocardial mechanical energy expenditure. The reciprocal of the slope of the regional VO_2-TAA relation may represent regional contractile efficiency. During increased regional myocardial contractility with dobutamine, the regional VO_2-TAA relation shifts upward in a parallel manner without a change in the slope. Thus, TAA may be a useful research tool to connect regional mechanics and regional energetics in the left ventricle. Recent advances in technology have allowed noninvasive measurements of both segment strain by magnetic resonance imaging using a myocardial tagging technique [86] and regional VO_2 by positron emission tomography [87]. These new methods merit further studies to apply the TAA concept to a clinical setting.

Acknowledgments. Supported in part by a grant-in-aid for Scientific Research from the Ministry of Education, Science, and Culture (02670418), a Research Grant for Cardiovascular Diseases from the Ministry of Health and Welfare of Japan (1A-1), and grants from the Japan Cardiovascular Research Foundation and from the Nissan Science Foundation.

We thank all coauthors in our previous publications for their technical assistance and helpful discussion, which enabled this article to be completed. We also thank Tad W. Taylor for his helpful comments in the preparation of this manuscript.

References

1. Sechtem U, Sommerhoff BA, Markiewicz W, White RD, Cheitlin MD, Higgins CB (1987) Regional left ventricular wall thickening by magnetic resonance imaging: evaluation in normal persons and patients with global and regional dysfunction. Am J Cardiol 59:145–151
2. Herman MV, Heinle RA, Klein MD, Gorlin R (1967) Localized disorders in myocardial contraction. Asynergy and its role in congestive heart failure. N Engl J Med 277:222–232
3. Ross J Jr (1986) Assessment of ischemic regional myocardial dysfunction and its reversibility. Circulation 74:1186–1190
4. Suga H, Sagawa K (1974) Instantaneous pressure-volume relationships and their ratio in the excised, supported canine left ventricle. Circ Res 35:117–126
5. Sagawa K, Maughan L, Suga H, Sunagawa K (eds) (1988) Cardiac contraction and the pressure-volume relationship. Oxford University Press, New York
6. Suga H (1990) Ventricular energetics. Physiol Rev 70:247–277

7. Goto Y, Suga H, Yamada O, Igarashi Y, Saito M, Hiramori K (1986) Left ventricular regional work from wall tension-area loop in canine heart. Am J Physiol 250:H151–H158
8. Goto Y, Igarashi Y, Yasumura Y, Nozawa T, Futaki S, Hiramori K, Suga H (1988) Integrated regional work equals total left ventricular work in regionally ischemic canine heart. Am J Physiol 254:H894–H904
9. Theroux P, Franklin D, Ross J Jr, Kemper WS (1974) Regional myocardial function during acute coronary artery occlusion and its modification by pharmacologic agents in the dog. Circ Res 35:896–908
10. Kaseda S, Tomoike H, Ogata I, Nakamura M (1984) End-systolic pressure-length relations during changes in regional contractile state. Am J Physiol 247:H768–H774
11. Lew WYW, Chen Z, Guth B, Covell JW (1985) Mechanisms of augmented segment shortening in nonischemic areas during acute ischemia of the canine left ventricle. Circ Res 56:351–358
12. Goto Y, Slinker BK, LeWinter MM (1989) Nonhomogeneous left ventricular regional shortening during acute right ventricular pressure overload. Circ Res 65:43–54
13. Serruys PW, Brower RW, Ten Katen HJ (1981) Regional wall motion from radiopaque marker after intravenous and intracoronary injections of nifedipine. Circulation 63:584–591
14. Schnittger I, Fitzgerald PJ, Gordon EP, Alderman EL, Popp RL (1984) Computerized quantitative analysis of left ventricular wall motion by two-dimensional echocardiography. Circulation 70:242–254
15. Gelberg HJ, Brundage BH, Glantz S, Parmley WW (1979) Quantitative left ventricular wall motion analysis: a comparison of area, chord, and radial methods. Circulation 59:991–1000
16. Sasayama S, Nonogi H, Fujita M, Sakurai T, Wakabayashi A, Kawai C, Eiho S, Kuwahara M (1984) Analysis of asynchronous wall motion by regional pressure-length loops in patients with coronary artery disease. J Am Coll Cardiol 4:259–267
17. Klausner SC, Blair TJ, Bulawa WF, Jeppson GM, Jensen RL, Clayton PD (1982) Quantitative analysis of segmental wall motion throughout systole and diastole in the normal human left ventricle. Circulation 65:580–590
18. Force T, Bloomfield P, O'Boyle JE, Khuri SF, Josa M, Parisi AF (1984) Quantative two-dimensional echocardiographic analysis or regional wall motion in patients with perioperative myocardial infarction. Circulation 70:233–241
19. Ginzton LE, Conant R, Brizendine M, Thigpen T, Laks MM (1986) Quantitative analysis of segmental wall motion during maximal upright dynamic exercise: variability in normal adults. Circulation 73:268–275
20. Sasayama S, Franklin D, Ross J Jr, Kemper WS, McKown D (1976) Dynamic changes in left ventricular wall thickness and their use in analyzing cardiac function in the conscious dog. Am J Cardiol 38:870–879
21. Osakada G, Hess OM, Gallagher KP, Kemper WS, Ross J Jr (1983) End-systolic dimension-wall thickness relations during myocardial ischemia in conscious dogs. Am J Cardiol 51:1750–1758
22. Aversano T, Maughan WL, Hunter WC, Kass D, Becker L (1986) End-systolic measure of regional ventricular performance. Circulation 73:938–950
23. Pandian NG, Skorton DJ, Collins SM, Falsetti HL, Burke ER, Kerber RE (1983) Heterogeneity of left ventricular segmental wall thickening and excursion in 2-dimensional echocardiograms of normal human subjects. Am J Cardiol 51:1667–1673

24. O'Boyle JE, Parisi AF, Nieminen M, Kloner RA, Khuri S (1983) Quantitative detection of regional left ventricular contraction abnormalities by 2-dimensional echocardiography. Am J Cardiol 51:1732–1738
25. Mattery RF, Slutsky RA, Long SA, Higgins CB (1983) In vivo assessment of left ventricular wall and chamber dynamics during transient myocardial ischemia using prospectively ECG-gated computerized transmission tomography. Circulation 67: 1245–1251
26. Feiring AJ, Rumberberger JA, Reiter SJ, Collins SM, Skorton DJ, Rees M, Marcus ML (1988) Sectional and segmental variability of left ventricular function: experimental and clinical studies using ultrafast computed tomography. J Am Coll Cardiol 12:415–425
27. Fisher MR, von Schulthess GK, Higgins CB (1985) Multiphasic cardiac magnetic resonance imaging: normal regional left ventricular wall thickening. Am J Raentogenology 145:27–30
28. Isoyama S, Maruyama Y, Ashikawa K, Sato S, Suzuki, H, Watanabe J, Shimizu Y, Ino-Oka E, Takishima T (1983) Effects of afterload reduction on global left ventricular and regional myocardial functions in the isolated canine heart with stenosis of a coronary arterial branch. Circulation 67:139–147
29. Lew WYW, Ban-Hayashi E (1985) Mechanisms of improving regional and global ventricular function by preload alterations during acute ischemia in the canine left ventricle. Circulation 72:1125–1134
30. Gallagher KP, Osakada G, Hess OM, Koziol JA, Kemper WS, Ross J Jr (1982) Subepicardial segmental function during coronary stenosis and the role of myocardial fiber orientation. Circ Res 50:352-359
31. Freeman GL, LeWinter MM, Engler RL, Covell JW (1985) Relationship between myocardial fiber direction and segment shortening in the midwall of the canine left ventricle. Circ Res 56:31–39
32. Thomas CE (1957) The muscular architecture of the ventricles of hog and dog hearts. Am J Anat 101:17–58
33. Forrester JS, Tyberg JV, Wyatt HL, Goldner S, Parmley WW, Swan HJC (1974) Pressure-length loop: a new method for simultaneous measurement of segmental and total cardiac function. J Appl Physiol 37:771–775
34. Tyberg JV, Forrester JS, Wyatt JL, Goldner SJ, Parmley WW, Swan HJC (1974) An analysis of segmental ischemic dysfunction utilizing the pressure-length loop. Circulation 49:748–754
35. Glower DD, Spratt JA, Snow ND, Kabas JS, Davis JW, Olsen CO, Tyson GS, Sabiston DC Jr, Rankin JS (1985) Linearity of the Frank-Starling relationship in the intact heart: the concept of preload recruitable stroke work. Circulation 71: 994–1009
36. Crozatier B (1982) Relations between myocardial blood flow and postextrasystolic potentiation in epicardial and endocardial left ventricular regions early after coronary occlusion in dogs. Circulation 66:938–944
37. Streeter DD Jr, Spotnitz HM, Patel DP, Ross J Jr, Sonnenblick EH (1969) Fiber orientation in the canine left ventricle during diastole and systole. Circ Res 24: 339–347
38. Guth BD, Tajimi T, Seitelberger R, Lee J, Matsuzaki M, Ross J Jr (1986) Experimental exercise-induced ischemia: drug therapy can eliminate regional dysfunction and oxygen supply-demand imbalance. J Am Coll Cardiol 7:1036–1046
39. Gaasch WH, Bernard SA (1977) The effect of acute changes in coronary blood flow on left ventricular end-diastolic thickness: an echocardiographic study. Circulation 56:593–598

40. Vogel WM, Apstein CS, Briggs LL, Gaasch WH, Ahn J (1982) Acute alterations in left ventricular diastolic chamber stiffness. Circ Res 51:465–478
41. Goto Y, Hiramori K, Suga H (1987) Quantitative evaluation of left ventricular regional work from wall tension-regional area loop in canine heart. Jpn Circ J 51:114–119
42. Sugawara M, Tamiya K, Nakano K (1985) Regional work of the ventricle. Wall tension-area relation. Heart Vessels 1:133–144
43. Nakano K, Sugawara M, Kato T, Sasayama S, Carabello BA, Asanoi H, Umemura J, Koyanagi H (1988) Regional work of the human left ventricle calculated by wall stress and the natural logarithm of reciprocal of wall thickness. J Am Coll Cardiol 12:1442–1448
44. Maruyama Y, Ashikawa K, Isoyama S, Satoh S, Suzuki H, Watanabe J, Shimizu Y, Ino-oka E, Takishima T (1984) Pressure-length loop in the ischemic segment during left circumflex coronary artery stenosis and its modification by afterload reducing in excised perfused canine hearts. Basic Res Cardiol 79:155–163
45. Yun KL, Fann JI, Rayhill SC, Nasserbakht F, Derby GC, Handen CE, Bolger AF, Miller DC (1990) Importance of the mitral subvalvular apparatus for left ventricular segmental systolic mechanics. Circulation 82(Suppl.4):IV-89–IV-104
46. Sagawa K (1967) Analysis of the ventricular pumping capacity as a function of input and output pressure loads. In: Reeve EB, Guyton AC (eds) Physical bases of circulatory transport: regulation and exchange. Saunders, Philadelphia, pp 141–149
47. Liedtke AJ, Nellis St H, Fultz CW, Dietz M (1983) Application of an end-systolic pressure-segment length relationship for measuring regional contractility. Basic Res Cardiol 78:384–395
48. Kaseda S, Tomoike H, Ogata I, Nakamura M (1985) End-systolic pressure-volume, pressure-length, and stress-strain relations in canine hearts. Am J Physiol 249: H648–H654
49. Lew WYW (1988) Time-dependent increase in left ventricular contractility following acute volume loading in the dog. Circ Res 63:635–647
50. Schipke JD, Alexander J Jr, Harasawa Y, Schulz R, Burkhoff D (1988) Interrelation between end-systolic pressure-volume and pressure-wall thickness relations. Am J Physiol 255:H679–H684
51. Funai JT, Thames MD (1988) Isochronal behavior in left ventricular systolic pressure-wall thickness relations. Am J Physiol 255:H1136–H1143
52. Goto Y, Igarashi Y, Yamada O, Hiramori K, Suga H (1988) Hyperkinesis without the Frank-Starling mechanism in a nonischemic region of acutely ischemic excised canine heart. Circulation 77:468–477
53. Goto Y, Futaki S, Ohgoshi Y, Yaku H, Kawaguchi O, Suga H (1990) Assessment of left ventricular regional work under ischemia. Front Med Biol Eng 2:201–205
54. Nakano K, Sugawara M, Ishihara K, Kanazawa S, Corin WJ, Denslow S, Biederman RWW, Carabello BA (1990) Myocardial stiffness derived from end-systolic wall stress and logarithm of reciprocal of wall thickness. Circulation 82: 1352–1361
55. Slinker BK, Glantz SA (1985) The accuracy of inferring left ventricular volume from dimension depends on the frequency of information needed to answer a given question. Circ Res 56:161–174
56. Sunagawa K, Maughan WL, Sagawa K (1983) Effect of regional ischemia on the left ventricular end-systolic pressure-volume relationship of isolated canine hearts. Circ Res 52:170–178

57. Aversano T, Maughan WL, Sunagawa K, Becher LC (1988) Effect of afterload resistance on end-systolic pressure-thickness relationship. Am J Physiol 254: H658–H663
58. Janz RF (1982) Estimation of local myocardial stress. Am J Physiol 242: H875–H881
59. Pouleur H, Rousseau MF, Van Eyll C, Charlier AA (1984) Assessment of regional left ventricular relaxation in patients with coronary artery disease: importance of geometric factors and changes in wall thickness. Circulation 69:696–702
60. Wong AYK, Rautaharju PM (1968) Stress distribution within the left ventricular wall approximated as a thick ellipsoidal shell. Am Heart J 75:649–662
61. Ghista DN, Sandler H (1969) An analytic elastic-viscoelastic model for the shape and the forces in the left ventricle. J Biomech 2:35–47
62. Mirsky I (1969) Left ventricular stresses in the intact human heart. Biophys J 9:189–208
63. Huisman RM, Sipkema P, Westerhof N, Elzinga G (1980) Comparison of models used to calculate left ventricular wall force. Med Biol Eng Comput 18:133–144
64. Suga H, Goto Y, Yamada O, Igarashi Y (1984) Is regional ventricular wall work determined from regional force and shortening always consistent with the law of conservation of energy? Jpn Circ J 48:1007–1016
65. Suga H, Hisano R, Hirata S, Hayashi T, Yamada O, Ninomiya I (1983) Heart rate-independent energetics and systolic pressure-volume area in dog heart. Am J Physiol 244:H206–H214
66. Suga H, Sagawa K, Shoukas AA (1973) Load independence of the instantaneous pressure-volume ratio of the canine left ventricle and effects of epinephrine and heart rate on the ratio. Circ Res 32:314–322
67. Goto Y, Ohgoshi Y, Yaku H, Kawaguchi O, Futaki S, Hata K, Takasago T, Suga H (1990) Linear relation between regional oxygen consumption and "tension-area" area reflects regional changes in myocardial contractility (abstract). Circulation 82:III–565
68. Goto Y, Yamada O, Igarashi Y, Suga H, Hiramori H, Saito M, Haze K, Sumiyoshi T, Fukami K (1985) Different effects of global and regional ischemia on left ventricular regional function. An analysis by wall tension-area relation (abstract). Jpn Circ J 49:863
69. Nakano J (1966) Effect of changes in coronary arterial blood flow on the myocardial contractile force. Jpn Heart J 7:78–86
70. Katz LN, Feinberg H (1958) The relation of cardiac effort to myocardial oxygen consumption and coronary flow. Circ Res 6:656–669
71. Weber KT, Janicki JS (1977) Myocardial oxygen consumption: the role of wall force and shortening. Am J Physiol 233:H421–H430
72. Sarnoff SJ, Braunwald E, Welch GH Jr, Case RB, Stainsby WN, Macruz R (1958) Hemodynamic determinants of oxygen consumption of the heart with special reference to the tension-time index. Am J Physiol 192:148–156
73. McDonald RH Jr (1966) Developed tension: a major determinant of myocardial oxygen consumption. Am J Physiol 210:351–356
74. Rooke GA, Feigl EO (1982) Work as a correlate of canine left ventricular oxygen consumption, and the problem of catecholamine oxygen wasting. Circ Res 50: 273–286
75. Weintraub WS, Hattori S, Agarwal JB, Bodenheimer MM, Banka VS, Helfant RH (1981) The relationship between myocardial blood flow and contraction by myocardial layer in the canine left ventricle during ischemia. Circ Res 48:430–438

76. Gayheart PA, Vinten-Johansen J, Johnston WE, Hester TO, Cordell AR (1989) Oxygen requirements of the dyskinetic myocardial segment. Am J Physiol 257: H1184–H1191
77. Gallagher KP, Matsuzaki M, Osakada G, Kemper WS, Ross J Jr (1983) Effect of exercise on the relationship between myocardial blood flow and systolic wall thickening in dogs with acute coronary stenosis. Circ Res 52:716–729
78. Forrester JS, Wyatt HL, Da Luz PL, Tyberg JV, Diamond GA, Swan HJC (1976) Functional significance of regional ischemic contraction abnormalities. Circulation 54:64–70
79. Suga H, Hisano R, Goto Y, Yamada O, Igarashi Y (1983) Effect of positive inotropic agents on the relation between oxygen consumption and systolic pressure volume area in canine left ventricle. Circ Res 53:306–318
80. Goto Y, Futaki S, Ohgoshi Y, Yaku H, Suga H (1989) A new measure of left ventricular regional oxygen consumption: systolic "tension-area" area (abstract). Circulation 80:II–154
81. Hisano R, Cooper G IV (1987) Correlation of force-length area with oxygen consumption in ferret papillary muscle. Circ Res 61:318–328
82. Edwards CH II, Rankin JS, McHale PA, Ling D, Anderson RW (1981) Effects of ischemia on left ventricular regional function in the conscious dog. Am J Physiol 240:H413–420
83. Lew WYW, LeWinter MM (1986) Regional comparison of midwall segment and area shortening in the canine left ventricle. Circ Res 58:678–691
84. Goto Y, Slinker BK, LeWinter MM (1988) Similar normalized E_{max} and O_2 consumption-pressure-volume area relation in rabbit and dog. Am J Physiol 255: H366–H374
85. Goto Y, Slinker BK, LeWinter MM (1990) Decreased contractile efficiency and increased nonmechanical energy cost in hyperthyroid rabbit heart. Relation between O_2 consumption and systolic pressure-volume area or force-time integral. Circ Res 66:999–1011
86. Buchalter MB, Weiss JL, Rogers WJ, Zerhouni EA, Weisfeldt ML, Beyar R, Shapiro EP (1990) Noninvasive quantification of left ventricular rotational deformation in normal humans using magnetic resonance imaging myocardial tagging. Circulation 81:1236–1244
87. Armbrecht JJ, Buxton DB, Brunken RC, Phelps ME, Schelbert HR (1989) Regional myocardial oxygen consumption determined noninvasively in humans with [1-^{11}C]acetate and dynamic positron tomography. Circulation 80:863–872

6

Myocardial Energetics of Hypertrophied Heart of Spontaneously Hypertensive Rat and Stroke-Prone Spontaneously Hypertensive Rat

KEIJIRO KUSUNOKI[1], YASUYUKI NAKAMURA[2], TAKASHI KONISHI[1], MASATO MATSUNAGA[3], CHUICHI KAWAI[1]

Summary. Left ventricular mechanical efficiency was examined in isolated working hearts of 7-month-old spontaneous hypertensive rats (SHR), stroke prone SHR (SHR-SP), and control Wistar-Kyoto rats (WKY). The heart was perfused with Krebs solution at 37°C and at three different afterloads (70 mmHg for WKY, 90 mmHg for SHR and 110 mmHg for SHR-SP) in order to maintain constant coronary perfusion per gram of the myocardium. Oxygen pressure was measured at the left atrium and the right ventricle which received coronary sinus flow. Mechanical efficiency was calculated as minute stroke work (Joules) divided by energy production by O_2 (Joules). Energy utilization was impaired in SHR and SHR-SP (WKY, 27 ± 6.9%; and SHR, 14 ± 3.8%, $P < 0.01$; SHR-SP, 13 ± 6.7%, $P < 0.01$, in comparison with control value) when the myocardial perfusion showed no significant difference. Therefore, the energy utilization in SHR and SHR-SP was impaired even when the coronary perfusion was sufficient. Our findings may contradict demonstrations of a shift in heavy chain myosin isozymes in hypertrophied small animal hearts, but may suggest that more drastic changes in the myocardium, which are disadvantageous to the myothermal economy, are present in the hypertrophied heart.

Key words: Energy utilization — SHR — SHR-SP — Hypertrophy

Introduction

What kind of mechanisms are responsible for the transition of a hypertrophied heart from the initial compensated phase to ultimate failure? This has been one of the classical questions in cardiology, and it still fascinates many investigators

[1]Third Division, Department of Internal Medicine, Faculty of Medicine, Kyoto University, Kyoto, Japan
[2]First Department of Medicine, Shiga University of Medical Science, Shiga, 520-21 Japan
[3]College of Medical Technology, Kyoto University, Kyoto, Japan

today. The study of hypertrophied heart energy efficiency in animal models may allow this question to be solved. Several investigations have been performed from this standpoint, but not all the results agree. One of the classic works was done by Gunning and Coleman [1], who described a relationship between paradoxically increased myocardial oxygen consumption and depressed contractility in pressure-hypertrophied myocardium, that is, the energy efficiency of the hypertrophied heart was found to be reduced. Cooper et al. [2] related this unusual finding to an altered myocardial calcium metabolism and mitochondrial calcium metabolism in pressure-induced hypertrophy. In contrast, Alpert and Mulieri [3] recently showed increased myothermal economy of isometric force generation in compensated hypertrophy induced by pulmonary artery constriction in the rabbit. Their findings may well link with the results of a study by Lompre et al. [4] that showed myosin isozyme redistribution and dominance of a myosin isoenzyme of a lower ATPase activity in chronic heart overload. The discrepancy of the results of the previous studies may stem from the difference in the model of hypertrophy used and the stage of hypertrophy in the hearts studied. Furthermore, relative ischemia, which has long been postulated to play a role in cardiac hypertrophy, may be one of the mechanisms causing depressed energy efficiency in some studies.

In this chapter, we will present the results of our recent study on energy utilization of the hypertrophied heart in spontaneously hypertensive rats (SHR) and stroke-prone spontaneously hypertensive rats (SHR-SP). These models of cardiac hypertrophy have never been used before in these kind of studies. A working rat heart system where coronary perfusion pressure is controlled was used in order to avoid relative ischemia in hypertrophy that can complicate interpretation of the results.

Models of Cardiac Hypertrophy

Experimental pressure-overloaded hypertrophy can be induced in animals by several methods: banding of the pulmonary artery [1–3, 5] or aorta [6–8], and induction of renal [9] or other hypertension. The SHR was developed by Okamoto and Aoki by repeated mating of Wistar strain rats with hypertension [10]. It provides a model for longitudinal studies of the natural progression of left ventricular hypertrophy and its function produced by a pressure overload [11–13]. Stroke-prone SHR is a sub-type of SHR that shows higher blood pressure and is prone to cerebral bleeding [14]. In the present study of myocardial energy efficiency, we used these two types of SHR rats and control Wistar-Kyoto rats (WYK), all 26–30 weeks old, with nine rats in each group. Figure 1 shows the body weight, left ventricular (LV) weight and right ventricular weight of these rats. The SHR and SHR-SP body weight is smaller than that of WKY, and the SHR and SHR-SP LV weight is heavier. Although the LV weight in SHR is not significantly different from that of WKY, the ratio LV weight/body weight in SHR is higher than that of WKY. The LV weight of

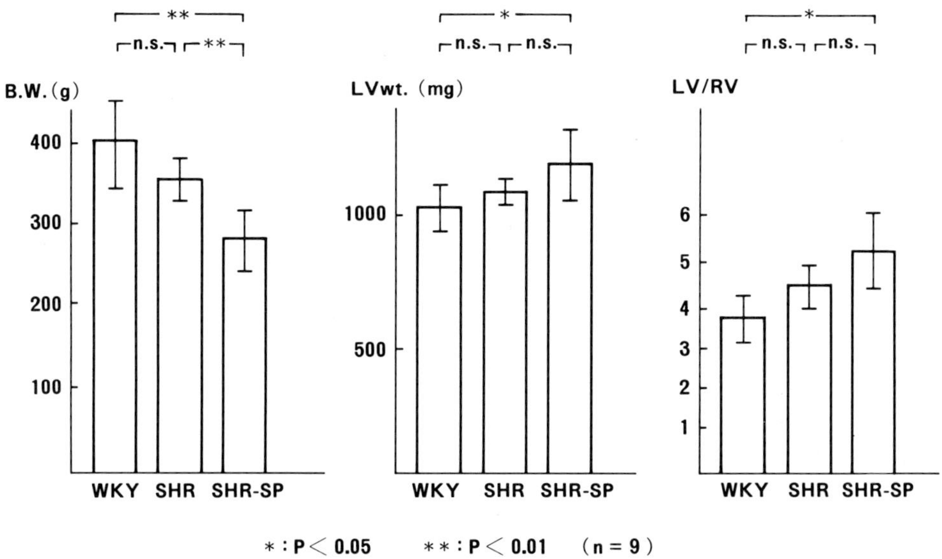

Fig. 1. Body weight, LV weight and LV/RV ratio of *WKY*, *SHR* and *SHR-SP*

SHR-SP itself without normalization by the body weight is heavier than that of WKY, indicating the degree of hypertrophy is more marked in SHR-SP.

1. Body weight (g) a) WKY, 401 ± 60 b) SHR, 362 ± 24 c) SHR-SP, 276 ± 36
2. Left ventricular weight (mg) a) WKY, 1054 ± 194 b) SHR, 1193 ± 49 c) SHR-SP, 1280 ± 250
3. LV/RV ratio a) WKY, 3.66 ± 0.75 b) SHR, 4.36 ± 0.64 c) SHR-SP, 5.18 ± 1.04

All the rats appeared well at the time of killing. One way to objectively describe whether rats are in heart failure or not is to measure the water content of tissues such as the lung and the liver. The wet weight of small tissue samples were measured after light blotting. The samples were placed in an incubator at 65°C for two days, and the dry weights were measured. These rats were not in overt heart failure as no significant differences were found among the groups:

1. Liver a) WKY, 32.8 ± 2.4 b) SHR, 33.7 ± 1.5 c) SHR-SP, 33.1 ± 1.1
2. Lung a) WKY, 22.3 ± 1.2 b) SHR, 20.9 ± 2.2 c) SHR-SP, 21.5 ± 2.4

Isolated Working Rat Heart Preparation

A technique for the preparation of isolated working rat hearts was originally developed by Neely et al. [15] to study function and metabolism, especially during ischemia. The Langendorf technique has also been used for the study of heart function and metabolism during ischemia and the other conditions. However, hearts prepared by Neely's technique eject perfusate, whereas hearts

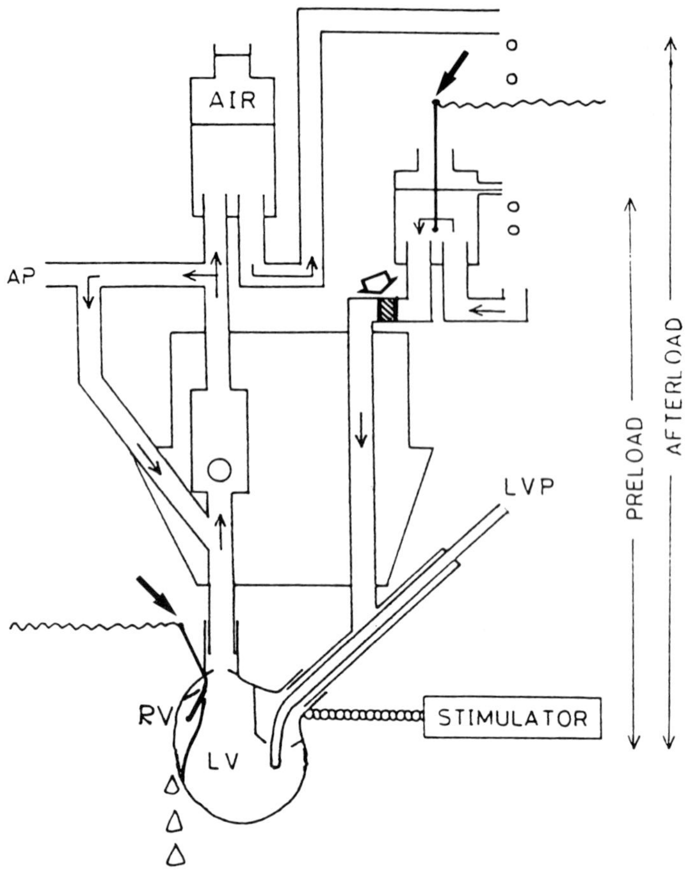

Fig. 2. Perfusion apparatus. Left ventricular pressure was monitored by a high fidelity tip manometer, which was threaded through the left atrial cannula. An oxygen pressure meter was placed in the chamber connected to the left atrium (LA) and the right ventricle (RV). Coronary flow was measured by collecting the fluid from the coronary sinus. The flow rate entering the left atrium was measure by an electromagnetic flow meter in order to obtain the stroke volume of the heart.

Thick arrows, probes of oxygen pressure meter; *white arrow*, probe of electromagnetic flow meter; *AP*, aortic pressure; *LVP*, left ventricular pressure; *LV*, left ventricle; *RV*, right ventricle

prepared by Langendorf's technique merely contract isovolumically. Hearts prepared by Neely's technique therefore have a more natural physiology, and the preload and afterload can be controlled at will. However, in the original Neely's isolated working rat heart system, only the aortic pressure is measured, and a precise evaluation of heart function cannot be made. Thus, we developed a modified system [16] in order to measure LV pressure and to allow electrocardiogram recordings. In the present study, we modified the system further to enable measurement of LV pressure, stroke work and oxygen consumption as described below and in Fig. 2.

Preparation of the Heart Using a Modified Version of Neely's Technique

Heparin (400 units) was injected intraperitoneally 30 min before the rats were decapitated and their hearts quickly excised. Cardiac arrest was induced by placing the organ in a beaker of iced Krebs-Henseleit solution. The isolated heart was attached by ligatures to an aortic cannula, and immediately supported by retrograde perfusion (as in Langendorf's technique) from a reservoir 70 cm above the heart. Continued support of the heart was provided until another cannula was inserted into the left atrium. The working rat heart system was then initiated by switching to the antegrade recirculating apparatus, as described by Neely et al. [15]. The atrial bubble trap was 14 cm above the left atrium throughout the experiment. LV contractions pumped fluid into the pressure chamber and out through the aortic outflow tube to the top of the oxygenation chamber above the heart. The coronary flow per gram of myocardium in the groups were made equal by varying the height of the chamber, so that there were three different afterloads depending on the strain of the rat: 70 mmHg for WKY, 90 mmHg for SHR and 110 mmHg for SHR-SP.

Left ventricular pressure was monitored by a high fidelity tip manometer, which was threaded through the left atrial cannula (Fig. 2). An oxygen pressure meter (M.T. Giken, Type POG-5000) was placed in the chamber and connected to the left atrium (LA) and the right ventricle (RV) (Fig. 2). Coronary flow was measured by collecting the fluid from the coronary sinus. The rate of flow into the left atrium was measured by an electromagnetic flow meter (Nihon Koden Inc.) in order to obtain the stroke volume of the heart (Fig. 2). The left ventricular pressure, aortic pressure, left atrial pressure, stroke volume and electrocardiogram were recorded on a recorder (Hewlett Packard, model 7758A) via transducers (Hewlett Packard, model 8826A) and amplifiers (Hewlett Packard, model 14060H, 14060K, 8811A). Electrocardiographic monitoring was carried out via bipolar electrodes inserted in the right ventricular free wall and the aortic cannula. Recordings were made intermittently at a paper speed of 100 mm/s.

The perfusate was Krebs-Henseleit solution (pH 7.4 at 37°C) containing NaCl, 118 mmol/l; KCl, 4.7 mmol/l; KH_2PO_4, 1.20 mmol/l; $CaCl_2$, 2.5 mmol/l; $MgSO_4$, 1.20 mmol/l; $NaHCO_3$, 25.50 mmol/l; glucose, 11.1 mmol/l. The solution was kept at 37°C, and a gas mixture of 95% O_2 and 5% CO_2 was bubbled through for oxygenation.

Coronary Flow, Work and Energy Efficiency

As stated above, the aortic pressure or the coronary perfusion pressure was set depending on the strain of the rats so that the coronary flow per gram of the myocardium of each strain was the same. The coronary sinus flow (ml/min per gram myocardium), shown in Fig. 3, showed no significant differences between the groups: WKY, 15.5 ± 3.3; SHR, 15.8 ± 3.6; SHR-SP, 17.1 ± 3.2 ml/min per gram.

The minute stroke work, calculated from the stroke volume and the mean left ventricular pressure during ejection, is shown in Fig. 4. There were no significant differences between the groups: WKY, 2.34 ± 0.60; SHR, 1.85 ± 0.33; SHR-SP, 2.27 ± 0.64 ml·mmHg/min.

The oxygen pressure of inflow fluid and coronary sinus were then measured to estimate the difference between them. We calculated oxygen consumption (g/min) from the oxygen difference and the coronary sinus flow, and the results are shown in Fig. 5. The oxygen consumption of the heart in SHR-SP was significantly higher than that in SHR and in WKY: WKY, 0.90 ± 0.36; SHR, 1.25 ± 0.21; SHR-SP, 1.98 ± 0.85 g/min.

The mechanical efficiencies of hearts (%) were calculated by the work (expressed in Joules) divided by energy consumption (expressed in Joules), and they are shown in Fig. 6: WKY, 27 ± 6.9; SHR, 14 ± 3.8; SHR-SP, 13 ± 6.7. The mechanical efficiency of SHR and of SHR-SP were lower than that of WKY despite the almost equal coronary flow per gram of myocardium.

The Reduced Energy Efficiency Mechanism of Pressure-Induced Hypertrophy

Abnormal cardiac function, myocardial energetics and metabolism in the hypertrophied heart that have been reported previously may be secondary to reduced coronary circulation or coronary reserve. Linzbach [17] postulated that heart failure in hypertrophy is caused by relative ischemia due to capillary growth that is not proportional to hypertrophy of the muscle fiber. Henquell et al. [18] measured intercapillary distance in hypertrophied rat hearts beating in situ, and found that the capillary reserve in hypertrophy was fully utilized and the mean functional intercapillary distance was greater than normal. They thought this was responsible for the focal necrosis and fibrosis observed in hypertrophy and for the development of circulatory failure. The observation in seven-month-old SHRs, almost the same age as the rats we studied, by Tomanek et al. [19] agree with previous studies in different models of hypertrophy. However, they found that capillary growth during stabilized hypertrophy in older SHRs was sufficient to reverse the decrement in capillary surface area, capillary density and the increase in minimal intercapillary distance observed in the earlier stage.

Reduced coronary reserve in hypertrophy is not only one of the mechanisms responsible for heart failure, but it can also cause some changes in the results of ex vivo studies, such as in isolated heart muscle studies. For instance, the average cross-sectional area of hypertrophied cardiac muscles whose energetics was studied by Cooper et al. in a diffusion bath was more than twice than that of the control muscles [2]. The observed change in energetics in cardiac hypertrophy may have been influenced by relative hypoxia due to limited oxygen diffusion in the thick muscles. In the present study, however, the myocardial perfusion in hypertrophy was adjusted to the almost same level as the controls, and therefore, we can rule out this possibility.

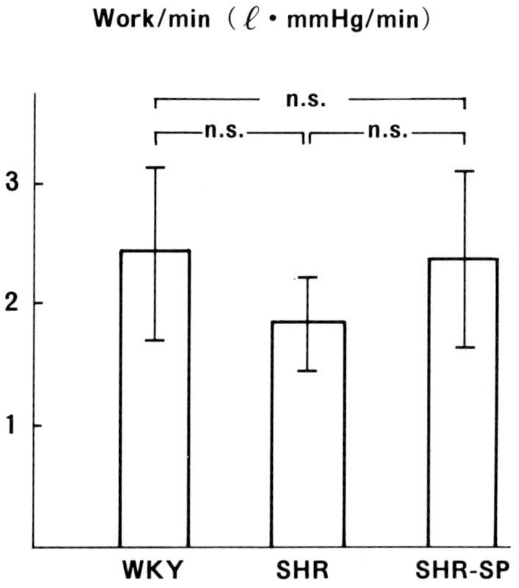

(n = 9)

Fig. 3. Work per minute of *WKY*, *SHR* and *SHR-SP*. Coronary sinus flow (ml/min per gram myocardium) of each groups. There were no significant differences between the groups

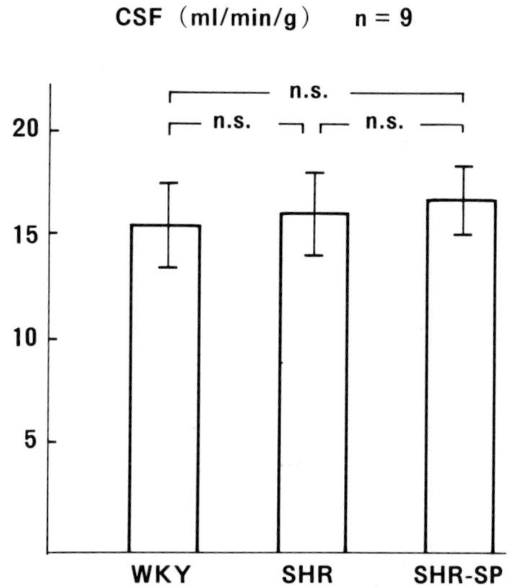

Fig. 4. Coronary sinus flow (*CSF*) of *WKY*, *SHR* and *SHR-SP*. The minute stroke work was calculated from the stroke volume obtained by the electromagnetic flow meter and the mean left ventricular pressure during ejection. There were no significant differences between the groups

Even after exclusion of the ischemic factor, our results agree with those of Cooper et al. [2], but contradict those of Alpert et al. [20]. In small animals, hypertrophy, whether due to a pressure overload or a volume overload, can cause a shift of heavy chain myosin isozymes, with an isozyme of a lower ATPase activity (V_3 type) predominating. This shift has been paralleled with a decrease in maximal speed of muscle shortening (V_{max}) and an increase in myothermal economy. A similar change has been reported in hypothyroid rat myocardium [20].

The fact that there is an overall reduction in myocardial energy efficiency in the hypertrophied heart, despite the possibly beneficial energy conservative changes in myosin isoenzymes, suggests that more drastic changes in the myocardium that are disadvantageous to myothermal economy are present in the hypertrophied heart. The altered myocardial and mitochondrial calcium metabolism may be one of the factors [2]. Another important change known to take place in the hypertrophied heart is depression of calcium uptake and calcium ATPase of the sarcoplasmic reticulum (SR) [21–22]. Recently, Komuro et al. found that the mRNA levels of calcium ATPase in the SR of pressure-overloaded hearts were decreased and that the expression of cardiac calcium-ATPase in SR is regulated by pressure overload [23]. This change in

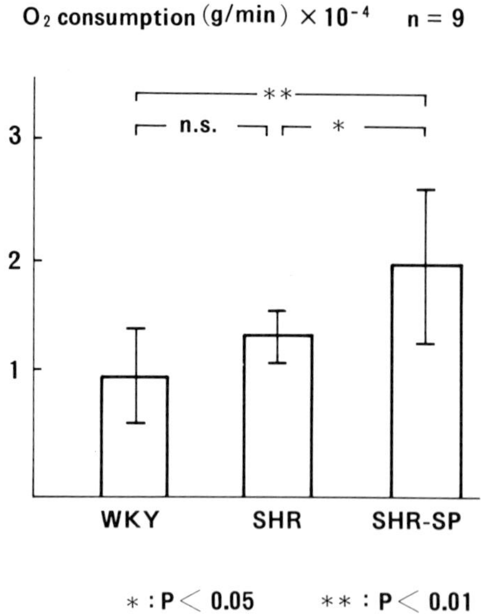

Fig. 5. O_2 consumption of *WKY*, *SHR* and *SHR-SP*. The oxygen consumption of the heart in SHR-SP was significantly higher than that in SHR and in WKY

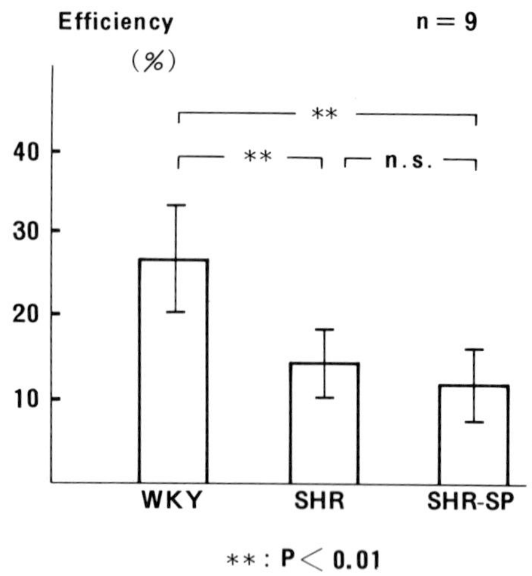

Fig. 6. Efficiency of external mechanical work of WKY, SHR and SHR-SP. We can calculate the mechanical efficiencies of hearts (%) by the work (expressed in Joules) divided by energy consumption (expressed in Joules). The mechanical efficiencies of *SHR* and of *SHR-SP* were lower than that of *WKY* in spite of the almost equal coronary flow per gram of myocardium

SR calcium ATPase may not only be responsible for the impaired relaxation in hypertrophy, but it also may cause greater accumulation of calcium in the mitochondria, and hence impairment of mitochondrial respiratory function and abnormal energetics in cardiac hypertrophy.

The reduced energy efficiency in the hypertrophied myocardium, independent of the diminished coronary reserve, may work against the compensation mechanisms and may play a role in the transition from compensation to ultimate failure in hypertrophy.

Acknowledgments. We are grateful to Drs. Kazuya Ogawa and Akihiko Tei, Kyoto University, for their technical assistance.

References

1. Gunning JF, Coleman HN (1973) Myocardial oxygen consumption during experimental hypertrophy and congestive heart failure. J Moll Cell Cardiol 5:25–38
2. Cooper G IV, Satava RM Jr, Harrison CE, Coleman HN III (1973) Mechanism for the abnormal energetics of pressure-induced hypertrophy of cat myocardium. Circ Res 33:213–223

3. Alpert NR, Mulieri LA (1982) Increased myothermal economy of isometric force generation in compensated cardiac hypertrophy induced by pulmonary artery constriction in the rabbit. A characterization of heat liberation in normal and hypertrophied right ventricular papillary muscles. Circ Res 50:491–500
4. Lompre AM, Schwartz K, d'Albis A, Lacombe G, Thiem NV, Swynghedauw B (1979) Myosin isozyme redistribution in chronic heart overload. Nature 282: 105–107
5. Spann JF Jr, Buccino RA, Sonnenblick EH, Braunwald E (1967) Contractile state of cardiac muscle obtained from cats with experimentally produced ventricular hypertrophy and heart failure. Circ Res 21:341–354
6. Bing OHL, Matsushita S, Fanburg BL, Levine HJ (1971) Mechanical properties of rat cardiac muscle during experimental hypertrophy. Circ Res 28:234–245
7. Sasayama S, Ross J Jr, Franklin D, Bloor CM, Bishop S, Dilley RB (1976) Adaptation of the left ventricle to chronic pressure overload. Circ Res 38:172–178
8. Gaasch WH, Zile MR, Hoshino PK, Apstein CS, Blaustein AS (1989) Stress-shortening relations and myocardial blood flow in compensated and failing canine hearts with pressure-overloaded hypertrophy. Circulation 79:872–883
9. Morioka S, Simon G (1982) Echocardiographic evidence for early left ventricular hypertrophy in dogs with renal hypertension. Am J Cardiol 49:1891–1898
10. Okamoto K, Aoki K (1963) Development of a strain of spontaneously hypertensive rats. Jpn Circ J 27: 282–293
11. Pfeffer MA, Pfeffer JM, Frohlich ED (1976) Pumping ability of the hypertrophying left ventricle of the spontaneously hypertensive rat. Circ Res 38:423–429
12. Bing OHL, Sen S, Conrad CH, Brooks WW (1984) Myocardial function structure and collagen in the spontaneously hypertensive rat: progression from compensated hypertrophy to haemodynamic impairment. Eur Heart J 5(Suppl F):43–52
13. Nakamura Y, Bing OHL, Wiegner AW, Konishi T, Apstein CS, Pfeffer MA, Kawai C (1986) Effects of hypertrophy and allylamine-induced fibrosis on mechanical properties of isolated rat heart muscles with references to the pumping function of the intact heart in the same models. Jpn Circ J 50:998–1006
14. Saito N, Matsunaga M, Hara A, Yamamota J, Yamori Y, Mukaino S, Ogino K, Kawai C (1975) Hypertensive vascular lesions and renin or lysosomal enzymes in rats. Jpn Circ J 39:551–558
15. Neely JR, Rovetto MJ, Whitmer JT, Morgan ME (1973) Effects of ischemia on function and metabolism of the isolated working rat heart. Am J Physiol 225: 651–658
16. Konishi T, Nakamura Y, Konishi T, Kawai C (1984) Accentuated negative inotropism of verapamil after ischemic intervention in isolated working rat heart. Cardiovasc Res 18:639–644
17. Linzbach AJ (1960) Heart failure from the point of view of quantitative anatomy. Am J Cardiol 5:370–382
18. Henquell L, Odoroff CL, Honig CR (1976) Intercapillary distance and capillary reserve in hypertrophied rat hearts beating in situ. Circ Res 41:400–408
19. Tomanek RJ, Searls JC, Lachenbruch PA (1982) Quantitative changes in the capillary bed during developing, peak, and stabilized cardiac hypertrophy in the spontaneously hypertensive rat. Circ Res 51:295–304
20. Holubarsch Ch, Goulette RP, Litten RZ, Martin BJ, Mulieri LA, Alpert NR (1985) The economy of isometric force development, myosin isoenzyme pattern and myofibrillar ATPase activity in normal and hypothyroid rat myocardium. Circ Res 56:78–86

21. Sordahl LA, McCollum WB, Wood WG, Schwartz A (1973) Mitochondria and sarcoplasmic reticulum function in cardiac hypertrophy and failure. Am J Physiol 224:497–502
22. Ito Y, Suko J, Chidsey CA (1974) Intracellular calcium and myocardial contractility. V. Calcium uptake of sarcoplasmic reticulum fractions in hypertrophied and failing rabbit hearts. J Mol Cell Cardiol 6:237–247
23. Komuro I, Kurabayashi M, Shibazaki Y, Takaku F, Yazaki Y (1989) Molecular cloning and characterization of a Ca^{2+} + Mg^{2+}-dependent adenosine triphophatase from rat cardiac sarcoplasmic reticulum. Regulation of its expression by pressure overload and developmental stage. J Clin Invest 83:1102–1108

7
Optimal Left Ventricle Versus Optimal Afterload

Kenji Sunagawa[1], Kiyoshi Hayashida[1], Masaru Sugimachi[1], Koji Todaka[1], Toru Kubota[1], Ryoichi Itaya[1], Chishaki Akiko[1], Akira Takeshita[1]

Summary. We investigated whether ventricular-arterial coupling is energetically optimized in animals when it is to be regulated. We evaluated the optimality of energy usage of ventricular-arterial coupling from the view point of the arterial system (i.e., afterload) and that of the heart (i.e., left ventricle). We defined the optimal afterload as the afterload which extracts maximum external work from a given heart under a fixed preload. We defined the optimal heart as the heart which requires minimum oxygen to support a fixed peripheral demand. A series of experiments demonstrated that external work of the left ventricle of dogs at rest was nearly maximum, external work remained nearly maximum during exercise and volume changes, in spite of tremendous changes in hemodynamics, and conversion efficiency of metabolic energy to generate cardiac output to meet peripheral demand was not compromised as long as the heart was capable of responding to the command of the regulatory system. Once the heart failed to respond normally to the regulatory system, however, the optimality of ventricular-arterial coupling as defined above was no longer maintained.

Key words: End-systolic pressure-volume relationship — Optimal afterload — Optimal heart — Ventricular-arterial coupling

Introduction

For any animals, adequate perfusion by the cardiovascular system of peripheral tissues is vital to maintain normal physiological activity. Since a given level of cardiac output can be achieved by various combinations of cardiac function and loading conditions, the animal must choose a unique combination of them on

[1] Research Institute of Angiocardiology and Cardiovascular Clinic, Kyushu University Medical School, Higashiku, Fukuoka, 812 Japan

the basis of some natural principle. If an animal is required to increase cardiac output, a new, unique combination of these parameters will be chosen. This consideration leads us to a fundamental question; what is the natural principle in adjusting the cardiovascular parameters which determines cardiac output?

The heart continues to eject blood to the peripheral tissues without interruption as long as animals are alive. This unavoidably makes the energy requirement of the heart enormous. Furthermore, since cardiac muscle per se is a biological converter of energy from a metabolic form to a mechanical form, it is conceivable that efficient usage of energy would be one of nature's major concerns when the heart pumps blood. As a matter of fact, the mean stroke power output of the isolated feline left or right ventricle was found to be maximum when the ventricle was loaded with normal arterial impedance [1–3]. This was also the case in the open chest cat [4–6]. In the canine left heart, external work was expected to be nearly maximum under normal loading conditions [7, 8]. This was also experimentally demonstrated [9–12]. Although all these studies indicated that the energy output of the ventricle is fairly maximized under normal conditions, it is not clear whether this is an intended outcome or not. It is also not clear how efficiently energy is converted from the metabolic to mechanical form.

To answer these questions, we investigated what parameters of ventricular-arterial coupling are optimized in animals when the ventricular-arterial system is to be regulated. We imposed four different stresses on animals and observed responses with a special reference to energy usage optimization of ventricular-arterial coupling. Those stresses included exercise, volume changes, left ventricular dysfunction and activation of baroreflex. Some of them are very common in the process of evolution, and thus the animals may well be able to adjust themselves against these stresses.

We evaluated the optimality of energy usage of ventricular-arterial coupling from the view point of the arterial system (i.e., afterload) and that of the heart (i.e., left ventricle). We defined the optimal afterload as the afterload which extracts maximum external work from a given heart [13–16]. We defined the optimal heart as the heart which requires minimum oxygen (i.e., minimum metabolic energy) to meet a peripheral demand [13, 15]. The derivation of these indices requires the concept of the end-systolic pressure-volume relationship, the framework of ventricular-arterial coupling and the relationship of the pressure-volume area vs. myocardial oxygen consumption. In the following sections, we briefly introduce the current background knowledge, and then formulate optimality indices, as outlined above. Finally, we introduce experimental results, some of which are still preliminary, and discuss their implications.

Ventricular-arterial Coupling

Characterization of the Ventricle

The end-systolic pressure-volume relationship (ESPVR) has been known to be reasonably linear and relatively insensitive to changes in loading conditions

[17–20]. The slope of the ESPVR represents end-systolic volume elastance (E_{es}), which is the elastic properties of the end-systolic ventricle, and indicates the inotropic state. Using this concept, end-systolic pressure (P_{es}) is expressed as

$$P_{es} = E_{es}(V_{es} - V_o) \tag{1}$$

where V_{es} is end-systolic volume and V_o is the volume-axis intercept of ESPVR. Using stroke volume (SV) and end-diastolic volume (V_{ed}), Eq. (1) can be rewritten as

$$P_{es} = E_{es}(V_{ed} - SV - V_o) \tag{2}$$

Therefore, for a given V_{ed}, P_{es} varies inversely and linearly with changes in stroke volume (P_{es}-SV relationship) (left of Fig. 1).

Characterization of the Arterial System

If, as we did for the ventricle, we characterize the mechanical properties of the afterload system in terms of the P_{es}-SV relationship (right of Fig. 1) [10, 20–23], an equilibrium stroke volume when both systems are coupled can be determined graphically as the point of intersection between the ventricular P_{es}-SV relationship and arterial P_{es}-SV relationship (bottom of Fig. 1). For this purpose Sunagawa and his associates [10, 20–23] proposed the concept of effective arterial elastance (E_a) which was defined as the ratio of end-systolic pressure to stroke volume. With E_a, end-systolic pressure of the arterial system is expressed as

$$P_{es} = E_a SV \tag{3}$$

If we approximate the end-systolic pressure by mean arterial pressure, Eq. (3) can be rewritten as

$$P_{es} = (R/T)SV \tag{4}$$

where R is arterial resistance and T is one cardiac cycle length. Thus E_a can be approximated by

$$E_a = R/T \tag{5}$$

Note that the effective arterial elastance is linearly proportional to the arterial resistance and inversely proportional to the cardiac cycle length. It does not directly relate at all to the physical elastic properties of the arterial system.

Ventricular-arterial Coupling

Once we have characterized both the ventricular system and arterial system in terms of the P_{es}-SV relationship (Fig. 1), we can determine the stroke volume that should result when the ventricle is coupled with the arterial system as the imtersection between the two P_{es}-SV relationships. The equilibrium stroke volume can be obtained analytically by simultaneously solving Eqs. (2) and (3) as

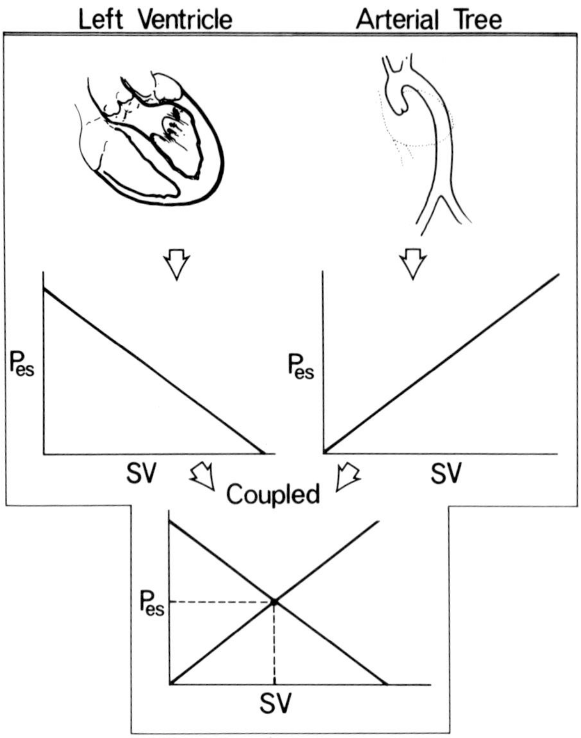

Fig. 1. Explanation of the proposed approach to coupling the ventricle with the arterial load. Both the ventricular system (*left panels*) and the arterial system (*right panels*) are characterized by the relationship of end-systolic pressure (P_{es}) to stroke volume (SV). The intersection between these two relationship lines (*bottom panel*) gives the stroke volume resulting from coupling of the two systems. (From [21] with permission of the American Physiological Society)

$$SV = \frac{E_{es}}{E_a + E_{es}} (V_{ed} - V_o) \tag{6}$$

To validate this framework, Sunagawa et al. [21] predicted stroke volumes for a known E_{es}, arterial resistance, heart rate and end-diastolic volume in isolated cross-perfused canine left ventricles. They then compared those predictions against measured values. Figure 2 shows an example of the relationship between the predicted and measured stroke volumes at various values of arterial resistance, compliance and end-diastolic volume. All the data in this plot were obtained from a single ventricle ejected into simulated arterial impedance [24]. Different symbols represent data with different combinations of arterial resistance and compliance. The correlation coefficient in this example was 0.993 ($P < 0.0001$). The slope of the linear regression equation was close to unity with a very small y-axis intercept, indicating the accuracy of prediction. The average correlation coefficient in the eight ventricles studied was 0.985. Thus the framework proposed by Sunagawa et al. [10, 20–23] was able to predict stroke volume reasonable well in all left ventricles studied.

Physical Implication of the Ventricular-arterial Coupling Framework

We demonstrated that the proposed framework to couple the left ventricle with the arterial system could accurately predict stroke volume. This coupling was

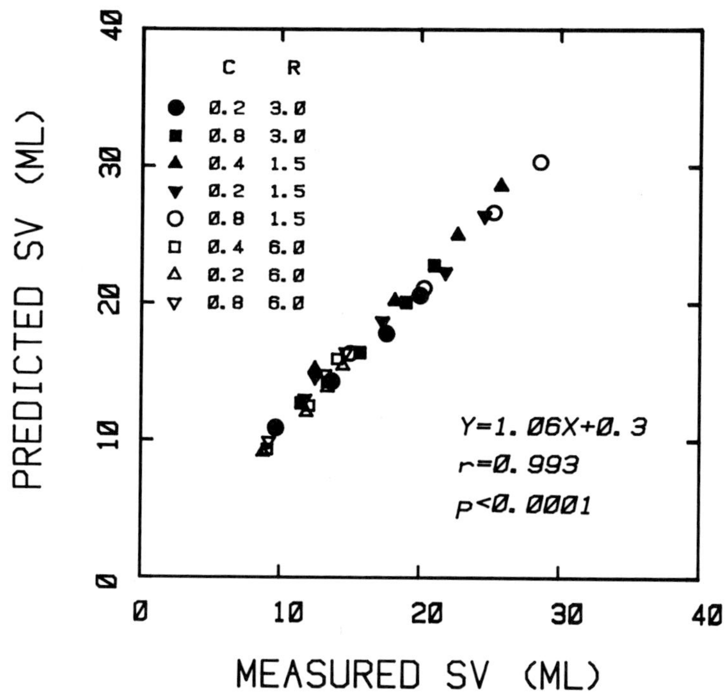

Fig. 2. Representative example of the relationship between predicted and measured stroke volume (*SV*) obtained in one ventricle. *C* represents compliance (ml/mmHg) and *R* is resistance (mmHg s/ml). Different *symbols* represent different loading conditions. Despite a wide range of loading conditions, the data were distributed close to the identity line (not shown), indicating accuracy of the prediction. (From [21] with permission of the American Physiological Society)

made possible by representing the function of both the ventricle and the arterial system in terms of their P_{es}-SV relationships. Since the slope of both of these P_{es}-SV relations have dimensions of volume elastance (mmHg/ml), we are treating the arterial system like an elastic chamber with a volume elastance E_a, just as we treat the ventricle like an elastic chamber with an end-systolic elastance, E_{es} (Fig. 3). Thus our prediction of stroke volume when the ventricle is coupled to the arterial system might be thought of as an answer to the question "How much volume will be transferred if one couples an elastic chamber (left ventricle) with a known volume elastance, dead volume and initial volume to a second elastic chamber (arterial system) with a known volume elastance?" Obviously, the distribution of the volume between the two chambers is determined by the ratio of their volume elastance values. The slope of the arterial P_{es}-SV relationship represents not the physical elastance or compliance of the arterial system but an "effective" arterial elastance. The effective arterial elastance changes more with changes in physical arterial resistance than with changes in arterial compliance.

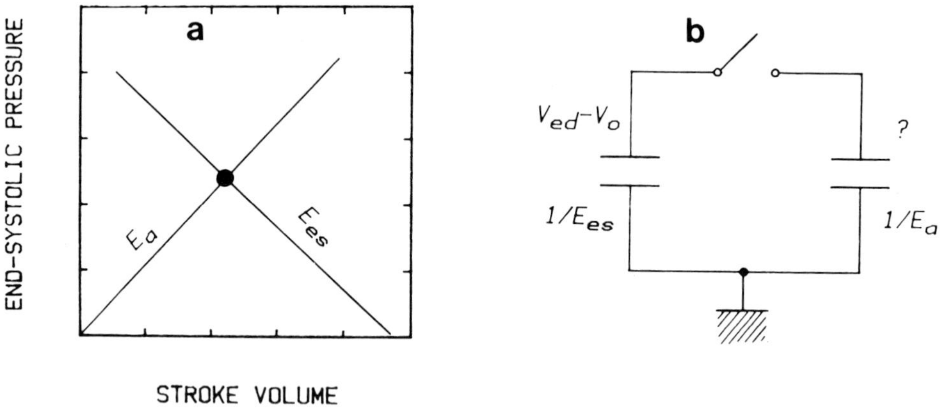

Fig. 3. **a** Graphical determination of the equilibrium stroke volume when the ventricle with a volume elastance, E_{es}, is coupled to the arterial system with an effective volume elastance, E_a. The stroke volume is obtained as the abscissal coordinate of the intersection of these two lines. **b** Physical meaning of the proposed ventricular-arterial coupling model. Both the ventricle and the arterial system are considered as elastic chambers with known volume elastances E_{es} and E_a, respectively. Stroke volume is determined as the amount of fluid transferred from the ventricle to the arterial system when the two are connected. (From [21] with permission of the American Physiological Society)

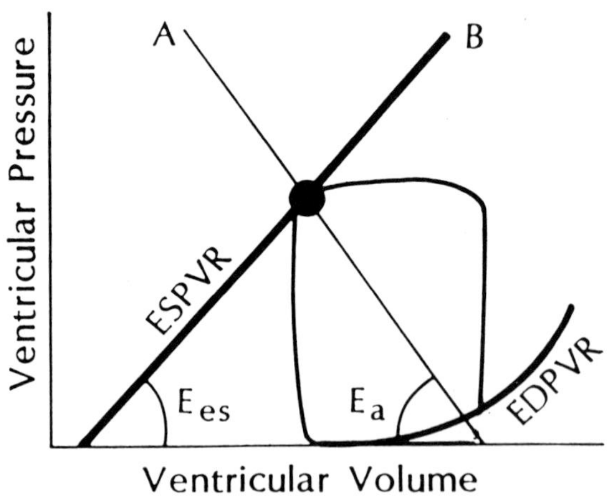

Fig. 4. The slope of the arterial end-systolic pressure-volume relationship (*ESPVR*) (*line A*) is E_a with the volume axis intercept of V_{ed}. *Line B* represents the ventricular *ESPVR*, with the volume axis intercept of V_o. End-systolic volume is given as the intersection between these two lines. Stroke volume is the difference between the end-diastolic volume (the *abscissal coordinate* of the *lower right corner* of pressure-volume loop) and end-systolic volume (the *abscissal coordinate* of the *upper left corner* of pressure-volume loop). *EDPVR* represents the end-diastolic pressure-volume relationship. (From [20] with permission of Oxford Press, New York)

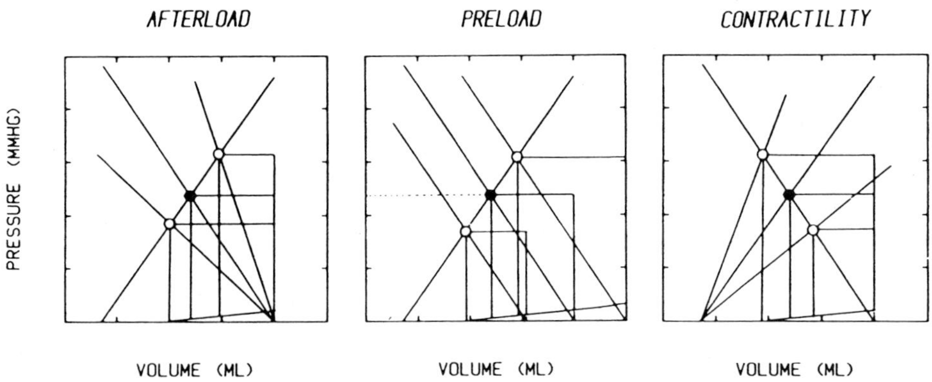

Fig. 5. Effects on stroke volume of changes in arterial resistance (*left panel*), end-diastolic volume (*middle panel*) and contractility (*right panel*). The *closed circle* represents the equilibrium end-systolic pressure-volume point under control conditions. (From [23] with permission of Springer-Verlag, New York)

A Graphical Analysis to Couple the Ventricle with the Arterial System

Although the fundamental concept of ventricular-arterial coupling is best explained by the P_{es}-SV relationship of both the ventricle and arterial system, specific contributions of the mechanical properties of the ventricle and those of the arterial system to stroke volume can be more easily identified in the pressure-volume diagram of the ventricle. Illustrated in Fig. 4 is the same framework for the coupling analysis as shown in Fig. 1, but in the ventricular pressure-volume plane instead of the pressure-stroke volume plane [20]. In this plane, the arterial system is characterized by the diagonal line labeled A (arterial end-systolic pressure-volume relationship). The slope of the arterial end-systolic pressure-volume relationship is E_a. The origin of the relationship line, that is, its volume axis intercept, is a given end-diastolic volume, V_{ed}. The stroke volume is represented on this ventricular volume axis as a distance to the left of this intercept. When the ventricle is coupled with the arterial system, the equilibrium is determined graphically as the intersection between the end-systolic pressure-volume relationship of the arterial system (Line A of Fig. 4) and that of the ventricle (Line B of Fig. 4).

Figure 5 presents examples of this graphical analysis under a variety of conditions [23]. The left panel of Fig. 5 illustrates the effect of changes in arterial resistance. The closed circle represents the equilibrium end-systolic pressure-volume point under the control conditions. If we increase arterial resistance while keeping contractility and preload constant, the slope of the arterial end-systolic pressure-volume relationship ($E_a = R/T$) is increased. This in turn decreases the stroke volume by shifting the intersection up and to the right. If we reduce arterial resistance, the intersection point shifts down and to the left, resulting in an increase in stroke volume.

The middle panel in Fig. 5 illustrates the effect of changes in preload on stroke volume while contractility and arterial resistance are constant. With an increase in end-diastolic volume, the origin of the arterial end-systolic pressure-volume relationship shifts to the right and stroke volume increases from the control value (the closed circle) to a new equilibrium value. If the end-diastolic volume decreases, the stroke volume decreases because the intersection between the ventricular and arterial end-systolic pressure-volume relationship shifts leftward.

If the contractility of the ventricle is augmented (i.e., if E_{es} increases), the slope of the ventricular end-systolic pressure-volume relationship increases without a change in its volume axis intercept as shown in the right panel of Fig. 5. The arterial end-systolic pressure-volume relationship does not change as long as the end-diastolic volume is held constant. Therefore, stroke volume increases from the control equilibrium value (the closed circle) to a new equilibrium value. A decrease in contractility results in a decrease in stroke volume.

Optimal Afterload

Optimal Effective Arterial Elastance

The vital function of a cardiovascular system is to provide necessary blood flow to peripheral tissues to maintain normal biological functions. As we indicated, a given level of cardiac output that maintains adequate peripheral perfusion can be achieved by various combinations of ventricular contractility, preload and afterload. Thus the regulatory system must choose a particular combination of them. It is not clear, however, how optimal functioning of the cardiovascular system is naturally defined, whether in terms of cardiac output, stroke volume, and/or external work, or alternatively, the efficiency of the ventricular ejection. In view of the vital function of the cardiovascular system, performance may well be more essential than efficiency, although the optimal loading conditions for performance and for efficiency may well be the same.

We defined the optimal afterload as that at which external work of the left ventricle becomes maximum [13–16]. With the framework of ventricular-arterial coupling, external work (EW) for normal, quasi-isobaric ejecting contraction can be approximated as

$$EW = \frac{E_a E_{es}^2}{(E_a + E_{es})^2}(V_{ed} - V_o)^2 \quad (7)$$

By differentiating Eq. (7) with respect to E_a, one can show that EW becomes maximum (EW_{max}) when E_{es} equals E_a. Substituting E_a in Eq. (7) yields

$$EW_{max} = \frac{E_{es}}{4}(V_{ed} - V_o)^2 \quad (8)$$

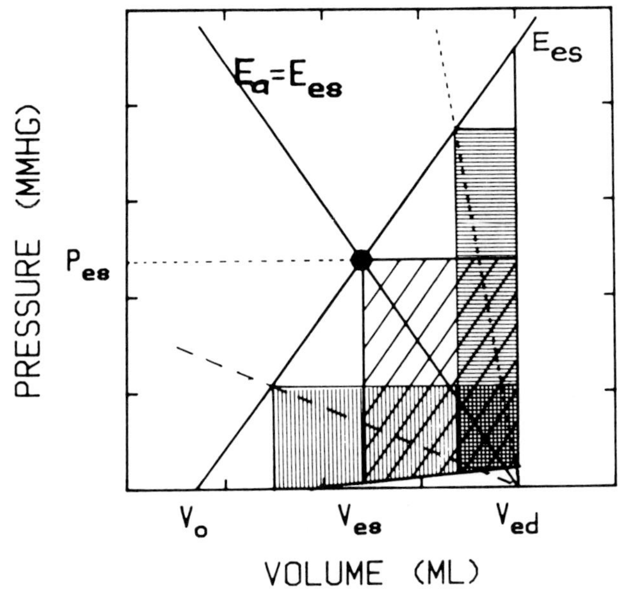

Fig. 6. Schematic representation of ventricular-arterial coupling in the pressure-volume plane. The *cross-hatched area* represents the maximal external work from a given end-diastolic volume (V_{ed}) under optimal coupling when the slopes of both ventricular and arterial P_{es}-SV relationships are the same. Under optimal conditions, the stroke volume is 50% of the effective preload (i.e., $V_{ed} - V_o$). (From [22] with permission of Pergamon Press)

Figure 6 illustrates the condition at which he external work (cross-hatched area) becomes maximum for a heart with a given E_{es} and end-diastolic volume. It is evident and intuitively obvious from the figure that the shaded area is largest when E_a equals E_{es}. Note that EW_{max} is 50% of the total pressure-volume area which is obtainable when the ventricle contracts isovolumically at the end-diastolic volume.

To test whether external work truly becomes maximum when E_a equals E_{es}, Sunagawa et al. predicted the effective arterial elastance values at which external work of the left ventricle became maximum and compared those predicted against measured ones using isolated canine heart preparation [10]. As shown in Fig. 7, despite changes in end-diastolic volume, contractility, arterial compliance or heart rate, external work of the left ventricle always became maximum when the ratio of E_a to E_{es} was unity. At the same time, the effective ejection fraction, defined as the ratio of stroke volume to $V_{ed} - V_o$, was found to be approximately 50% when external work was maximum. Thus the proposed framework of coupling is simple but very useful to predict the coupling condition at which external work of the left ventricle becomes maximum.

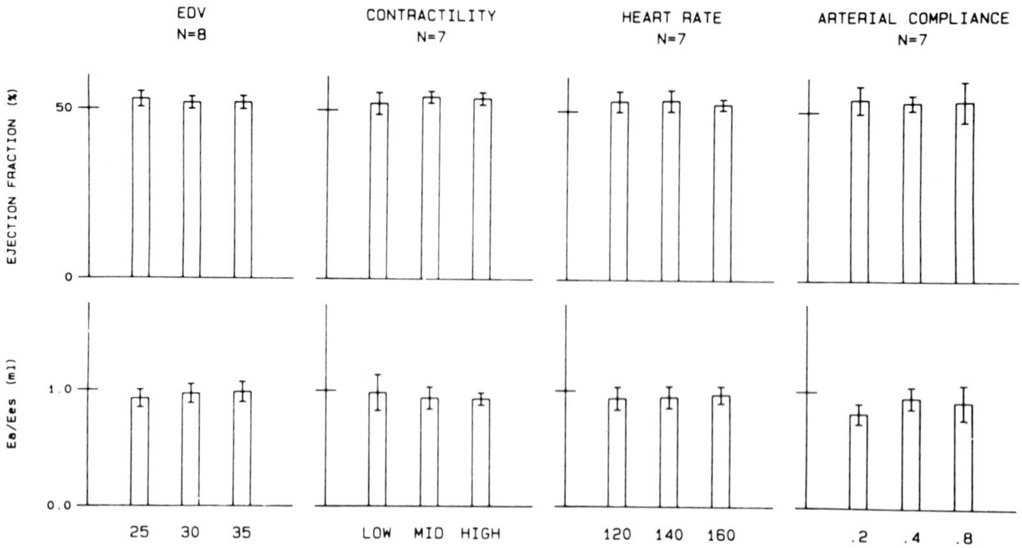

Fig. 7. Effects of changes in end-diastolic volume (*EDV*) (ml), contractility, heart rate (bpm), and arterial compliance (ml/mmHg) on ejection fraction and E_a/E_{es}. Ejection fraction is defined as the ratio of stroke volume to $V_{ed} - V_o$. As shown in the *top panel*, ejection fraction remains virtually constant at 50% under the optimal arterial load. The ratio of effective arterial elastance (E_a) to ventricular end-systolic elastance (E_{es}) remains constant at matched conditions, irrespective of end-diastolic volume, contractility, heart rate and arterial compliance. (From [10] with permission of the American Heart Association)

Optimality of the Afterload

The framework of ventricular-arterial coupling makes it possible to estimate maximum external work as well as optimal effective arterial elastance when ventricular end-systolic elastance is known. Thus, we defined the optimality of the afterload (Q_{load}) as the ratio of external work to its maximum value [13–16], i.e.,

$$Q_{load} = \frac{EW}{EW_{max}} \tag{9}$$

Substituting EW and EW_{max} in Eq. (9) with Eqs. (7) and (8) yields

$$Q_{load} = \frac{4E_aE_{es}}{(E_{es} + E_a)^2} \tag{10}$$

Note that Q_{load} varies from zero to unity. Q_{load} becomes unity (maximum) when E_a equals E_{es}. This is the condition at which external work becomes maximum. If Q_{load} is 0.5 it means that the afterload elastance extracts only 50% of potential external work of a given left ventricle. Q_{load} represents mechanical optimality of the ventricle as a pump.

Optimal Heart

Optimal Left Ventricle

We define the optimal left ventricle as the heart which requires minimum metabolic energy per unit time to support a peripheral demand [13, 15]. The peripheral demand is characterized by a fixed cardiac output and fixed arterial resistance. One can experimentally determine a particular combination of ventricular contractility, heart rate and end-diastolic volume at which metabolic demand of the heart becomes minimum if one systematically and exhaustively varies these parameters. However, it is impractical, if not impossible, to carry out such an experiment. Since we can precisely predict end-systolic pressure, stroke volume, external work, and cardiac output, once ventricular end-systolic elastance and arterial resistance or elastance are known, one may estimate the metabolic cost of the heart accurately if the relationship between mechanical behavior and metabolic cost of the ventricle is precisely known.

End-systolic Pressure-volume Area and Oxygen Consumption of the Ventricle

Suga and his associates [25–28] demonstrated a tight linear correlation between the end-systolic pressure-volume area (PVA) and oxygen consumption

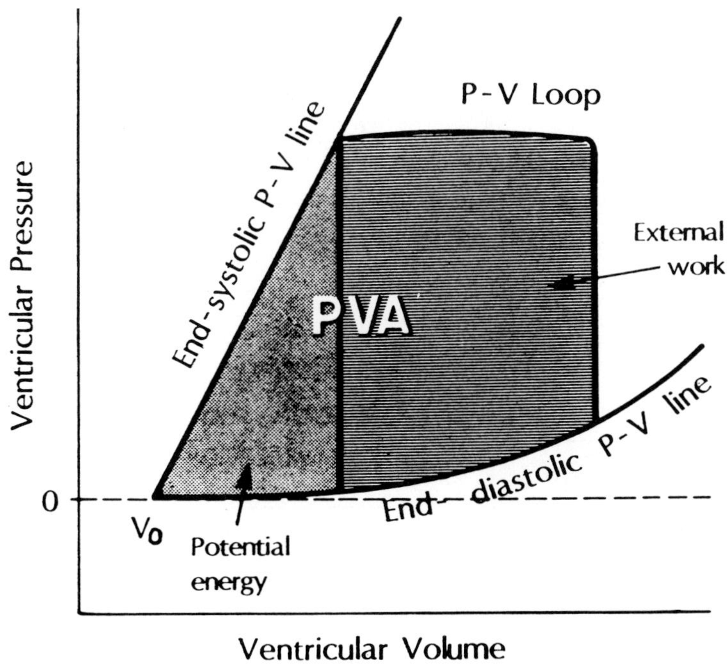

Fig. 8. Pressure-volume area (*PVA*), consisting of external work and end-systolic elastic potential energy. *P*, pressure; *V*, volume. (From [20] with permission of Oxford Press, New York)

(VO_2) (equivalent to metabolic demand) of the left ventricle. Shown in Fig. 8 is the PVA, which is defined as the area circumscribed by the ESPVR, the end-diastolic pressure-volume relationship and the systolic segment of the pressure-volume trajectory. Changes in contractility hardly affected the slope of the PVA-VO_2 relationship, but it altered the intercept significantly [25–29]. The oxygen consumption per beat is expressed as

$$VO_2 = A\mathrm{PVA} + B\mathrm{E_{es}} + C \tag{11}$$

where A, B and C are experimentally determined constants. Equation (11) relates oxygen consumption to mechanical work of the left ventricle, which is precisely predictable from ventricular contractility and loading conditions using the framework of ventricular-arterial coupling.

Optimality of the Left Ventricle

As we defined above, the optimal heart requires minimum oxygen per unit time to support a given peripheral demand. By combining the framework of ventricular-arterial coupling and that of the PVA-VO_2 relationship, one can estimate oxygen consumption of the heart for various combinations of contractility, preload and afterload. Figure 9 illustrates the estimated relationship between oxygen consumption (VO_2), E_{es} and heart rate (HR) obtained for a constant cardiac output and arterial resistance. Each of the curvilinear lines is obtained for a different heart rate with changing E_{es}. As can be seen for a given heart rate, VO_2 becomes minimum at a particular E_{es}. On the

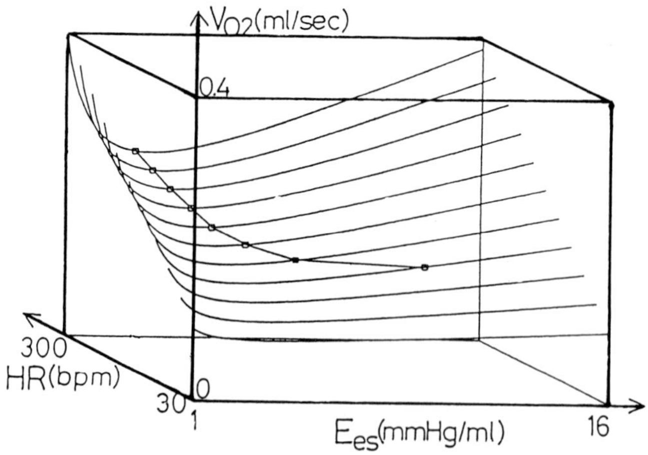

Fig. 9. Estimated ventricular oxygen consumption per unit time (*VO_2*) as a function of heart rate (*HR*) and end-systolic elastance (*E_{es}*) to generate a required amount of cardiac output and arterial pressure. *Parallel curvilinear lines* represent *VO_2* for a given *HR* as a function of *E_{es}*. Note that, although for any given *HR*, the minimum *VO_2* always exists at a particular *E_{es}* value, decreasing *HR* monotonically decreases *VO_2* for any given *E_{es}*. The *curvilinear line* which connects *open squares* represents *VO_2* for a given preload as a function of *HR* and *E_{es}*. Under this condition, we now have a unique combination of *E_{es}* and *HR* which minimizes *VO_2* (*closed square*)

other hand, lowering heart rate monotonically lowers VO_2 at the expense of increased preload. If end-diastolic volume is fixed, for a given heart rate, E_{es} is uniquely determined to meet the peripheral demand. This is shown as the curvilinear line which connects the open squares. Under these conditions, there is a particular combination of E_{es} and HR which minimizes VO_2 to meet a fixed peripheral demand (as indicated by the closed square).

We defined the optimality of the heart (Q_{heart}) as the ratio of minimum oxygen consumption (VO_{2min}) to actual oxygen consumption (VO_2) [13, 15], i.e.,

$$Q_{heart} = \frac{VO_{2min}}{VO_2} \tag{12}$$

Q_{heart} varies between zero and unity. Unity Q_{heart} implies that the heart requires minimum oxygen to meet a peripheral demand. If Q_{heart} is 0.5, the heart requires twice as much oxygen relative to the most efficient heart to meet the same peripheral demand. Q_{heart} represents metabo-mechanical efficiency of the heart.

Effect of Exercise on the Optimality of Load and Heart

We evaluated how exercise stress affected optimality of the load and heart in chronically instrumented dogs [13–16]. We used six chronically instrumented mongrel dogs preconditioned to run on a treadmill. Under sterile conditions, thoracotomies were carried out at the fourth left intercostal space under artificial ventilation. After pericardotomy, a high-fidelity pressure transducer was inserted into the left ventricle through a small incision at the apex. An electromagnetic flow probe was placed around the ascending aorta. The left atrium and left internal mammalian artery were cannulated for arterial pressure measurement and for calibration of the left ventricular pressure transducer. We then closed the chest and allowed the dogs to recover for about 10 days. After complete recovery from the surgery for instrumentation, we imposed on the dogs exercise loads of various degrees with the treadmill. The exercise stress varied stepwise in random order from complete standstill to maximum speed (up to 7 km/h) with a 20% slope. When the hemodynamic condition was judged to reach a steady state for a given exercise stress level, we recorded hemodynamic variables.

With exercise, both cardiac output and heart rate were nearly doubled, arterial pressure was slightly increased and arterial resistance was decreased. Figure 10 shows changes in E_{es} and E_a in response to exercise. E_{es} increased from 7.5 at rest to 10.9 mmHg/ml at peak exercise ($P < 0.001$) (left of Fig. 9) and E_a tended to increase from 4.9 to 6.7 mmHg/ml (middle of Fig. 9), while the ratio of E_a to E_{es} remained fairly constant (from 0.69 ± 0.26 to 0.63 ± 0.21, n.s.) (right of Fig. 9).

With reference to Fig. 11, optimality of the afterload, as assessed by Q_{load}, was 0.93 ± 0.08 at rest and 0.92 ± 0.09 at peak exercise (left of Fig. 10). Hence, it was reasonable to say that the afterloading condition chosen by the regulatory system always maximized external work from a given heart not only

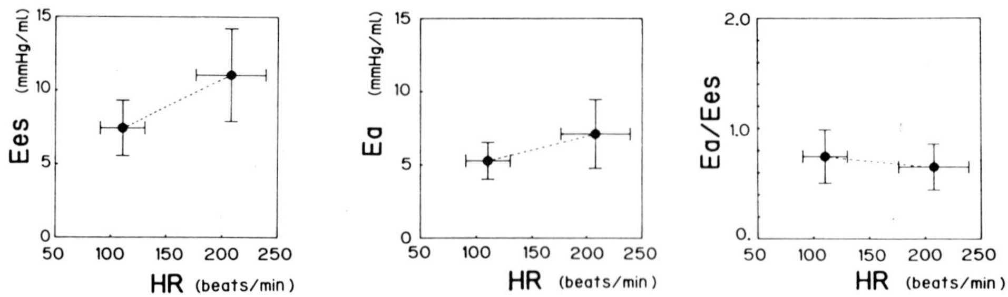

Fig. 10. *Left panel*: Effect of exercise on the left ventricular end-systolic elastance (E_{es}). With increases in exercise load, E_{es} increased from 7.4 to 11.1 mmHg/ml ($P < 0.001$). *Middle panel*: Effect of exercise on the effective arterial elastance (E_a). With increases in exercise load, increases in heart rate overrode the decreases in arterial resistance, which in turn increased E_a from 5.3 to 7.1 mmHg/ml. *Right panel*: Effect of exercise on the ratio of E_a to E_{es} (E_a/E_{es}). The ratio was not significantly altered by exercise. (From [14] with permission of CRC)

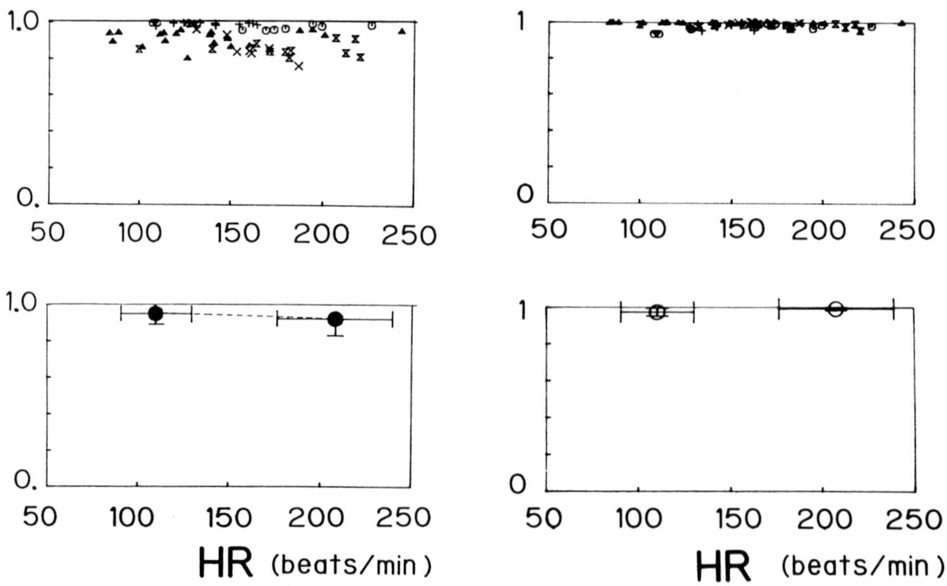

Fig. 11. *Left panels*: Effect of exercise on optimal load (Q_{load}). Q_{load} is nearly unity at all exercise levels (*upper panel*). Different symbols represent different animals. Averaged Q_{load} remained close to unity regardless of exercise stress (*lower panel*). *Right panels*: Effect of exercise on the optimality of the heart (Q_{heart}). Q_{heart} is nearly unity at all exercise levels (*upper panel*). Averaged Q_{load} remained close to unity regardless of exercise stress (*lower panel*). (Modified from [16])

at rest but also at peak exercise. Similarly, optimality of the heart, as assessed by Q_{heart}, was 0.98 ± 0.02 at rest and 0.99 ± 0.01 at peak exercise (right of Fig. 10). This means that ventricular contractility and heart rate chosen by the regulatory system minimized oxygen consumption of the heart despite tremendous changes in peripheral demand associated with exercise.

Effect of Volume Change on the Optimality of Load and Heart

Using similarly prepared chronically instrumented conscious dogs, we evaluated how changes in blood volume affects the optimal afterload and heart function [30]. We infused dextran stepwise up to 30 ml/kg, and we hemorrhaged stepwise up to 30 ml/kg. For each level of changes in blood volume, we recorded the hemodynamic variables when they reached steady states.

Decreases in blood volume up to 30 ml/kg decreased arterial pressure by 18 mmHg and decreased cardiac output by 40%, but increased heart rate up to 120 beat/min. Arterial resistance was also increased by 43%. Increases in blood volume up to 30 ml/kg significantly increased cardiac output by 86% with an increase in arterial pressure by 20 mmHg. Heart rate was also increased up to 120 beat/min in response to the volume load.

Decreases in blood volume significantly increased effective arterial elastance by 78%, while changed end-systolic elastance a little. The ratio of effective arterial elastance to end-systolic elastance increased from 0.8 to 1.55. The optimality of the load, Q_{load}, remained unchanged (from 0.97 ± 0.03 to 0.96 ± 0.02, n.s.) (left of Fig. 12). The optimality of the heart, Q_{heart}, decreased (from 0.92 ± 0.04 to 0.80 ± 0.04, $P < 0.01$) (right of Fig. 12).

Increases in blood volume slightly lowered effective arterial elastance without significant changes in ventricular end-systolic elastance. The ratio of effective arterial elastance to ventricular end-systolic elastance remained fairly constant. The volume load altered neither Q_{load} (from 0.93 ± 0.07 to 0.94 ± 0.04, n.s.) (left of Fig. 12) nor Q_{heart} (from 0.92 ± 0.09 to 0.92 ± 0.06, n.s.) (right of Fig. 12).

Thus, it appeared that the conscious dogs were capable of extracting maximum external work from the left ventricle and minimize its oxygen consumption despite wide ranges of changes in blood volume. With extreme hemorrhaging (30 ml/kg), the dogs still managed to maintain arterial pressure to perfuse vital organs by increasing arterial resistance. This response inevitably increased the oxygen consumption, but the external work remained close to maximum for a given preload.

Effect of Left Ventricular Dysfunction on Optimality of Load and Heart

Both stresses, exercise and changes in volume, are rather common ones for animals. The animals may have experienced such stresses in the process of evolution. However, what will happen if the ventricle per se is no longer

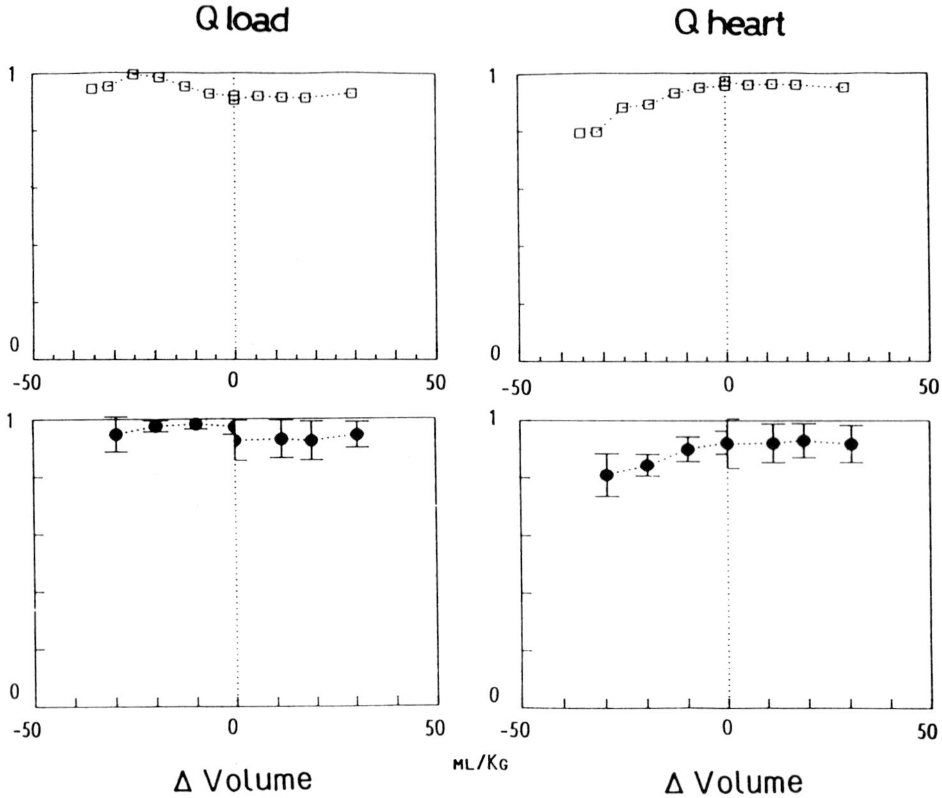

Fig. 12. *Left panels*: Effect of volume changes on the optimality of the load (Q_{load}) in one dog (*upper panel*). Q_{load} is nearly unity despite decreases or increases in volume. Averaged Q_{load} remains close to unity (*lower panel*). *Right panel*: Effect of volume changes on the optimality of the heart (Q_{heart}) in one dog (*upper panel*). Q_{heart} is nearly unity regardless of changes in volume. Averaged Q_{heart} remains close to unity (*lower panel*). (Modified from [30])

capable of responding to the command of the regulatory system? Is the heart capable of generating maximum external work for a given level of function? Is the heart capable of meeting the peripheral demand with minimum oxygen consumption? To answer these questions we investigated how ventricular dysfunction affects the optimality of the load and heart [31].

Using chronically instrumented dogs, we created left ventricular dysfunction by microembolization of the coronary artery. We injected repetitively, under anesthesia, 15-μ microspheres into the left main coronary artery until left atrial pressure reached 30 mmHg. One or two days after the microembolization, we measured hemodynamics in the conscious state and compared them against those obtained under control conditions.

The microembolization of the coronary artery decreased cardiac output by 20%, while minimally affecting arterial pressure, indicating increases in arterial resistance. Heart rate increased by 40%. Left ventricular end-systolic elastance did not significantly decrease but the effective arterial elastance significantly increased, which in turn increased the ratio of effective arterial elastance to end-systolic elastance (from 0.7 to 1.5, $P < 0.01$). Although we were not certain why the end-systolic elastance did not significantly decrease in the presence of decreased cardiac output, increased heart rate and increased arterial resistance, all of which were compatible with left ventricular dysfunction, we speculated that the left ventricular dysfunction was mild enough to be masked by the compensatory mechanism.

The mild left ventricular dysfunction did not significantly decrease Q_{load} (from 0.95 ± 0.08 to 0.96 ± 0.05, n.s.). Assuming that the insulted heart still obeys the PVA-VO_2 relationship as expressed in Eq. (11), we estimated Q_{heart}. Unlike Q_{load}, Q_{heart} significantly decreased from 0.98 ± 0.02 to 0.88 ± 0.05 ($P < 0.001$).

We also observed how a positive inotropic agent, dobutamine, influenced optimality of the load and heart. In the normal hearts, an infusion of dobutamine decreased Q_{load} to 0.83 ± 0.08 ($P < 0.01$), whereas in the diseased hearts, it increased both Q_{load} (0.99 ± 0.01, $P < 0.01$) and Q_{heart} (0.96 ± 0.03, $P < 0.01$).

Thus, from these studies, we concluded that the left ventricle with mild dysfunction could maintain nearly maximum external work. The oxygen consumption of the ventricle, however, was no longer minimum as evidenced by the decreased Q_{heart}. The positive inotropic agent improved both the optimality of the afterload and heart in the ventricle with dysfunction. The afterload was not able to extract maximum external work from the normal ventricle with increased contractility by dobutamine.

Effect of Baroreflex on the Optimality of Load and Heart

To investigate what makes it possible to maintain optimality of the load and heart in the presence of various stresses, we evaluated how the carotid sinus baroreflex affected the optimality of ventricular-arterial coupling [32]. We isolated the bilateral carotid sinuses in anesthetized dogs, and measured aortic pressure, aortic flow and left ventricular pressure, while randomly perturbing carotid sinus pressure using a specially designed servo-pump. We used a Gaussian white noise for carotid sinus pressure perturbation because it allowed us to estimate the unbiased linear transfer characteristics of the system even from that with significant nonlinearity [33, 34]. After a beat-to-beat estimation of left ventricular end-systolic elastance and effective arterial elastance, we determined the transfer function from the carotid sinus pressure to end-systolic elastance and to effective arterial elastance over the frequency range of 0.002 to 0.25 Hz using a multichannel autoregressive model [35].

Both transfer functions were reasonably linear and showed characteristics of the second order delay system with the identical corner frequency of 0.02 Hz. The gain below 0.02 Hz was about 0.08 mmHg/ml per mmHg for both of them.

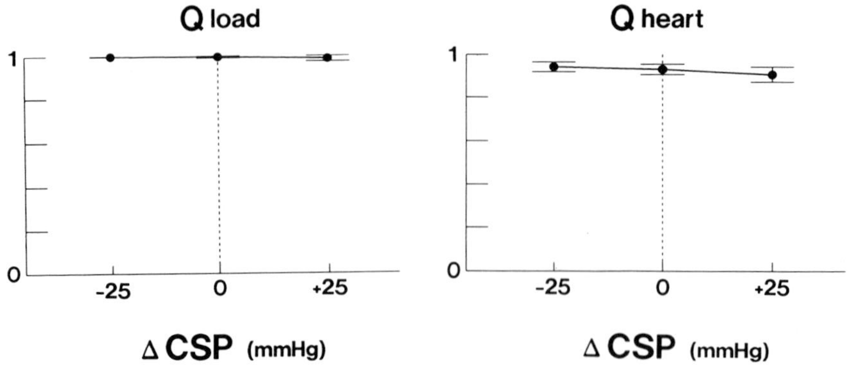

Fig. 13. Using the transfer function experimentally estimated, we evaluated the optimality of the load (Q_{load}) and heart (Q_{heart}) in response to a step change in carotid sinus pressure (*CSP*). Changes in *CSP* neither significantly affected Q_{load} nor Q_{heart}

That is, a 50 mmHg decrease of carotid sinus pressure results in an increase in end-systolic elastance and effective arterial elastance by 4.0 mmHg/ml. The estimated instantaneous ratio of changes in effective arterial elastance to those in end-systolic elastance in response to step changes in carotid sinus pressure was not significantly different from unity. This implies that whenever the baroreflex altered ventricular elastance, it was always coupled with a change in effective arterial elastance. As the net effect, the baroreflex did not change the ratio of effective arterial elastance to ventricular end-systolic elastance.

Since external work of the left ventricle becomes maximum when effective arterial elastance equals and-systolic elastance, the carotid sinus baroreflex appeared to be preprogrammed to regulate the ventricular and arterial properties so as to maintain optimality of the load. Figure 13 shows the estimated response, against the step change in carotid sinus pressure, of the optimality of the load and heart. As anticipated, Q_{load} remains close to unity. At the same time, the baroreflex hardly affected the optimality of the heart, Q_{heart}, indicating that the baroreflex maintains arterial pressure without compromising energy efficiency of the left ventricular-arterial coupling.

Discussion

Effect of Various Stresses on the Optimality of Ventricular-arterial Coupling

We have shown that the left ventricle, for a given level of preload, generates maximum external work at rest and under various levels of exercise stresses. External work was nearly maximum under volume loading and hemorrhage.

The ventricle generates cardiac output to meet peripheral demand with minimum metabolic energy cost irrespective of the level of physical activity or volume changes. Only extreme volume reduction sizably increases oxygen costs to meet the same peripheral demand. We believe that exercise and volume changes were one of the major natural stresses when animals evolved. Thus, from a view point of teleology, animals are expected to optimize ventricular-arterial coupling so as to maximize external work and minimize oxygen cost. Simultaneous optimization of the load and heart would be desirable. This appears to be the case for normal ventricular-arterial coupling. On the other hand, with extreme hemorrhaging, minimization of oxygen demand failed. In order to survive, minimization of oxygen consumption would no longer be the major concern, as maintenance of blood pressure in vital organs is more important. Thus, this response is again teleologically sound.

When the left ventricular function was depressed, the heart was unable to respond normally to the command of the regulatory system. Indeed, under these conditions, even though the external work of the ventricle was still close to maximum, the metabolic energy required to meet the peripheral demand at rest was no longer at a minimum. It appears that in case of left ventricular dysfunction, even though the ventricular contractility was rather well compensated in our experiment, the associated changes in heart rate and arterial resistance made oxygen consumption larger. The increase in heart rate and in resistance would be crucial to maintain arterial blood pressure, and thus perfusion of vital organs. But the regulatory system achieved the goal at the expense of increases in the metabolic cost of the heart.

It appears that optimality of ventricular-arterial coupling, as defined by the optimal load and heart, is rather well maintained under stresses if the heart is capable of responding to the command of the regulatory system. If the heart is unable to respond to the command of the regulatory system, the compensatory response of the regulatory system against stresses may well have deleterious effects on the optimality of ventricular-arterial coupling.

The above is further supported by an experiment where we investigated the effect of baroreflex on the optimality of ventricular-arterial coupling. The transfer functions from the carotid sinus pressure to end-systolic elastance of the left ventricle and to effective arterial elastance were remarkably similar. That is to say, in response to changes in arterial pressure, both end-systolic elastance and effective arterial elastance change similarly even under transient conditions. As a result, the baroreflex changes ventricular-arterial coupling so as to maximize external work and to minimize the oxygen cost of the ventricle. Thus, if the ventricle was unable to respond to the baroreflex and only the effective arterial elastance responded to maintain arterial pressure, external work of the left ventricle would no longer be at a maximum. Oxygen cost of the ventricle was also no longer be at a minimum. Although there would be other mechanisms by which the animals regulate ventricular-arterial coupling, even the baroreflex system alone would have significant deleterious effects on it if the target organ was unable to respond to the regulatory command.

Significance of the Ratio of E_a to E_{es} in Determining Optimalities of the Load and Heart

As we have already indicated, external work of the ventricle becomes maximum for a given preload when E_a equals E_{es}. Thus, the optimality of the load becomes unity when E_a equals E_{es}. Illustrated in Fig. 14 is Q_{load} as a function of E_a/E_{es}. As anticipated, Q_{load} becomes unity when E_a/E_{es} is unity.

How, then, does the oxygen consumption of the heart relate to E_a and E_{es}? Using the framework of ventricular-arterial coupling and that of pressure-volume area vs. oxygen consumption, one can derive the optimality of the heart as a function of E_a/E_{es} (Fig. 14). As can be seen, Q_{heart} becomes unity when E_a/E_{es} is slightly above 0.5. If the ratio is lowered below 0.5, Q_{load} decreases sharply.

Note that both Q_{load} and Q_{heart} are close to unity if the ratio of E_a to E_{es} is somewhere between 0.5 to 1.0. Indeed, the ratio E_a to E_{es} in conscious normal dogs varies between 0.5 to 1.0. Thus, both Q_{load} and Q_{heart} remain at almost unity. Furthermore, even when the animals exercised, the E_a/E_{es} remained within a narrow range (between 0.42 and 0.84). Again, in this range of E_a/E_{es}, both Q_{load} and Q_{heart} are very high. Changes in volume varies E_a/E_{es} rather widely. For the volume loading, the ratio remains within the normal range. On the other hand, for extreme hemorrhaging, E_a/E_{es} can reach as high as 1.55, and this in turn decreases Q_{heart} while maintaining Q_{load}. When cardiac function deteriorates, E_a/E_{es} increase. As shown in Fig. 14, E_a/E_{es} ranges between

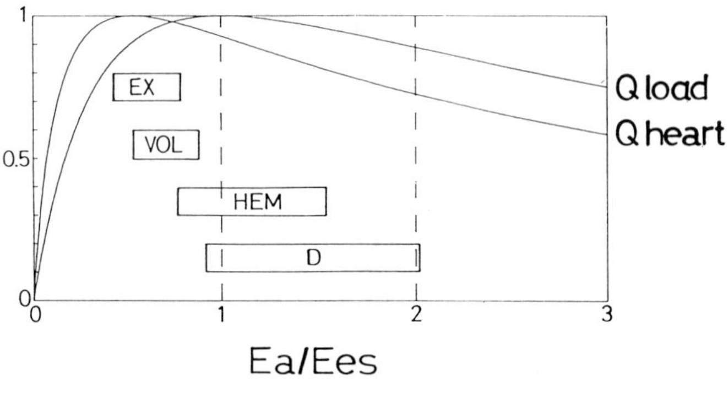

Fig. 14. Changes in optimality of the load (Q_{load}) and heart (Q_{heart}) as a function of E_a/E_{es}. Q_{load} becomes unity when E_a/E_{es} is unity. Q_{heart} becomes unity when E_a/E_{es} is slightly above 0.5. During exercise (*EX*), E_a/E_{es} varies between 0.42 and 0.84 (mean+SD and mean−SD, respectively). Within this change in E_a/E_{es}, both Q_{load} and Q_{heart} are close to unity. In response to volume load (*VOL*), E_a/E_{es} varies between 0.50 and 0.90. Thus both Q_{load} and Q_{heart} are close to unity. In case of volume depletion (*HEM*), E_a/E_{es} rises as high as 1.55. Now we see a significant decrease in Q_{load} and Q_{heart}. Q_{heart} decreases more than Q_{load} does. When left ventricular function is deteriorated (*D*), E_a/E_{es} increases up to 2.0. Both Q_{load} and Q_{heart} decrease significantly. That is, under left heart dysfunction, the left ventricle neither generates maximal external work for a given preload nor minimizes its oxygen consumption to meet peripheral demand

0.95 and 2.0 in the diseased heart. Under these conditions, Q_{heart} decreases whereas Q_{load} remains rather high.

The fact that both Q_{load} and Q_{heart} near unity when E_a/E_{es} varies between 0.5 and 1.0 makes it possible for the animal to simultaneously maximize external work for a given preload and minimize oxygen consumption of the heart to meet the peripheral demand. Whether these are intended results by the regulatory system or a simple coincidence is unknown. Nevertheless, it is fair to say that the ventricular-arterial coupling of conscious animals was very efficient from a view point of energy usage.

Alternative Definition of Optimalities

In this review article, we defined two indices of optimality, i.e., Q_{load} and Q_{heart}. Obviously, there are many alternative ways to define optimality. Instead, in order to see these somewhat abstract parameters, one can directly deal with optimal values of effective arterial elastance, resistance, heart rate and end-systolic elastance. Although these parameters give us the difference between actual operating points in terms of individual parameters, they do not provide us with the overall deviation of the operating points in terms of specific optimization criteria. These two are certainly not mutually exclusive, but rather complimentary.

Some investigators define the optimality of ventricular-arterial coupling by analyzing energy efficiency per beat. Namely, they looked for a condition at which the ratio of external work to oxygen consumption per beat becomes minimum [7, 11, 16, 36]. Conceptually, this resembles Q_{heart}. The major difference, however, is that in Q_{heart}, we derive the ventricular-arterial coupling parameters at which the oxygen consumption per unit time becomes minimum. The minimization of oxygen consumption per beat does not necessarily give the minimum oxygen consumption per unit time. What is important for the oxygen supply system to the heart is not the amount of oxygen consumption per beat but that of per unit time. This is why we used the myocardial oxygen consumption per unit time. Minimization of oxygen consumption per beat takes place when E_a/E_{es} is close to 0.5 [7, 16, 36], whereas that of per unit time takes place when E_a/E_{es} is slightly higher than that but lower than unity.

Pathophysiological Significance

We have shown that the left ventricle of conscious animals generated maximum external work for a given preload at rest and during exercise. The external work was also nearly maximum despite tremendous changes in volume. If the relationship between the end-systolic pressure-volume area of the left ventricle and its oxygen consumption is maintained under these stressed conditions, the ventricle did meet the altered peripheral demand while minimizing its oxygen consumption.

On the other hand, if ventricular contractility fails to increase in response to exercise, as in patients with heart failure, increasing heart rate and increased resistance inevitably increase effective arterial elastance. Thus, under these conditions, the ratio of E_a to E_{es} becomes significantly high. As shown in Fig. 14, the increased ratio of E_a to E_{es} decreases both optimality of the load and that of the heart assuming that the heart still obeys the PVA — VD_2 relation. This deterioration of the optimality of the load and heart would be best illustrated when we express these indices as a function of the effective ejection fraction. As shown in Fig. 15, Q_{load} and Q_{heart} for a heart with an effective ejection fraction of 15% are 0.5 and 0.35, respectively. This means that at this ejection fraction, the ventricle generates only 50% of its maximum potential external work and consumes three times more oxygen than the normal heart to meet peripheral demand. Note that Q_{heart} is more sensitive than Q_{load} to the decrease in ventricular function. The deterioration of optimality of the load (mechanical optimality) in the ventricle with poor contractility has been demonstrated in animals by Myhre et al. [12] and in patients with left ventricular dysfunction [37].

When we treat patients with heart failure, we often use positive inotropic agents and vasodilators in addition to diuretics. From the view point of the optimal load and heart, positive inotropic agents with minimum chronotropic effects would decrease the ratio of effective arterial elastance to end-systolic elastance. This would in turn increase the effective ejection fraction, which ultimately increases optimality of the load and heart. In the case of pure vasodilators, they would primarily decrease effective arterial elastance, which would lead to a decrease in the ratio of effective arterial elastance to end-

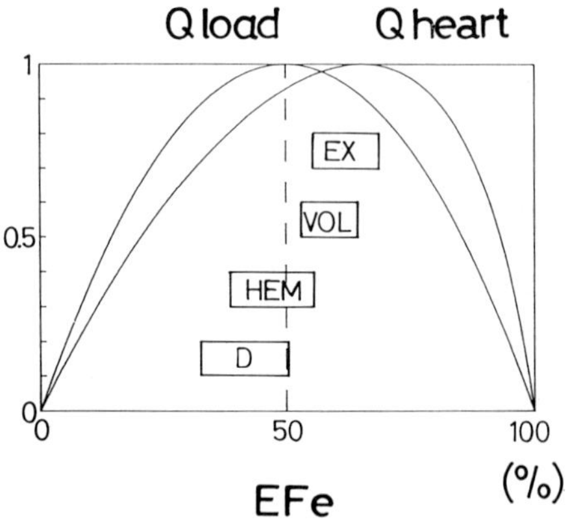

Fig. 15. Changes in optimality of the load (Q_{load}) and heart (Q_{heart}) as a function of effective ejection fraction (i.e., EFe = $SV/(V_{ed} - V_o)$). Q_{load} becomes unity when *EFe* is 50%. Q_{heart} becomes unity when *EFe* is about 65%. During exercise (*EX*), *EFe* varies between 55 and 70% (mean+SD and mean−SD, respectively). In this range of *EFe*, both Q_{load} and Q_{heart} are close to unity. In response to volume load (*VOL*), *EFe* varies between 53 and 65%. Again, both Q_{load} and Q_{heart} are close to unity. In the case of volume depletion (*HEM*), *EFe* decreases up to 38%. Now we see a significant decrease in Q_{load} and Q_{heart}. Q_{heart} decreases more than Q_{load} does. When left ventricular function is deteriorated (*D*), *EFe* varies between 33% and 50%. Both Q_{load} and Q_{heart} decrease significantly

systolic elastance. This would result in increases in the effective ejection fraction and thus improvements in the optimalities of the load and heart.

When the left ventricle is hypertrophied due to increases in afterload, such as in patients with hypertension, the end-systolic elastance of the left ventricle increases [38]. Since this increase in E_{es} is associated with an increase in arterial resistance, the resultant ratio of E_a to E_{es} may remain unchanged. This is supported by the fact that the ejection fraction of patients with hypertension and hypertrophy is not necessarily low unless heart failure exists. Under this condition, optimality of the load is well maintained. Numeric analyses indicated that even if increases in E_{es} are a consequence of increased myocardial mass, Q_{heart} remains high as long as the inotropic state of the myocardium is unchanged.

In the case of hypertrophic cardiomyopathy without outflow obstruction, supernormal systolic function as evidenced by systolic obliteration of the cavity has been demonstrated [39]. Since the increase in E_{es} is unrelated to the afterload, the resultant ratio of E_a to E_{es} would decrease. If the effective ejection fraction is as high as 90%, the ventricle delivers only one-third of external work of its potential. To support the same peripheral demand, such a heart requires 30% more oxygen than the normal heart. The use of beta-blockers or calcium channel antagonists for these patients depresses systolic function, and thus, improves both optimality of the load and ventricle. Hence, it seems that these treatments are reasonable from a view point of efficiency of energy usage.

Conclusion

We conclude that (1) external work of the left ventricle of dogs at rest is nearly maximum, (2) external work remains nearly maximum during exercise and volume changes in spite of tremendous changes in hemodynamics, and (3) conversion efficiency of metabolic energy to generate cardiac output to meet peripheral demand was not compromised as long as the heart is capable of responding to the command of the regulatory system during, the stresses above described. Once the heart fails to respond normally to the regulatory system, the optimality of ventricular-arterial coupling would not be maintained.

These unique features of ventricular-arterial coupling are teleologically sound. However, we are still not certain whether these optimizations are intended by the cardiovascular regulatory system or a simple coincidence. Needless to say, further investigations are required to scrutinize the mechanism of these observations.

References

1. Piene H, Sund H (1979) Flow and power output of right ventricle facing load with variable input impedance. Am J Physiol 237(Heart Circ Physiol 6):H125–H130
2. Elzinga G, Piene H, Jong JP (1980) Left and right ventricular pump function and consequences of having two pumps in one heart. A study on the isolated cat heart. Circ Res 46:564–574

3. Piene H, Sund T (1982) Does normal pulmonary impedance constitute the optimum load for the right ventricle? Am J Physiol 242:H154–H160
4. Van den Horn GJ, Westerhof N, Elzinga G (1985) Optimal power generation by the left ventricle. A study in the anesthetized open thorax cat. Circ Res 56:252–261
5. Van den Horn GJ, Westerhof N, Elzinga G (1986) Feline left ventricle does not always operate at optimum power output. Am J Physiol 250(Heart Cric Physiol 19):H961–H967
6. Toorop GP, Gerardus J, Van den Horn GJ, Elzinga G, Westerhof N (1988) Matching between feline left ventricle and arterial load: optimal power or efficiency. Am J Physiol 254(Heart Circ Physiol 23):H279–H285
7. Burkhoff D, Sagawa K (1986) Ventricular efficiency predicted by an analytical model. Am J Physiol 250(Regulatory Integrative Comp Physiol 19):R1021–R1027
8. Tanaka N, Yasumura Y, Nozawa T, Futaki S, Uenishi M, Hiramori K, Suga H (1988) Optimal contractility and minimal oxygen consumption for constant external work of heart. Am J Physiol 254(Regulatory Integrative Comp Physiol 23): R933–R943
9. Wilcken DEL, Charlier AA, Hoffman JIE, Guz A (1964) Effects of alterations in aortic impedance on the performance of the ventricles. Circ Res 14:283–293
10. Sunagawa K, Maughan WL, Sagawa K (1985) Optimal arterial resistance for the maximal stroke work studied in isolated canine left ventricle. Circ Res 56:586–595
11. Suga H, Igarashi Y, Yamada O, Goto Y (1985) Mechanical efficiency of the left ventricle as a function of preload, afterload, and contractility. Heart and Vessel 1:3–8
12. Myhre ESP, Johansen A, Bjornstad, Piene H (1986) The effect of contractility and preload on matching between the canine left ventricle and afterload. Circulation 73:161–171
13. Sunagawa K, Sugimachi M, Todaka K, Nakamura M (1989) Ventricular matching with the arterial system in chronically instrumented dogs. In: Hori M, Suga H, Baan J, Yellin EL (eds) Cardiac mechanics and function in the normal and diseased heart. Springer, Tokyo, pp 207–210
14. Sunagawa K, Hayashida K, Sugimachi M, Noma M, Ando H, Tajimi T, Tomoike H, Nose Y, Nakamura M (1989) Ventriculoarterial matching in exercising dogs. In: Sideman S, Beyer R (eds) Analysis and simulation of the cardiac system-ischemia. CRC, Boca Raton, pp 89–98
15. Sugimachi M, Todaka K, Sunagawa K, Nakamura M (1990) Optimal afterload for the heart vs. optimal heart for the afterload. Front Med Biol Eng 2:217–221
16. Hayashida K, Sunagawa K, Noma M, Sugimachi M, Ando H, Nose Y, Nakamura M (1987) Mechanical matching of the left ventricle with the arterial system in exercising dogs. Automedica 9:31
17. Suga H, Sagawa K, Shoukas AA (1973) Load independence of the instantaneous pressure-volume ratio of the canine left ventricle and effects of epinephrine and heart rate on the ratio. Circ Res 32:314–322
18. Suga H, Sagawa K (1974) Instantaneous pressure-volume relationships and their ratio in the excised, supported canine left ventricle. Circ Res 35:117–126
19. Sagawa K (1978) The ventricular pressure-volume diagram revisited. Circ Res 43:677–687
20. Sagawa K, Maughan WL, Suga H, Sunagawa K (1988) Cardiac contraction and the pressure-volume relationship. Oxford, New York
21. Sunagawa K, Maughan WL, Burkhoff D, Sagawa K (1983) Left ventricular interaction with arterial load studied in isolated canine ventricle. Am J Physiol 245(Heart Circ Physiol 14):H773–H780

22. Sunagawa K, Sagawa K, Maughan WL (1984) Ventricular interaction with the loading system. Ann Biomed Eng 12:163–189
23. Sunagawa K, Sagawa K, Maughan WL (1986) Ventricular interaction with the vascular system. In: Yin FCP (ed) Ventricular interaction. Springer, New York, pp 210–239
24. Sunagawa K, Burkhoff D, Lim K, Sagawa K (1982) Impedance loading servo-pump system for excised canine ventricle. Am J Physiol 234(Heart Circ Physiol 12): H346–H350
25. Suga H (1979) Total mechanical energy of a ventricle model and cardiac oxygen consumption. Am J Physiol 236(Heart Circ Physiol 5):H498–H505
26. Khalafbeigui F, Suga H, Sagawa K (1979) Left ventricular systolic pressure-volume area correlates with oxygen consumption. Am J Physiol 237(Heart Circ Physiol 6):H566–H569
27. Suga H, Hayashi T, Shirahata M (1981) Ventricular systolic pressure-volume area as predictor of cardiac oxygen consumption. Am J Physiol 240(Heart Circ Physiol 9):H39–H44
28. Suga H, Yamamura Y, Nozawa T (1987) Prospective prediction of O_2 consumption from pressure volume area (PVA) in dog heart. Am J Physiol 252(Heart Circ Physiol 21):H1258–H1268
29. Burkhoff D, Yue DT, Oikawa RY, Franz MR, Schaefer J, Sagawa K (1985) Influence of contractility on ventricular oxygen consumption (abstract). Circulation 72:III–298
30. Todaka K, Sugimachi M, Sunagawa K, Ando H (1989) Do the heart and arterial system of conscious dogs operate at the optimal point in hemorrhage and volume load? (abstract) Circulation 80:II–248
31. Sugimachi M, Sunagawa K, Todaka K, Hayashida K, Noma M, Egashira S, Nose Y (1988) Ventriculo-arterial matching in conscious dogs with left ventricular dysfunction (abstract). Circulation 78:II–523
32. Kubota T, Alexander J Jr, Itaya Y, Todaka K, Sugimachi M, Sunagawa K (1990) Dynamic matching of the left ventricle with the arterial system by carotid sinus baroreflex (abstract). Circulation 82:III–695
33. Sugimachi M, Imaizumi T, Sunagawa K, Hirooka Y, Todaka K, Takeshita A, Nakamura M (1990) A new method to identify dynamic transduction properties of the aortic baroreceptors. Am J Physiol 258(Heart Circ Physiol 27):H887–H895
34. Suyama A, Sunagawa K, Hayashida K, Sugimachi M, Todaka K, Nose Y, Nakamura M (1988) Random exercise stress test in diagnosing effort angina. Circulation 78:825–830
35. Kubota T, Itaya R, Alexander J Jr, Todaka K, Sugimachi M, Sunagawa K (to be published) (1991) Autoregressive analysis of aortic input impedance: comparison with Fourier transform. Am J Physiol 260 (Heart Circ Physiol 29):H998–H1002
36. Jones SR, de Tombe PP, Burkhoff D, Kass D (1990) Optimization of total ventricular efficiency studied in isolated canine hearts (abstract). Circulation 82:III–695
37. Asanoi H, Sasayama S, Kameyama T (1989) Ventriculoarterial coupling in normal and failing heart in humans. Circ Res 65:483–493
38. Sasayama S, Franklin D, Ross J Jr (1977) Hyperfunction with normal inotropic state of the hypertrophied left ventricle. Am J Physiol 232(Heart Circ Physiol): H418–H422
39. Raizner AE, Chahine RA, Ishimon T, Audec M (1977) Clinical correlates of left ventricular cavity obliteration. Am J Cardiol 40:303–309

8
Coupling Between Ventricluar and Arterial Properties

Shigetake Sasayama[1], Hidetsugu Asanoi[1]

Summary. The ventricle transfers the mechanical energy of contraction to blood accumulated in the ventricular chamber to provide adequate cardiac output for peripheral perfusion and to generate adequate pressure in the ascending aorta. The ventricle is generally considered matched to a given load if it allows a maximal amount of external work against that load, while the matching between the ventricle and arterial system can also be defined from the principle of economical fuel consumption or mechanical efficiency.

Ventriculo-arterial coupling will deviate from the optimal condition through changes in elastance of either ventricle or artery. Ventricular and arterial properties are substantially modified by aging, arteriosclerosis, and hypertension together with myocardial hypertrophy.

When the ventriculo-arterial coupling is investigated in humans in terms of end-systolic elastance of the ventricle and effective input elastance of the arterial tree, it is normally set toward higher left ventricular work efficiency, whereas in patients with moderate cardiac dysfunction, this coupling is adjusted to maximize stroke work at the expense of the work efficiency. Neither the stroke work nor the work efficiency is near maximum for patients with severe cardiac dysfunction.

Key words: Aging — Arterial elastance — Arteriosclerosis — Hypertrophy — Mechanical efficiency — Myocardial oxygen consumption — Ventricular elastance

Introduction

The ventricle transfers the mechanical energy of contraction to blood accumulated in the ventricular chamber to provide adequate flow to peripheral tissues. Cardiac flow output and myocardial oxygen consumption are deter-

[1] The Second Department of Internal Medicine, Toyama Medical and Pharmaceutical University, Toyama, 930-01 Japan

mined by the interaction between the heart and arterial system, and ventricular performance is optimized when ventricular properties and arterial impedance system properties are matched [1]. The term "matching" means in engineering science the loading conditions under which a power generator yields maximum output power to the load. However, in the intact beating heart, there have been considerable disputes concerning the criteria for such optimal coupling.

Optimal Coupling Between the Heart and Arterial System

Optimization of Power

Elzinga and his associates [2–4] used anesthetized cats with open chest to investigate "matching" of ventricle and load at which no further increase in work output was allowed at a given end-diastolic volume, contractile state and prevailing heart rate. They characterized the heart by the pump function graph which inversely relates mean left ventricular pressure (Plv) and mean flow (F). They determined the apparent source resistance (Rs) as follows:

$$\bar{P}lv = \bar{P}_{max}(1 - \bar{F}^2/\bar{F}^2{}_{max}) \tag{1}$$

where $\bar{P}_{max}$ and F_{max} are the pressure axis and flow axis intercepts of the pump function graph, and

$$Rs = (\bar{P}_{max} - \bar{P}lv)/\bar{F} = \bar{F} \cdot \bar{P}_{max}/\bar{F}^2{}_{max} \tag{2}$$

They also described the arterial system by the relationship between mean aortic pressure (Pao) and mean flow from which they calculated peripheral resistance (Rp).

$$Rp(\bar{F}) = \bar{P}ao/\bar{F} \tag{3}$$

Mean external power (Wext) is defined as:

$$\bar{W}ext = \frac{1}{T}\int_0^T P(t)F(t)dt \tag{4}$$

Steady power is calculated from mean values of either aortic (Waost) or left ventricular (Wlvst) pressure and flow:

$$Waost = \bar{P}ao \cdot \bar{F} \tag{5}$$

$$Wlvst = \bar{P}lv \cdot \bar{F} \tag{6}$$

From Eqs. (1) and (6)

$$Wlvst(\bar{F}) = \bar{P}_{max} \cdot (\bar{F} - \bar{F}^3/\bar{F}^2{}_{max}) \tag{7}$$

Figure 1 shows an example of the fit of the curve described from Eq. (7) using the same values of P_{max} and F_{max} to the actual left ventricular steady power data.

Maximal left ventricular power is obtained when the derivative of Eq. (7) with respect to mean flow is zero:

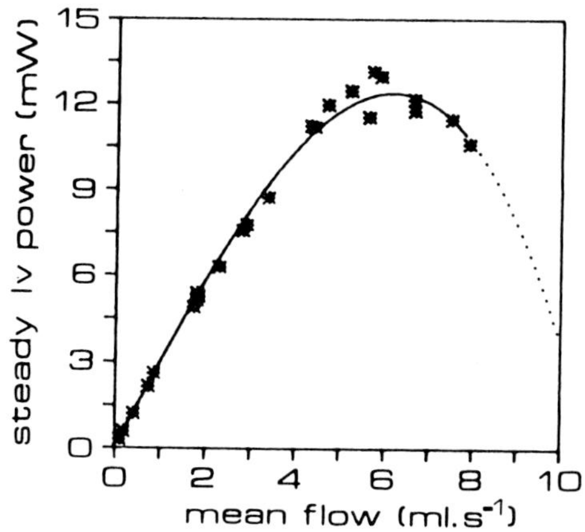

Fig. 1. Left ventricular steady power derived as a function of mean flow. (From [4] with permission)

$$d[Wlvst(\bar{F})]/d\bar{F} = \bar{P}_{max} \cdot (1 - 3\bar{F}^2/\bar{F}^2{}_{max}) = 0 \tag{8}$$

Optimal left ventricular power and the mean flow value (reached for flow Fw_{max}) is:

$$\bar{F}w_{max} = \bar{F}_{max}/\sqrt{3} \tag{9}$$

Figure 2 shows a pump function graph from nine experiments carried out by van den Horn et al. [4]. The working point is indicated by $\bar{W}$ and the mean flow value for which external power transfer by the heart would be optimal (Fw_{max}) is indicated by the dotted lines. van den Horn et al. [4] showed that optimal power is transferred when the ratio of peripheral and apparent source resistance equals twice the ratio of mean aortic and mean left ventricular pressure. The power optimum and the working point were shown to coincide, and they concluded that under normal conditions, the heart operates at optimal external power.

Optimization of Stroke Work

The ventricle is generally considered matched to a given load if it allows a maximal amount of external work against that load. Sunagawa et al. [5, 6] proposed the framework for coupling of the ventricle with arterial load by modeling the left ventricle as an elastic chamber which periodically increases its volume elastance to a value equal to the slope of the linear end-systolic pressure-volume relation, and the arterial load property as an effective arterial elastance represented by the slope of the arterial end-systolic pressure-stroke volume relation (Ea). The left ventricular end-systolic pressure (Pes)-volume (Ves) relation is approximately linear over a physiologic range, with slope Ees and constant volume axis Vo. The Ees varies in response to changes in ventricular contractility. According to this relationship, the end-systolic pressure (Pes) varies inversely with stroke volume (SV) for a given end-diastolic volume (Ved):

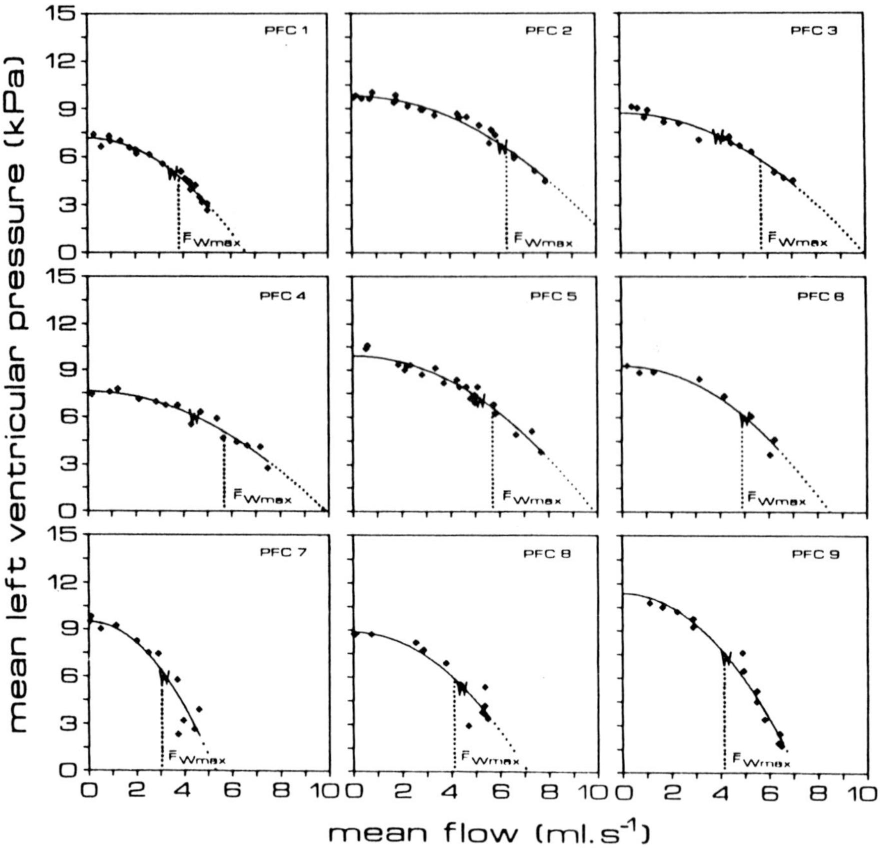

Fig. 2. Pump function graphs obtained from experiments in nine cats. *W*, working point; *dotted lines*, the mean flow value at optimal left ventricular steady power. (From [4] with permission)

$$\begin{aligned} \text{Pes} &= \text{Ees(Ved} - \text{SV} - \text{Vo)} \\ &= \text{Ees(Ves} - \text{Vo)} \end{aligned} \tag{10}$$

Arterial system properties can be expressed by a Pes-SV relationship, and the SV can be given analytically as follows:

$$\text{Pes} = \text{EaSV} \tag{11}$$

$$\text{SV} = (\text{Ved} - \text{Vo})/(1 + \text{Ea/Ees}) \tag{12}$$

Assuming that the time-averaged ventricular ejection pressure is close to Pes, ventricular stroke work (SW) can be derived as follows:

$$\begin{aligned} \text{SW} &= \text{SV} \times \text{Pes} \\ &= \text{Ees(Ved} - \text{Vo)}^2[(\text{Ea/Ees})/(1 + \text{Ea/Ees})^2] \end{aligned} \tag{13}$$

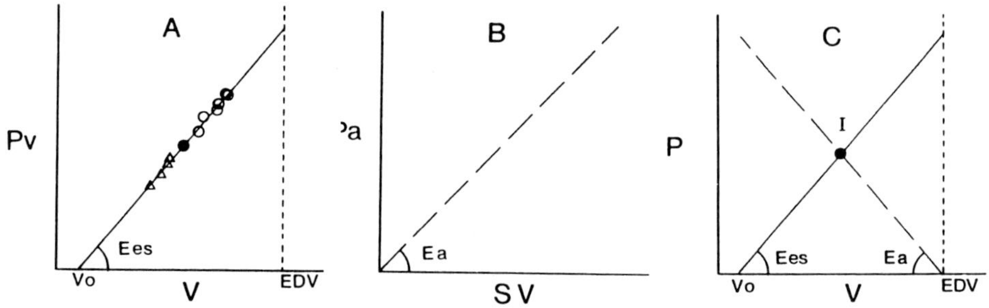

Fig. 3. The framework of analysis for coupling the ventricle with the arterial load. *Pv*, left ventricular end-systolic pressure; *V*, left ventricular volume; *Pa*, arterial end-systolic pressure; *SV*, stroke volume; *Ees* and *Vo*, slope and volume axis intercept of ventricular end-systolic pressure-volume relation; *Ea*, slope of arterial end-systolic pressure-stroke volume relation; *EDV*, end-diastolic volume. The Pa-V relation can be superimposed on the Pv-V relation in the same pressure (P)-V plane with the equilibrium end-systolic pressure and volume at the intersection (*I*) between these two P-V relation lines. (From [7] with permission)

The interaction between the ventricular and arterial Pes-SV relation is shown diagramatically in Fig. 3 [7]. Equation (11) indicates that the greater the SV ejected into the arterial system, the greater is the generated Pes. This relation can be superimposed on the ventricular end-systolic pressure-volume relationship by simply reversing the volume axis so that the SV is plotted with zero reference to some specified end-diastolic volume. The stroke volume that the ventricle can eject from a given Ved can be obtained from the intersection of these two end-systolic pressure-volume relations. Within the framework of this coupling concept, Sunagawa et al. [5, 6] demonstrated that the ventricle does maximal external work to the arterial load when the ventricular and arterial elastances are equalized. An increase in Ved induced rightward shift of the arterial Pes-SV relation without a change in the ventricular Pes-Ves relation, and therefore the optimal loading was achieved with the same arterial elastance value. Enhancement of contractility was associated with an increase in the slope of the ventricular Pes-Ves relation together with an increase in the arterial elastance by increasing arterial resistance to similar extents. Therefore, a graphical coupling has been shown to be useful in understanding the major mechanisms determining SV, and under various loading conditions and different inotropic states, the ratio of the optimal effective arterial elastance to the given ventricular elastance remained nearly unity.

Optimization of Ventricular Efficiency

Another criterion for optimal coupling between an energy source and its load is the principle of economical fuel consumption or mechanical efficiency, which is defined as the ratio of stroke work to myocardial oxygen consumption per beat [8–10]. Burkhoff and Sagawa [8] derived a simple analytic model that relates the properties of the vascular system and the left ventricle to the mechanical work done by the heart and the amount of chemical energy consumed by the heart.

Recently Suga and colleagues [11, 12] have demonstrated that the total mechanical work performed by the ventricle with each cardiac cycle can be estimated by the pressure-volume area (PVA) defined as the sum of the external stroke work and the unexpressed mechanical potential energy stored in the ventricle at the end of ejection (PE):

$$\mathrm{PE} = \mathrm{Pes}(\mathrm{Ves} - \mathrm{Vo})/2 \tag{14}$$

Substituting Eqs. (10) and (12) into Eq. (14), PE can be expressed as

$$\mathrm{PE} = \mathrm{Ees}(\mathrm{Ved} - \mathrm{Vo})^2[(\mathrm{Ea}/\mathrm{Ees})^2/2]/(1 + \mathrm{Ea}/\mathrm{Ees})^2 \tag{15}$$

PVA is the sum of SW and PE, therefore it is approximated by

$$\mathrm{PVA} = \mathrm{Ees}(\mathrm{Ved} - \mathrm{Vo})^2[(\mathrm{Ea}/\mathrm{Ees})/(1 + \mathrm{Ea}/\mathrm{Ees})^2][1 + (\mathrm{Ea}/\mathrm{Ees})/2] \tag{16}$$

According to the linear relation between PVA and myocardial oxygen consumption (MVO_2),

$$\mathrm{MVO}_2 = A[\mathrm{PVA}] + B \tag{17}$$

Ventricular efficiency (Eff) is, by definition, the ratio between external SW and MVO_2. Accordingly, the following analytic equation is obtained by combining Eqs. (13), (16), and (17).

$$\mathrm{Eff} = 1/[A(1 + \mathrm{Ea}/2\mathrm{Ees}) + B(1 + \mathrm{Ea}/\mathrm{Ees})^2/\mathrm{Ea}(\mathrm{Ved} - \mathrm{Vo})^2] \tag{18}$$

Figure 4 shows an example of the predictions of equations (13), (17), and (18), in which SW, MVO_2 and efficiency are plotted as a function of effective arterial elastance (Ea) [8].

With increases in Ea, SW initially increases, reaches a plateau and then decreases. As shown by Sunagawa [6], the maximum SW occurs when arterial and ventricular properties are equalized. This matched condition is indicated by the dashed line at Ea = 7 mmHg/ml.

Ventricular efficiency (defined as the ratio between external SW and MVO_2) initially rises with increases in Ea, reaches a maximum and then decreases. Optimum efficiency occurs when Ea is less than Ees (at Ea = 3.4 in this case) as indicated by the dotted lines. Therefore, with this model analysis, Burkhoff and Sagawa [8] demonstrated that SW is maximum when Ea equals Ees, but the afterload that results in the greatest efficiency is always less than that which provides the maximum SW. They suggested that cardiovascular properties are set more toward optimization of ventricular efficiency than stroke work under physiological conditions.

Ventriculo-arterial Coupling in the Human Heart

We have extended this concept of ventriculo-arterial interaction for the first time in a study on humans and evaluated physiological matching of cardiac

Fig. 4. Relation between arterial elastance (*Ea*) and (**a**) stroke work (*SW*), (**b**) myocardial oxygen consumption (MVO_2) and (**c**) ventricular efficiency derived from an analytic model. (From [8] with permission)

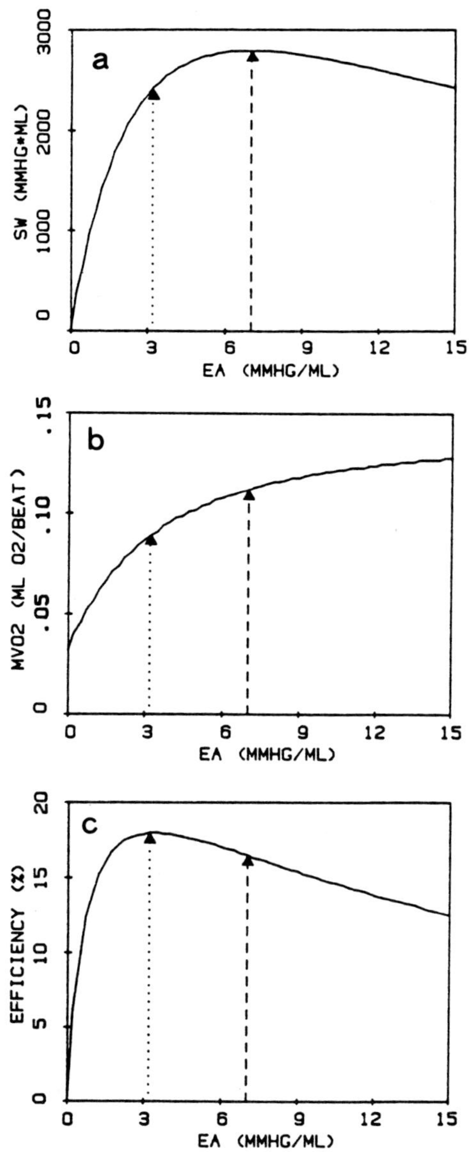

performance with arterial load in terms of the above mentioned ventricular and arterial volume elastance [7].

Eight normal subjects with no symptoms and signs of cardiac disease, four patients with atypical chest pain, and 16 patients with cardiac dysfunction formed the study group. All patients had supporting clinical, chest radiographic, and echocardiographic evidences of impaired left ventricular function. Severity of cardiac disease ranged from class II to class III by the New York Heart Association functional classification.

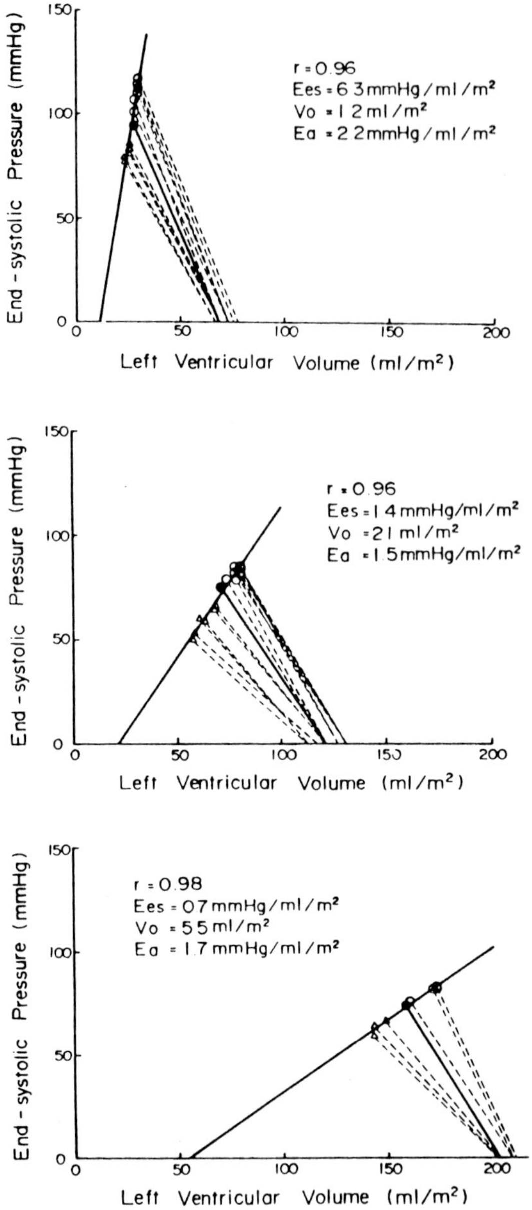

Fig. 5. Left ventricular end-systolic pressure-volume relation and arterial end-systolic pressure-stroke volume relation in three representative cases with normal (*top*), mildly depressed (middle) and severely depressed ventricle (*bottom*). *Ees*, slope; *Vo*, volume axis intercept of ventricular end-systolic pressure-volume relation; *Ea*, slope of arterial end-systolic pressure-stroke volume relation. (From [7] with permission)

Subjects were divided into three groups based on their resting left ventricular ejection fraction (EF). Group A consisted of 12 subjects with a left ventricular EF of 60% or more. Group B consisted of seven patients with mild left ventricular dysfunction in whom EF was 40%–59%. Group C consisted of nine patients with more marked left ventricular dysfunction in whom EF was less than 40%.

A 19-gauge cannula was inserted percutaneously into a brachial artery and connected to a strain-gauge manometer. After control recordings at rest, the systolic pressure was changed by about 40 mmHg by intravenous infusion of phenylephrine and nitroprusside. Two-dimensional targeted M-mode echocardiograms of the left ventricular cavity were recorded simultaneously with arterial pressure. Left ventricular volume was determined using the formula proposed by Teichholz et al. [13]. Left ventricular end-systolic pressure was approximated from the arterial dicrotic pressure, which is considered to be caused by aortic valve closure.

Left ventricular contractile properties were again defined by the slope of the end-systolic pressure-volume relation Ees and Vo. Similarly, the properties of the arterial system were defined by Ea. SW was calculated as Pes(Ved − Ves). Pes and Ves are the graphically determined data points at which two end-systolic pressure-volume relation lines intersect with each other. We studied the ratio of SW to the systolic pressure-volume area (PVA), which has been defined as the total mechanical energy of ejecting contraction.

Figure 5 shows representative ventricular Pes-Ves relationship and arterial Pes-SV relationships at baseline (solid line) and after pressure manipulation (dashed line) for patients in groups A, B and C. Linear relationships between corresponding end-systolic pressure and volume are observed in these patients.

Ees was 4.5 mmHg/ml/m^2 in group A, and this value substantially decreased as the heart failed, to 2.5 mmHg/ml/m^2 in group B and 1.5 mmHg/ml/m^2 in group C. With a reduction of ejection fraction, Ved and Vo were progressively augmented and Ea tended to increase. In group A, Ea/Ees was 0.50, Ea tended to increase, and Ees was nearly twice as much as Ea. In group B, Ea/Ees was 0.97 and Ees was nearly equal to Ea, while in group C, Ea/Ees increased to 2.29 and Ees was far less than Ea (Fig. 6).

Pump efficiency is highest in group A (82 ± 5%) and progressively fell with a reduction of ejection fraction to 69 ± 5% in group B and 50 ± 10% in group C (Fig. 7). SW is near its maximum in group B patients with moderate cardiac failure, with the ventricle providing a maximal transfer of mechanical energy of contraction to the arterial system (Fig. 7).

Thus, the normal coupling condition in group A is surprisingly similar to the data of Burkhoff and Sagawa [8], and cardiovascular interaction in normal subjects appears to be set to optimize left ventricular work efficiency in the resting state. The moderately depressed hearts maximize SW as demonstrated by Sunagawa [5, 6] but they generate a greater potential energy with resultant reduction in work efficiency. Severely depressed hearts are no longer capable of maintaining SW or work efficiency properly.

Mechanisms

The nature of the error detector for the ventriculo-arterial coupling described above is unclear. Despite the distinctive difference between normal and variably depressed ventricles in terms of the matching concept, it was surprising that arterial pressure was appropriately maintained in all patients [14]. There-

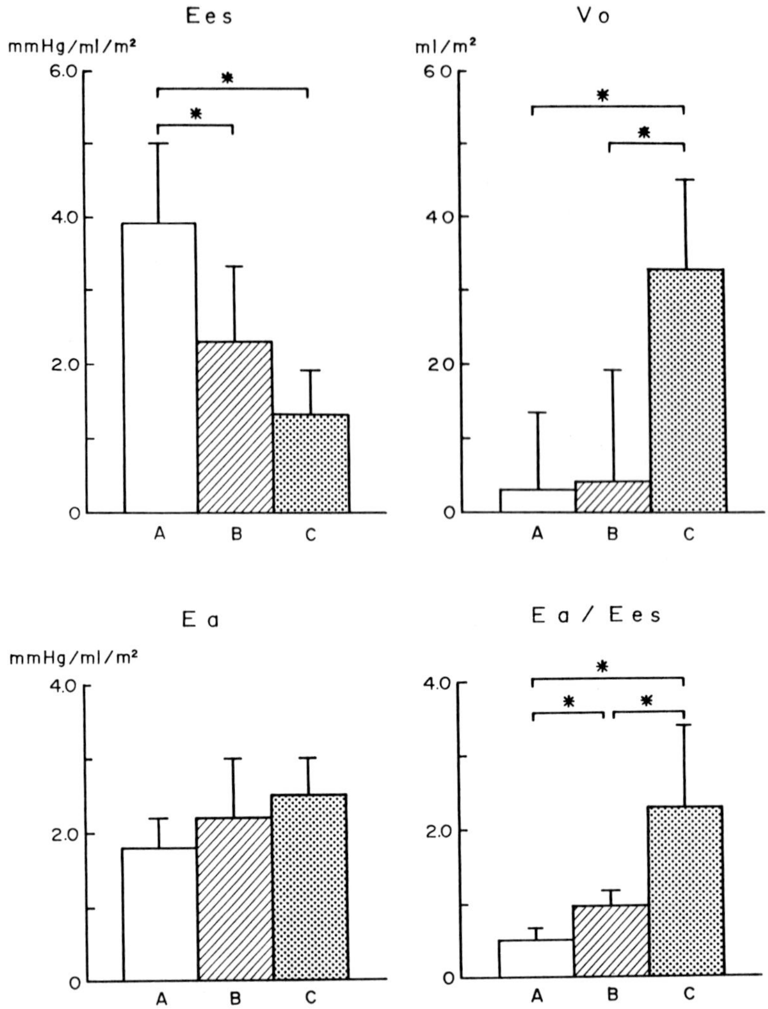

Fig. 6. Group mean values for slope (*Ees*) and volume axis intercept (*Vo*) of left ventricular end-systolic pressure-volume relation, slope of arterial end-systolic pressure-stroke volume relation (*Ea*) and Ea to Ees ratio for subjects with normal (*A*), mildly depressed (*B*) and severely depressed ventricle (*C*). *, $P < 0.05$

fore, we postulated that the body senses the arterial pressure and modulates coupling conditions to maintain the arterial pressure. This is achieved in heart failure by an increase in systemic resistance mediated in part by a greatly increased activity of the sympathetic nervous system. To test this, we assessed the autonomic regulation of ventriculo-arterial coupling in conscious dogs.

The dogs were chronically instrumented with a high-fidelity micromanometer and a conductance catheter. This experimental model permitted the analysis of the left ventricular pressure (P)-volume (V) relation on a beat-to-beat basis.

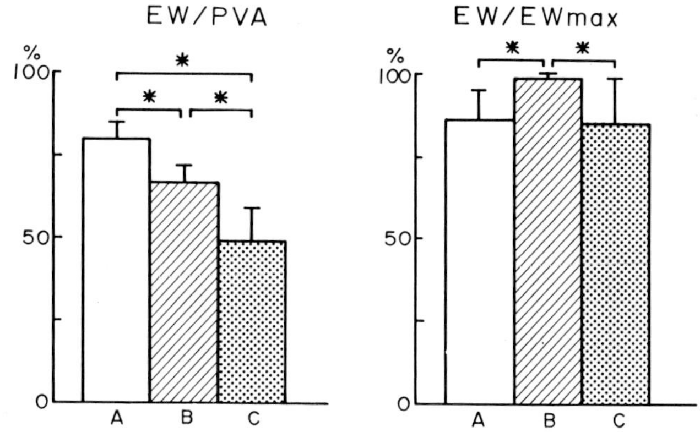

Fig. 7. Group mean values for left ventricular pump efficiency expressed as the ratio of external work to pressure volume area (*EW/PVA*) and the ratio of actual external work to the maximal external work obtainable if Ea were equal to Ees (EW/EW_{max}). Subjects with normal (*A*), mildly depressed (*B*) and severely depressed ventricle (*C*). *, $P < 0.05$

All the experiments were carried out in the conscious state with an intact autonomic nervous system [15].

When venous return was transiently interrupted by inflating the pneumatic cuffs placed around the venae cavae, peak left ventricular pressure gradually reduced. In the resting state and for several cardiac cycles during this pressure change, the slope of the LV end-systolic pressure-volume relation (Ees) was analyzed from superimposed PV loops. The slope of the arterial end-systolic pressure-stroke volume relation (Ea) was also determined in the same manner as mentioned before. In conscious dogs with an intact autonomic reflex, the Ea/Ees ratio was 1.4.

Nitroprusside was then slowly infused to provoke reflex activation of sympathetic nervous system. This resulted in a substantial reduction of end-systolic pressure associated with an increase in heart rate. Ees was augmented by 42% without any significant change in Ea, and the Ea/Ees ratio decreased accordingly to 0.8 (Fig. 8).

When the autonomic nervous system was blocked completely with atropine and hexamethonium, Ees became nearly equal to Ea, resulting in an Ea/Ees ratio of 0.9. Nitroprusside infusion under autonomic blockade reduced arterial blood pressure to the same extent, but the Ea/Ees ratio remained unchanged (Ea/Ees = 0.9). These findings indicate that when neural control of the cardiovascular system is abolished, ventricular and arterial properties are so matched as to maximize stroke work at the expense of the work efficiency. However, impaired autonomic regulation of the blood pressure will lead to a failure to perfuse the tissues adequately.

The body appears to monitor the adequacy of tissue perfusion, and the resting human's matching of the ventricular properties with arterial load pro-

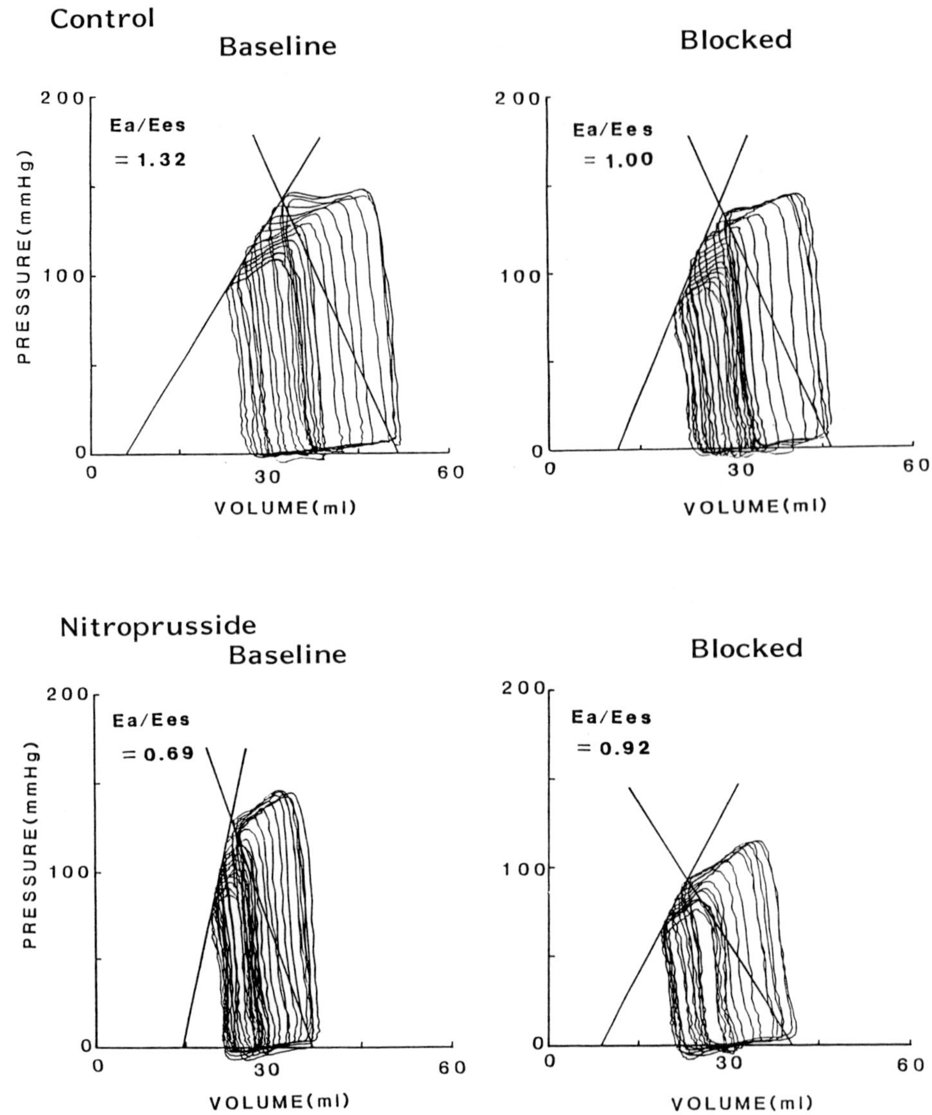

Fig. 8. Left ventricular end-systolic pressure-volume relation and arterial end-systolic pressure-stroke volume relation and their ratio (*Ea/Ees*) recorded by micro-manometer and conductance catheter in the conscious dog. Data were obtained at autonomically intact baseline (*left*) and after autonomically blocked states (*right*) in the control (*above*) and during nitroprusside infusion (*below*)

perties is set to maintain adequate blood pressure under autonomic regulation through the basoreflex arc and from higher centers.

Effect of Vasodilator Therapy on Ventriculo-arterial Coupling

There is ample evidence that vasodilator therapy corrects afterload mismatch and augments stroke volume in the failing heart. Most afterload reducing agents have little or no direct effect on cardiac contractility. If mixed venous and arteriolar dilators are employed, there is usually an accompanying reduction in mean circulatory pressure and venous return. Thus, the resultant decrease in end-diastolic volume attenuates the magnitude of augmentation of cardiac output along with the decrease in adjustment through the Frank-Starling mechanism [16]. The proposed coupling concept provides a convenient framework for the evaluation of the specific roles of preload and afterload in determining the stroke volume during infusion of nitroprusside.

In 13 patients with moderate congestive heart failure (ejection fraction 32 ± 3%), a left ventricular echocardiogram was obtained with simultaneous recordings of direct arterial pressure. Infusion of nitroprusside produced a 9% reduction in end-diastolic volume with unaltered stroke volume and an 18% fall in end-systolic pressure. In order to separate the pure preload effect from this balanced action of the drug on the arteriolar and venous beds, we applied a negative pressure chamber on the lower half of the body which produced the desired decrease in end-diastolic volume by regulating venous return. Using lower body negative pressure (LBNP), an equivalent reduction in end-diastolic volume (−8%) was produced in the same patients. End-systolic pressure was maintained unchanged but stroke volume substantially decreased (−22%). Changes in end-diastolic volume or pressure did not alter the slope of the end-systolic pressure-volume relationship (Ees), while the arterial elastance value (Ea) achieved considerable changes (being decreased by decreasing afterload and increased by decreasing preload) to meet the stroke volume. The ratio of Ea to Ees (Ea/Ees) fell by nitroprusside (−26%) and rose by LBNP (+21%). Both nitroprusside and LBNP decreased external stroke work (EW) (−16% and −28%, respectively). This effect may be mediated primarily by a decrease in left ventricular end-systolic pressure with the former and by a decrease in stroke volume with the latter. Accordingly, work efficiency of the ventricle expressed as the ratio of EW to pressure volume area was significantly augmented (by 12%) by nitroprusside, while it was decreased by LBNP (−9%). Thus, we concluded that vasodilator therapy restored the more optimal ventriculo-arterial coupling in patients with congestive heart failure. This response was mediated largely by a reduction in afterload rather than preload (Fig. 9) [17].

The capability of vasodilators to optimize stroke work or mechanical efficiency apparently depends on the baseline inotropic state for each patient. If we assume that ventricular contractility remains unchanged with vasodilators, efficiency is always maximized at a lower level of end-systolic pressure than the pressure necessary for external work to be maximized. Therefore, a severely

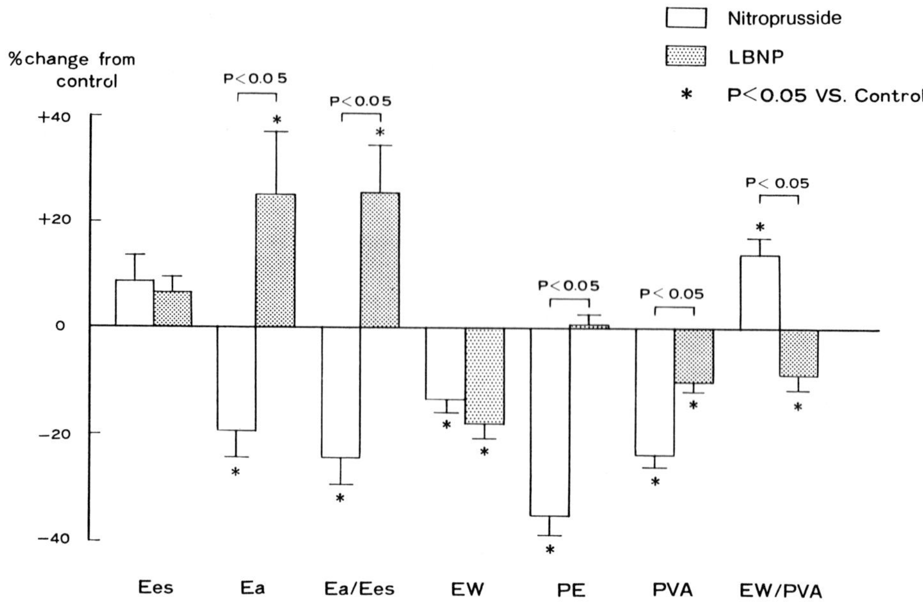

Fig. 9. Effect of nitroprusside (*open bars*) and comparable reduction of preload by applying lower body negative pressure (*shaded bars*) on the slope of the ventricular end-systolic pressure-volume relation (*Ees*), the slope of the arterial end-systolic pressure-stroke volume relation (*Ea*), *Ea*/*Ees* ratio, left ventricular external work (*EW*), potential energy (*PE*), pressure-volume area (*PVA*), and left ventricular pump efficiency (*EW*/*PVA*). With a similar reduction in preload, *Ea* decreased with nitroprusside, while it increased with lower body negative pressure. The *Ea*/*Ees* ratio also changed in the same direction because *Ees* remained unchanged by both maneuvers and pump efficiency was augmented only by nitroprusside. (From [17] with permission)

depressed heart cannot maintain adequate systemic circulation at a level of arterial pressure at optimal efficiency. On the other hand, in a patient with less compromised cardiac function whose ventricular contractility is nearly equal to arterial input impedance, optimal efficiency can be attained by afterload reduction without deterioration of systemic circulation. This concept may provide a rational basis for preventive use of vasodilator agents in patients with symptomatic cardiac dysfunction (Fig. 10).

Effects of Inotropic Stimulation on Ventriculo-arterial Coupling

The failing heart is unable to meet the demands for blood flow, and treatment is directed to recruit the energetic reserve of the heart most efficiently and economically to restore normal circulation.

With the proposed coupling concept, we also evaluated the specific roles of contractility change in determining the stroke volume in nine patients with heart failure (ejection fraction 33 ± 11) [18]. To determine the end-systolic

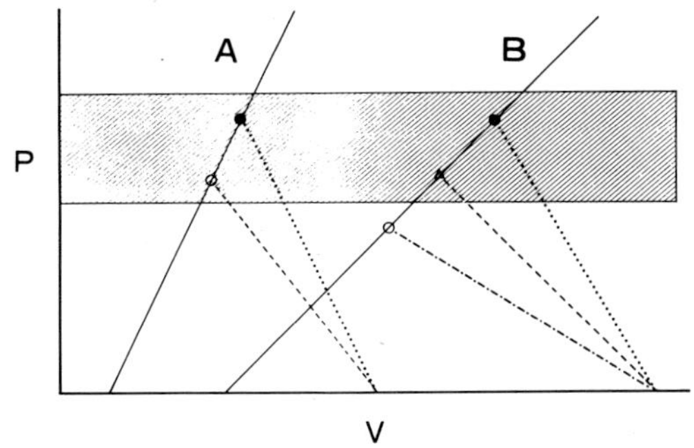

Fig. 10. Effects of afterload reduction on ventriculo-arterial coupling. *Shaded area* represents the normal range of arterial pressure. In patients with mildly depressed ventricular function (*A*), the Ea/Ees ratio is nearly one in the baseline state (*solid circle*). This ratio equals the ratio which optimizes the external stroke work (*open triangle*). With afterload reduction, ventricular efficiency is augmented within the normal range of systemic pressure (*open circle*). In patients with severely depressed ventricular function (*B*), Ea is always greater than Ees in the baseline state (*solid circle*) with smaller stroke work than when Ea is equal to Ees (*open triangle*). Afterload reduction achieves maximal stroke work for a given contractility and preload but cannot maintain the level of arterial pressure which optimizes pump efficiency. (From [17] with permission)

pressure-volume relationship, linear regression analysis was applied to several data points collected under varying afterloads induced by phenylephrine or nitroprusside. In the resting state, the Ea/Ees ratio was 1.4. With dobutamine, the left ventricular end-systolic volume significantly decreased (−20%) and Ees increased by 44% when the volume intercept (Vo) of the end-systolic pressure volume relation remained unchanged. When the ejection preceded at a constant pressure, the slope of the arterial end-systolic pressure volume relation (Ea) decreased (−22%) (Fig. 11). Thus, the ratio of Ea/Ees was reduced to 0.8, indicating that the heart achieved higher work efficiency by generating a smaller potential energy relative to the external work. The mechanical efficiency is the product of work efficiency (SW/PVA) and PVA/myocardial oxygen consumption (MVO_2). Inotropic intervention shifts up the linear relationship between PVA and MVO_2 without changing the slope [11]. This non-zero positive intercept for PVA = 0 is assumed to represent the oxygen consumption for basal metabolism and for activation of the contractile machinery. Consequently, with the enhanced contractile state, PVA/MVO_2 is reduced for a given PVA, which reduces the increase in mechanical efficiency relative to the extent of the increase in SW/PVA. Taking all of these factors into account, we concluded that an enhancement of the inotropic state adjusts the ventriculo-arterial coupling toward optimizing ventricular work efficiency.

Exercise stress also increases cardiac contractility by excessive sympathetic stimulation [19]. The cardiovascular system can adjust to a moderate degree of exercise sufficiently to supply oxygen to working muscle. When oxygen avail-

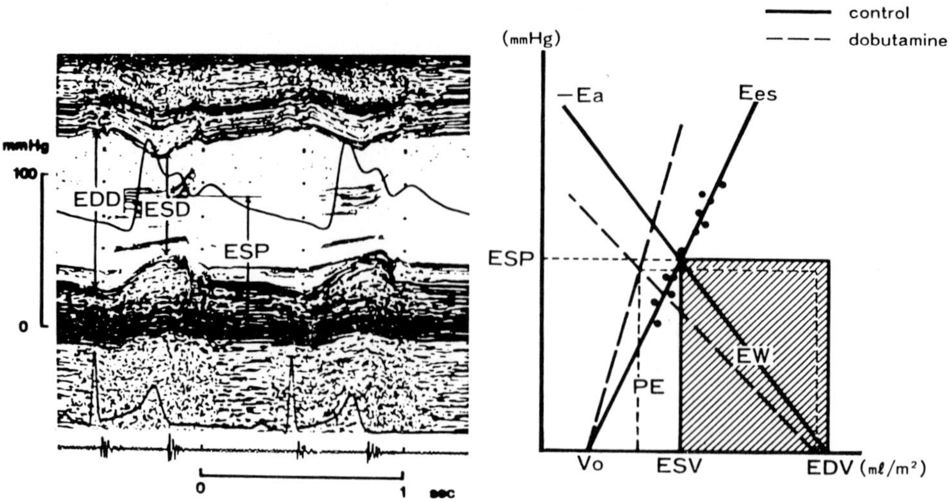

Fig. 11. Changes in ventriculo-arterial coupling by increasing contractility with dobutamine. *Left* End-systolic pressure-volume relation was obtained by simultaneous recordings of direct arterial pressure and left ventricular M-mode echocardiogram. *EDD*, end-diastolic dimension; *ESD*, end-systolic dimension; *ESP*, end-systolic pressure; *Right Shaded area* represents external work (*EW*). Augmented contractility is indicated by an increase in Ees and a decrease in Ea (*dotted lines*). Therefore pump efficiency defined as the ratio of *EW* to pressure volume area is substantially augmented. *PE*, potential energy; *ESV*, end-systolic volume; *EDV*, end-diastolic volume. (From [18] with permission)

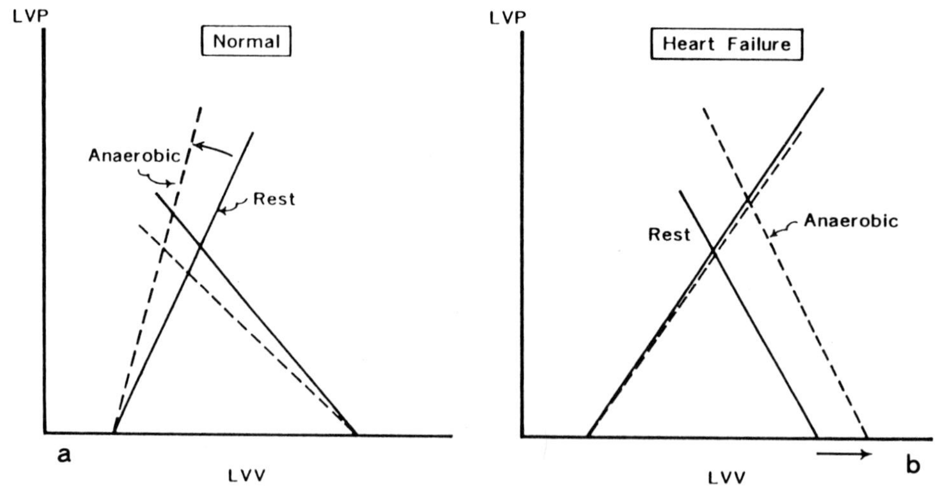

Fig. 12. Schematic representation of ventriculo-arterial coupling at rest (*solid line*) and during anaerobic exercise (*dashed line*) in the normal (**a**) and failing heart (**b**). In the normal heart, stroke volume is augmented from essentially unchanged end-diastolic volume by enhanced contractility, with a resultant increase in Ees and a decrease in Ea. In contrast, in the failing heart, an increase in stroke volume during anaerobic exercise is mediated by an increase in preload without detectable changes in Ees and Ea. *LVP*, left ventricular pressure; *LVV*, left ventricular volume; *Ees*, ventricular end-systolic elastance; *Ea*, arterial elastance

ability to the tissues becomes inadequate with more strenuous exercise, the anaerobic threshold is reached.

In normal subjects, stroke volume increases during exercise, either due to an increase in preload or an increase in the contractile state. Though the preload effect is more important during low levels of exercise, the contractility change comes into play at high levels of exercise, leading to a reduction in the left ventricular end-systolic dimension. This response is represented by an increase in Ees and a decrease in Ea, and therefore mechanical efficiency has been markedly augmented (Fig. 12, left panel).

In patients with severe cardiac dysfunction, stroke volume is generally augmented during anaerobic exercise by an increase in end-diastolic volume rather than a decrease in end-systolic volume. Ees and Ea remained unchanged both during aerobic and anaerobic exercise (Fig. 12, right panel). The failure of Ees to rise during anaerobic exercise despite an excessive sympathetic stimulation is a result of reduced contractile reserve in these hearts. Thus, in advanced heart failure, the regulation of stroke volume during exercise shifts from a catecholamine-mediated reduction in end-systolic volume to a greater reliance on the Frank-Starling mechanism [20].

Effect of Hypertrophy on Ventricular Elastance

Ventricular and arterial load interaction is greatly modified if arterial properties are so altered that mean aortic systolic pressure is increased and mean diastolic pressure is reduced in relation to mean pressure throughout the cardiac cycle. Increases in the steady-state and/or pulsatile components of vascular load lead to ventricular hypertrophy.

Shroff et al. [21] compared the effects of myocardial hypertrophy on performance of the ventricle coupled to the arterial loading using 25-week-old, spontaneously hypertensive rats (SHR) and matched controls of Wistar-Kyoto rats (WKY). They recorded LV pressure and aortic flow for steady state ejection beats followed by an isovolumic beat obtained by transient occlusion of the ascending aorta in diastole, and calculated ventricular elastance E(t), and resistance R(Po), using the following equation [22]:

$$E(t)[V(t) - Vd] - R(Po)\dot{V}(t) = P(t) \tag{19}$$

where P(t), V(t), $\dot{V}(t)$ and Vd are instantaneous ventricular pressure, volume, flow and absolute residual volume, respectively. Volume ejected up to the time t[Ve(t)] is calculated as

$$Ve(t) = \int_0^t \dot{V}(t)dt \tag{20}$$

Therefore Eq. (19) can be rewritten as

$$A\,Po(t)Ve(t) + B\,Po(t)[1 - A\,Ve(t)]\dot{V}(t) = Po(t) - P(t) \tag{21}$$

where Po(t) = isovolumetric pressure

$$APo(t) = E(t)$$
$$A = 1/(\text{end-diastolic volume} - Vd)$$
$$BPo(t)\,[1 - AVe(t)] = R(Po)$$

Therefore, E(t) and R(Po) are obtained from *A* and *B* calculated using the least square parameter estimation technique.

From this analysis, Shroff et al. [20] documented that the maximum elastance (Ees) was 1100 ± 163 mmHg/ml in SHR and 577 ± 88 mmHg/ml in WKY. The higher ventricular elastance in SHR was accounted for by the increased left ventricular muscle mass (916 ± 69 in SHR, and 571 ± 49 mg in WKY). Therefore, when Ees was normalized by LV mass, this difference was shown to be greatly attenuated (1.19 ± 0.12 mmHg/ml mg for SHR and 1.01 ± 0.13 mmHg/ml mg for WKY).

Previously, we assessed the end-systolic pressure volume relation in the hypertrophied ventricle in patients with systemic hypertension [23]. The study groups consisted of ten normal subjects and 15 hypertensive patients. Left ventricular echocardiograms were obtained, together with simultaneous measurement of brachial arterial pressure by direct puncture. Systolic arterial pressure averaged 119 mmHg in the control group, and 183 mmHg in the hypertensive group. Posterior wall thickness at end-diastole averaged 0.7 cm in the normal subjects, and 1.1 cm in hypertensive patients with a 53% increase in the cross-sectional area of the LV wall over the normal value. There was no difference in mean circumferential shortening velocity (VCF) in these groups. In the normal group, following the recording at the basal state, methoxamine was given intravenously to elevate the peak systolic pressure by about 30% over the control value. In the hypertensive group, nitroprusside was slowly infused until the peak arterial pressure was decreased to the levels matching the control pressure in the normal group.

The left panel of Fig. 13 shows the plots of end-systolic points in each subject throughout the course of afterload change. Each response for a given patient was connected by a solid line. The pressure-diameter relation at the end of ejection obtained during a single pressure elevation in each individual forms a linear relation. The left ventricular diameter was significantly less at each matched level of systolic pressure in the hypertensive group as compared to normal controls. Thus, the pressure-diameter relation at end-systole was clearly shifted to the left of those in the normal group with a steeper slope (81.9 ± 10.1 vs. 114.2 ± 25.2 mmHg/cm, $P < 0.001$).

We then calculated wall stress (WSt) by the equation

$$\begin{aligned} WSt &= PRi^2/(Ro^2 - Ri^2) \\ &= PD/4h(D + h) \end{aligned} \qquad (22)$$

where P is peak arterial pressure, Ri is LV internal radius, Ro is LV external radius, D is LV diameter measured by echocardiography and h is LV wall thickness. This is an exact expression for the average meridional wall stress which may be defined as the force per unit area acting at the equatorial plane of the ventricle in the direction of the apex-to-base axis. This method of wall

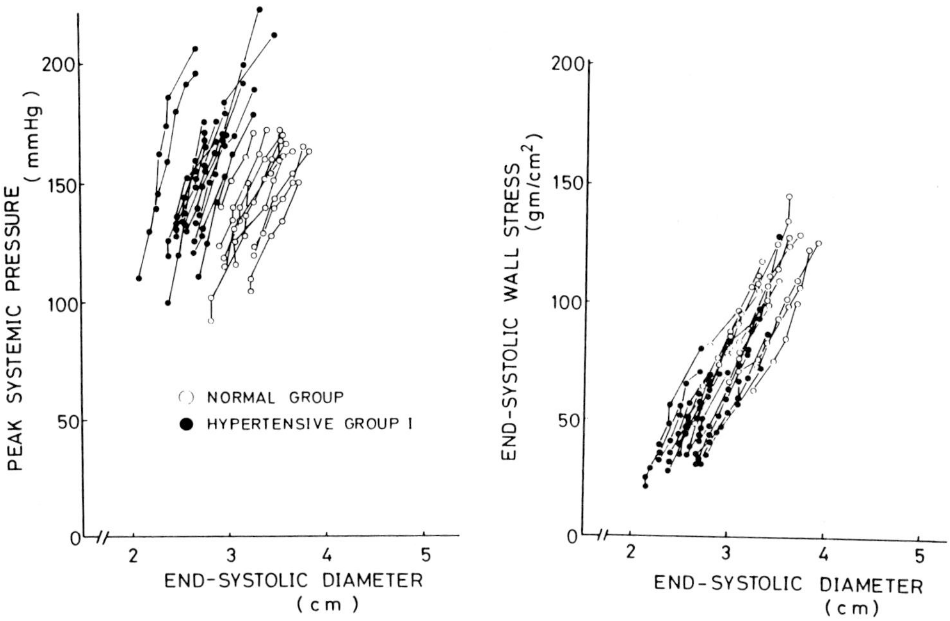

Fig. 13. Relations between peak arterial pressure (*left*) or end-systolic wall stress (*right*) and left ventricular end-systolic diameter in normal subjects (*open circle*) and the hypertensive patients with moderate hypertrophy (*solid circle*). (From [23] with permission)

stress calculation has the advantage that the expression is independent of the long axis of the chamber. End-systolic wall stress was approximated with data on the dimension at end-systole and peak arterial pressure, which was based on the assumption that during normal contraction, changes in peak arterial systolic pressure generally reflect similar changes in LV systolic pressure and that peak systolic pressure is sustained until the end of ventricular ejection. Although the cause has not been determined, the pulse wave clearly undergoes several characteristic transformations as it traverses to the periphery, and peak systolic pressure in the brachial artery usually exceeds that in the central aorta. Nevertheless, a comparison of relative changes in peak systolic pressure can be made from the peripheral arterial pressure pulse so long as these changes are measured in a consistent fashion.

The right panel of Fig. 13 shows the end-systolic wall stress-diameter relation in the same series of beats as the pressure-diameter relation. End-systolic wall stress was significantly less in the hypertrophied group at the same pressure levels than in the normal group, as a consequence of the smaller end-systolic chamber size together with increased wall thickness due to hypertrophy. Therefore, wall stress-diameter relations at end ejection of the hypertrophied ventricle overlap those in the normal group. These data emphasized that the moderately hypertrophied ventricle exhibited hyperfunction as a pump (increase in ventricular elastance) but it does not appear to result in an intrinsic change in the properties of the ventricular myocardium.

In Shroff's study [20], though the cardiac indexes of SHR and WKY were similar, the slope of the resistance-isovolumetric pressure relation (B) was shown to be higher in SHR (0.206 ± 0.034 sec/ml) than in WKY (0.096 ± 0.018 sec/ml), indicating that the extrapolated maximum flow, V_{max}, ($1/B$) was significantly reduced for SHR. Therefore, they hypothesized that increased Ees and reduced V_{max} counteract and preserve pump function in compensated hypertrophy. They presumed that if ventricular resistance continued to increase without a proportional increase in Ees, cardiac failure would result.

Gunther and Grossman [24] observed a close inverse correlation between midwall circumferential wall stress and ejection fraction in 14 patients with aortic stenosis and various degrees of left ventricular failure.

In these patients, normal values for ejection fraction are associated with normal levels of wall stress, while increasing levels of wall stress are associated with decreasing values for ejection fraction. Values for normal controls fall on or near the regression line for the aortic stenosis group. Thus, they concluded that the intrinsic contractility of hypertrophied myocardium is not necessarily depressed and poor cardiac performance in some patients with pressure overloading may be due to inadequate hypertrophy rather than to depression of myocardial contractility.

The stress-diameter relation in a severely hypertensive group with a marked increase in wall thickness, however, was clearly shifted to the right in the normal or compensated hypertrophy, with a reduced Ees slope, indicating depression of myocardial contractility [23].

These observations are consistent with the sequential transition observed in the animal experiments from the earlier stable stage of normal myocardial function to a later stage of progressive deterioration with massive hypertrophy resulting in an overt failure, presumably due to pathologic and biochemical disturbances, including changes in myosin isoenzymes or in collagen composition.

In summary, ventricular elastance plays an important role in determining the overall ventricular function. The viscous-like behavior of the left ventricle can be represented as ventricular resistance. Changes in resistance due to structural, or geometric changes as well as biochemical alterations significantly affect the average performance of the ventricle coupled to the arterial load.

Effect of Aging on Left Ventriculo-arterial Coupling

The coupling in health can be substantially modified by the changes in ascending aortic impedance. Aging and atherosclerosis disturb ideal ventriculo-arterial coupling by elevating mean pressure through an increase in arteriolar tone or by increasing pulse pressure through a decrease in aortic distensibility.

With aging, there are progressive increases in wall thickness and vessel diameter. In the large arterial walls, collagen fibers, unsheathing elastic lamellae, and smooth muscle cells are embedded in a non-fibrous matrix. Collagen fibers bear most of the stress force at high pressures, and elastic lamellae and fibers serve to distribute the force uniformly [25]. When the arterial pressure and the diameter increase, the circumferential wall stress from the readily stretched elastin fibers is progressively transferred to the highly inextensible collagen fibers [26]. Collagen and elastin are complexed with an amorphous substance formed of macroprotein which is not itself elastic but contributes to the elastic properties of the artery. The stiffness of the aorta expressed in terms of elastic modulus, the distensibility of arteries characterized by the logarithmic slope of relative pressure and by the distension ratio (ratio of external radius at a given pressure to that at 100 mmHg) are all found to rise with age [27–30] in in vitro studies using isolated arteries.

We also studied static mechanical properties of arteries in the unexposed condition in 39 normal subjects aged between 6 and 81 years, using a newly-developed ultrasonic phase-locked echo tracking system to measure arterial diameter [31].

Measurement of the Distensibility of Arterial Walls

The transverse displacements of the arterial walls of the lower abdominal aorta, the carotid, brachial, and femoral arteries were recorded non-invasively by an ultrasonic phase-locked echo tracking system equipped with a real time linear array scanner. This technique was based on a phase-locked loop method which enables the zero crossing phase of the echoes reflected from the arterial wall to be tracked. A typical pulsatile arterial wall displacement recorded with the echo track is shown in Fig. 14. The central frequency of the ultrasonic probe used in this method was selected to be either 3.5, 5.0 or 7.5 MHz according to the acoustic condition of the individual arteries.

Brachial arterial pressure, which was substituted for the blood pressure of the respective arteries, was automatically measured by the conventional cuff method using a linear wide band pressure transducer fixed under the cuff, a cuff pressure controller, and a microcomputer. The time varying wave form from the transducer was fed directly into the microcomputer, which then provided a digital display of the maximum and minimum pressure.

Arterial pressure waves undergo characteristic transformations with more prominent peaks as they traverse to the periphery. The peak systolic pressure in the femoral or brachial arteries reaches values 15–20 mmHg higher than those in the central aorta. However, the pulse pressure of the brachial artery is usually about 10%–15% higher than that of the common carotid artery or of the lower abdominal aorta. This difference in pressure is almost within the total tolerance of our measuring system in a clinical setting. Moreover, a comparison of the relative changes in local distensibility can be made from the brachial arterial pressure as long as these changes are measured in a consistent fashion. Consequently, our fundamental results for the pressure-diameter relation are not affected by the lack of precision in the pressure data.

The distensibility or stiffness of vascular walls has been analyzed using the pressure-diameter relation by Hayashi and colleagues [30, 32]. On the assump-

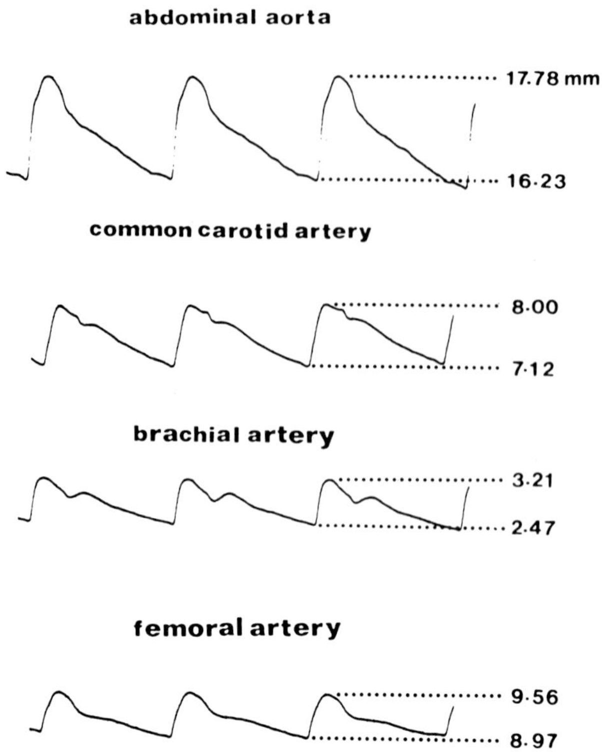

Fig. 14. Typical tracings of pulsatile changes in diameter of abdominal aorta, common carotid artery, brachial artery and femoral artery in a representative case. (From [31] with permission)

tion that an artery consists of homogeneous incompressible material and is isotropic in the cross-sectional plane, they analyzed the stress-strain relation from the pressure-diameter data by using the finite deformation theory to characterize static elastic deformation for an axisymmetric cylinder constrained at a constant length. From this analysis and their experimental data, they assumed that a simple exponential relation exists between the relative pressure and the distention ratio.

According to the experimentally obtained relations between the intraluminal pressures and the external radii, they defined the distention ratio (λ) as the arterial diameter (Dx) at a given pressure (Px), normalized by the diameter (Do) at a standard pressure (Po). When the distension ratio was plotted against the logarithmic value of the relative pressure (Px/Po, a given pressure normalized by standard pressure of 100 mmHg), a linear relation was observed in the physiological range of pressure. This relation is expressed as:

$$\ln \frac{Px}{Do} = \beta(\lambda - 1) \tag{23}$$

$$\ln \frac{Px}{Do} = \beta\left(\frac{Dx - Do}{Do}\right) \tag{24}$$

The index β represents the stiffness of the vascular walls. However, since the diameter (Do) at standard pressure (100 mmHg) cannot be measured clinically, we extrapolated these concepts to the clinical setting by trying to modify Eq. (24).

If the artery is assumed to be subject to systolic pressure (Ps), and diastolic pressure (Pd), where the external diameter is Dd at diastole and Ds at systole, Eq. (24) can be written as:

$$\ln Ps - \ln Po = \beta\left(\frac{Ds - Do}{Do}\right) \tag{25}$$

$$\ln Pd - \ln Po = \beta\left(\frac{Dd - Do}{Do}\right) \tag{26}$$

By subtracting Eq. (26) from Eq. (25), β is then given as:

$$\beta = \frac{\ln \dfrac{Ps}{Pd}}{\dfrac{Ds - Dd}{Do}} \tag{27}$$

$$= \frac{\ln \dfrac{Ps}{Pd}}{\dfrac{Ds - Dd}{Dd}} \left(\frac{Do}{Dd}\right) \tag{28}$$

$$\beta = \beta' \left(\frac{Do}{Dd}\right) \tag{29}$$

Eq. (29) can be rearranged as:

$$\frac{\beta}{\beta'} = 1 + \left(\frac{Do - Dd}{Dd}\right) \tag{30}$$

Here, we note that changes of diameter during a cardiac cycle do not usually exceed 10% in all arteries of subjects over 20 years of age. In a normotensive subject, the following relations are observed:

$$\frac{Do - Dd}{Dd} < \frac{Ds - Dd}{Dd} << 1 \tag{31}$$

$$\beta \approx \beta' = \frac{\ln \dfrac{Ps}{Pd}}{\dfrac{Ds - Dd}{Dd}} \tag{32}$$

Thus, β is approximately equal to β′, and so we can calculate β from pressure and dimensional data obtained non-invasively. However, in a subject of under 20 years in whom the diameter extension (Ds − Dd) of the aorta and the common carotid arteries is relatively large, the values of β derived from the above approximation would give values 5%–10% less than the actual ones. Such variations in the calculated β values do not significantly affect our conclusions.

Age-related Changes in Arterial Stiffness

With advancing age, there are certain geometrical changes. All arteries dilated and the stroke excursion of arterial diameter tended to decrease. The mean end-diastolic diameter of the abdominal aorta and the common carotid artery increased by 37% and by 33%, respectively in the old group of over 60 years compared to the young group of under 20 years. The mean stroke excursion of these arteries decreased by 42% and by 52%, respectively in the old group.

The aging process was associated with an increase in β values in all arteries. However, in the brachial and femoral arteries, there was considerable variation in the individual values for a given age due to their vasoactive nature. The mean data for four age groups, 1–19 years, 20–39 years, 40–59 years and over 60 years, are 4.29 ± 1.40, 6.05 ± 1.01, 7.45 ± 1.23, and 9.83 ± 2.07, respectively for the abdominal aorta, and 4.32 ± 1.00, 5.90 ± 1.29, 7.75 ± 1.66, and 11.31 ± 2.01, respectively for the carotid artery (Fig. 15).

The stiffness index β is relatively low in the abdominal aorta and the common carotid artery compared with the brachial or femoral arteries [8.56 and 9.41, respectively for young subjects (<20 years) and 13.73 and 15.31 respectively for old subjects (>60 years)].

Learoyd and Taylor [27] measured the amount by which a segment of artery shortened on removal from the body, and found that this retraction increases towards the periphery. Arndt et al. [33] also documented using angiography the decreases in aortic diameter and distensibility in relation to distance from the aortic root in unexposed thoracic aorta of cats. These regional differences in distensibility may be ascribed to the relative paucity of elastic fibers in the medial layers of the distal arteries.

Age-related changes in elastic properties of the arterial system were first studied as early as in 1880 [34]. More recently, Berry et al. [35] studied the static mechanical properties of the rat aorta as defined by an incremental elastic modulus, and found that this modulus increased in the early weeks of life, accompanied by an apparently rapid decline in relative wall thickness as the wall became less cellular. Subsequently, there was no significant change with age in the incremental elastic modulus. At age 85 years, the tangential elastic modulus of the human thoracic aorta approaches that of collagen fibers so that the aorta becomes almost a rigid tube [28]. The concentration of elastin in the entire vessel apparently decreases as age increases to adulthood, after which the concentration remains constant [26]. The frayed appearance of elastin with age has also been reported as evidence of its degeneration [36].

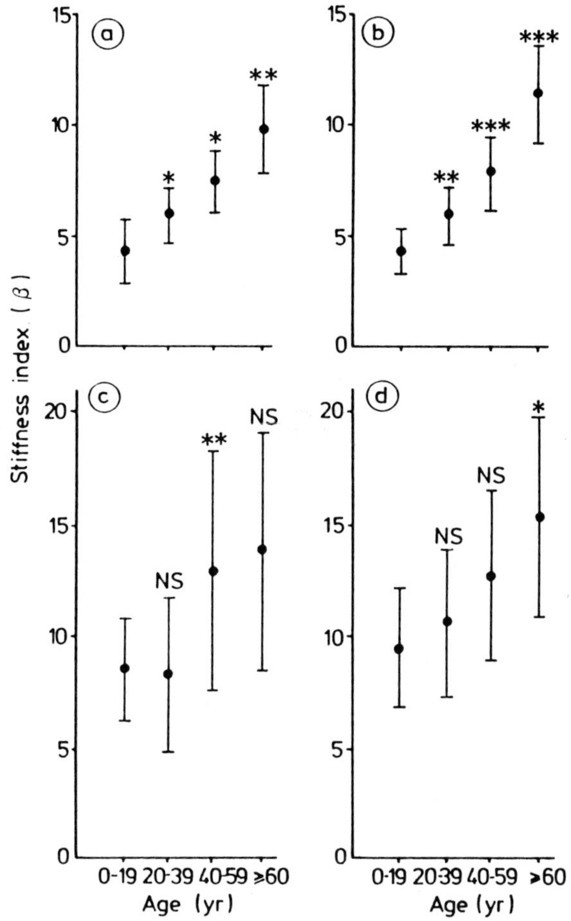

Fig. 15. Group mean values (± standard deviation) of stiffness index β in (**a**) abdominal aorta, (**b**) common carotid artery, (**c**) brachial artery and (**d**) femoral artery for four age groups. Significant difference from the preceeding group: $^{*}P < 0.05$, $^{**}P < 0.01$, $^{***}P < 0.001$. (From [31] with permission)

Elastic fibers in the wall may be stiffened by calcium deposits. With aging, the concentration of elastin apparently decreases, largely owing to a rapid increase in the concentration of collagen [26]. Collagen increases most rapidly initially, and then continues to increase throughout development, though less rapidly. On the other hand, many studies have indicated that the relative content of each connective tissue remains unchanged at all ages, despite the apparent increase in its elastic modulus with age [37, 38]. These studies suggest that age-related changes in the mechanical properties of the vessel are mainly due to some qualitative deficiency of the wall elements and not to changes in the proportions of collagen and elastin.

The Role of Relative Wall Thickness in Left Ventricular Arterial Load

The increase in stiffness of arteries with age has been suggested to be a result not only of changes in the structure and content of the wall scleroprotein, but also of an augmented relative wall thickness due to increases in caliber and wall thickness [27]. The increase in aortic volume is considered to be a useful mechanism of compensating for the decreased buffering capacity of the arterial system associated with increasing stiffness, thus keeping the volume elasticity (dP/dV) at the same low level. However, as a result of the increased stiffness and the enlarged caliber of the aorta, a larger blood volume fills the aged aorta at end diastole. This increases inertial forces against ventricular ejection and considerably affects myocardial performance.

Classical elastic theory describes the relations between applied forces and the resulting deformations. In a perfectly elastic or Hookean substance, there is a constant proportionality between stress and strain and this relation is expressed in Young's elastic modulus (E), the ratio of applied forces per unit area to relative change in dimension. The Young's modulus of an isotropic tube is given as follows:

$$E = (1 - \sigma^2)\frac{\Delta P}{\Delta R} \cdot \frac{R^2}{h} \tag{33}$$

where ΔR is the change in internal radius (R) following a pressure change ΔP. σ is Poisson's ratio, which is the ratio of transverse to longitudinal strain, all material becoming narrower when they are stretched in length. If $\sigma = 0.5$, no change in the volume of the material occurs for a very small strain. h is the wall thickness of the vessel.

In the clinical setting, Young's ratio of arteries in the physiological state was calculated by measuring the relative wall thickness at minimal pressure (hd/Rd) where the vessel wall is most static.

$$D = (1 - \sigma^2) \cdot \frac{(Ps - Pd)}{(Rs - Rd)} \cdot \frac{(Rs + Rd)Rd}{2hd} \tag{34}$$

The E value at a reference pressure of 100 mmHg (Eo) can be obtained from the differentiation of Eq. (24):

$$\frac{d}{dRx}[\ln Px] = \frac{1}{Px} \cdot \frac{dPx}{dRx} = \frac{\beta}{Ro} \tag{35}$$

Rearranging Eq. (33) gives

$$Ex = (1 - \sigma^2) \cdot \frac{\beta PxRx^2}{Rohx} \tag{36}$$

E at 100 mmHg (Eo) can be given by

$$Eo = (1 - \sigma^2) \cdot \beta Po \left(\frac{Ro}{ho}\right) \tag{37}$$

According to the assumption that a vessel is an isotropic tube which does not change in length on inflation, and with the cross-sectional area of the vessel wall remaining constant

$$Roho = Rdhd = Rshs \tag{38}$$

From Eq. (24), the ratio of changes in logarithmic pressure to changes in radius (α) is given by

$$\alpha = \left(\frac{\beta}{Ro}\right) = \frac{\ln Ps/Pd}{Rs - Rd} \tag{39}$$

Thus,

$$Ro = Rd + \frac{\ln Po/Pd}{\alpha} \tag{40}$$

From Eqs. (38), (39), and (40)

$$Eo = (1 - \sigma^2)\alpha Po \frac{\left(Rd + \frac{\ln Po/Pd}{\alpha}\right)^3}{Rdhd} \tag{41}$$

We recorded echo signals from the outer and inner layers of the vessel wall of the common carotid artery by an ultrasonic phase-locked echo-tracking system using a 10 MHz single probe. Wall thickness was obtained by cepstrum analysis with a maximum entropy method of these signals [39]. The wall thickness of arteries also changes progressively with age. The end-diastolic thickness of old subjects (over 40 years) was significantly larger than that of young subjects (under 40 years) (0.69 ± 0.08 vs. 0.55 ± 0.09 mm). End-diastolic diameter was also augmented in old subjects (7.5 ± 0.8 vs. 6.4 ± 0.5 mm, $P < 0.01$) and the relative wall thickness tended to increase from 8.7 ± 1.4 to 9.5 ± 1.2 (Table 1).

In a fluid-filled elastic pipe of some length, the ratio of pulsatile pressure to flow is termed the characteristic impedance if only centrifugal waves are present at the origin or if created at the terminations of the system [34]. This characteristic impedance (Zo) is defined as

Table 1. Comparison of systemic pressure, arterial dimension and stiffness parameters between young and old age groups

	Young group N = 26 (0–39 yr)	Old group N = 22 (40–80 yr)
Ps mmHg	107 ± 13	124 ± 14*
Pd mmHg	61 ± 8	74 ± 7**
Dd mm	6.35 ± 0.55	7.46 ± 0.77**
ΔD mm	0.69 ± 0.20	0.41 ± 0.11**
hd mm	0.55 ± 0.09	0.69 ± 0.08**
hd/Dd %	8.7 ± 1.4	9.5 ± 1.2 n.s.
K (X 10^6 dyne/cm^2)	0.30 ± 0.11	0.64 ± 0.20
Beta	5.35 ± 1.56	9.70 ± 2.45**
E (X 10^6 dyne/cm^2)	2.65 ± 0.96	5.37 ± 2.06**
Eo (X 10^6 dyne/cm^2)	4.10 ± 1.00	5.83 ± 1.66*

Values are given as mean ± SD. Ps, systolic pressure; Pd, diastolic pressure; Dd, diameter at diastole; Δd, diameter change; hd, wall thickness at diastole; K, volume elastic modulus; E, Young's modulus; Eo, Young's modulus at 100 mmHg. *$P < 0.05$, **$P < 0.01$

$$Zo = \frac{PCo}{\pi\gamma^2} \tag{42}$$

where P = blood density
Co = pulse wave velocity
γ = the lumen radius

Pulse wave velocity (Co) is related to the physical property of the vessel by the following equation:

$$Co = \sqrt{\frac{Eh}{2P}} = \sqrt{\frac{VdP}{PdV}} \tag{43}$$

where E = Young's modulus of elasticity of wall material
h = wall thickness of vessel
V = arterial volume
dP = pulse pressure
dV = change in arterial volume

From these equations, it is apparent that an increase in relative wall thickness results in an increase in pulse wave velocity and characteristic impedance.

Young's modulus of elasticity is essentially a measure of the intrinsic elastic properties of a given material independent of the amount or thickness of that material. Farrar et al. [40] observed during progression of experimental atherosclerosis induced by a high cholesterol diet in cynomolgus monkeys that E was not significantly different after 18 months of atherosclerosis induction and suggested that the average material in 18-month atherosclerotic and control arteries is roughly equivalent in elasticity in spite of greatly different morphology. Pulse wave velocity and the pressure-strain elastic modulus, which is the measure of E, and the amount and configuration of the material increased at 18 months. Thus, they postulated that these increases are due almost entirely to increases in h/R rather than to changes in E.

In our previous study, we demonstrated significant age-related increases in E of the common carotid artery both at the physiological state (E) and at a relative pressure of 100 mmHg (Eo) (Fig. 16) [41]. In young subjects (under 40 years), E was $2.7 \pm 0.8 \times 10^6$ dynes/cm^2 and Eo was $4.1 \pm 1.0 \times 10^6$, while in old subjects (over 40 years), E was augmented to $5.4 \pm 1.9 \times 10^6$ and Eo was to $5.8 \pm 1.6 \times 10^6$ (Table 1). Therefore, an increase in arterial stiffness with age explains to a large degree the increase in left ventricular arterial load, the change in the impedance spectrum of the ascending aorta and the change in pressure pulse wave contour [42]. These changes occur independently of changes that are attributed to atherosclerosis, and the cause of the increase in arterial load with age can be inferred from changes in average arterial wall elastic characteristics as described by Young's modulus of elasticity.

Impairment of Ventriculo-arterial Coupling by Atherosclerosis

Arteriosclerotic changes are characterized by smooth muscle proliferation, deposition of lipid and lipoprotein, and accumulation of collagen, elastin and

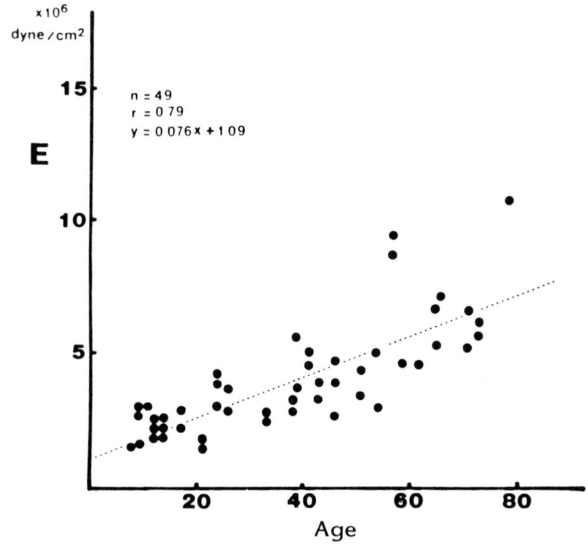

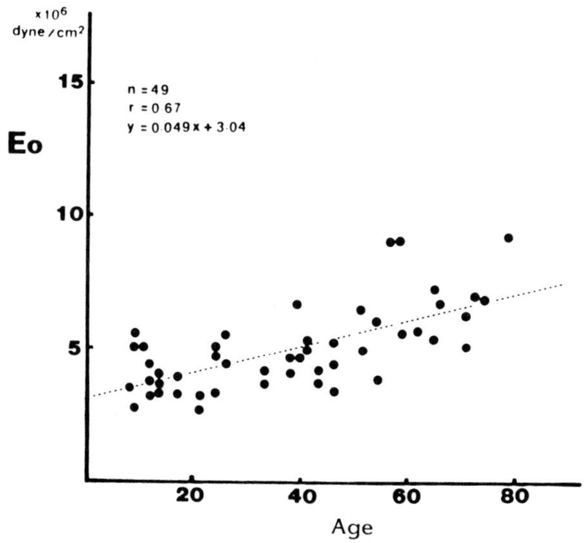

Fig. 16. Young's modulus of elasticity of common carotid artery measured at the physiological state (E) and at relative pressure of 100 mmHg (Eo) for 49 subjects aged between 8 and 79 years. (From [41])

proteoglycan in intima and subintimal regions of arterial walls [43, 44]. There are fibrotic, ulcerated or calcified lesions in advanced cases. Changes in the ratio of collagen to elastin structurally affect the elastic behavior of arterial walls. The former is much stiffer than the latter, the elastic modulus (Young's modulus) being about 1000×10^6 dynes/cm^2 at 100% elongation in collagen and only 3×10^6 dynes/cm^2 in elastin [45, 46].

These changes are more exaggerated in the pathological state than would be expected for any given age. The stiffness index β for the abdominal aorta and the common carotid artery was calculated in 49 patients with myocardial

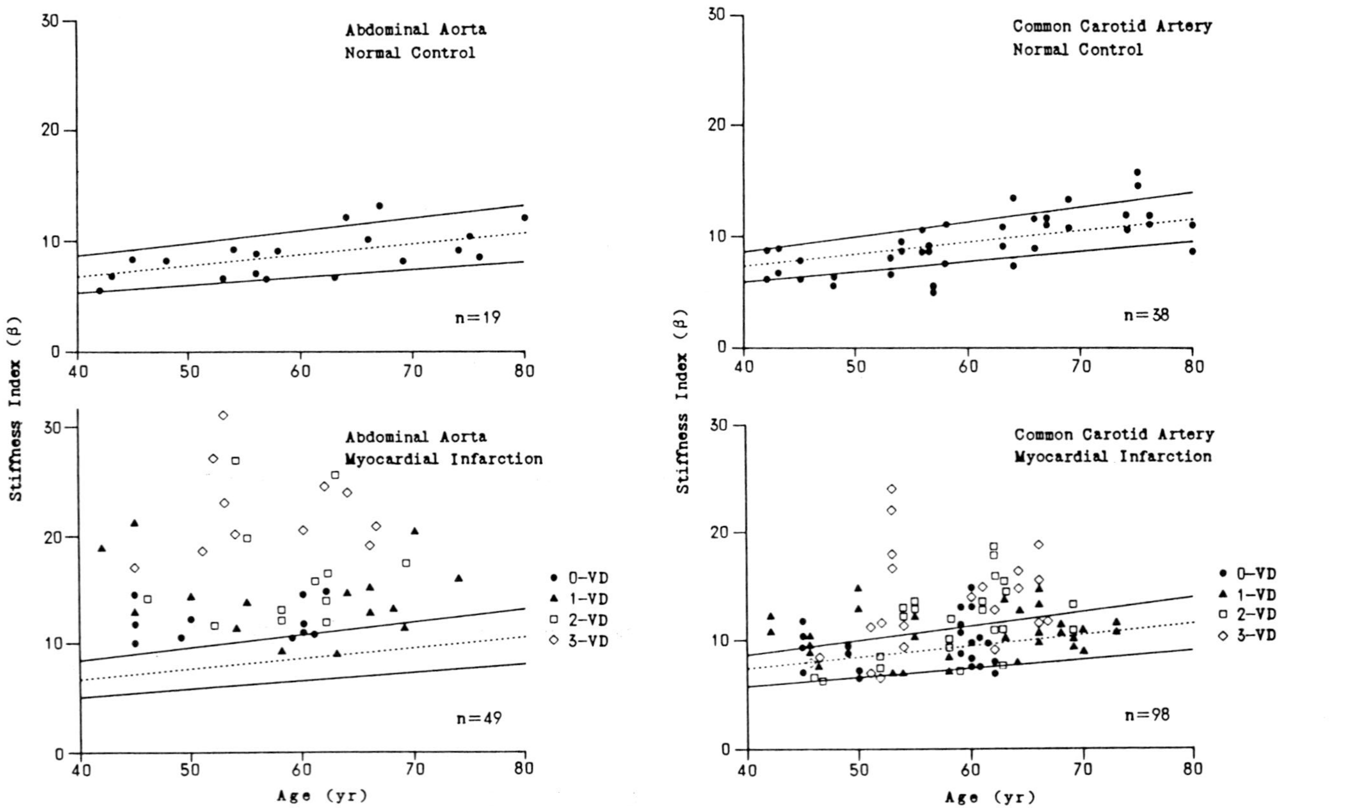

Fig. 17. Normogram of stiffness index β in abdominal aorta (*left*) and common carotid artery (*right*). *Dotted lines* indicate the actual regression line, and *solid lines*, the 95% confidence limits for normal data. *Upper panel*, normal control subjects, *lower panel*, myocardial infarction group. In the later group, patients were classified as those with no significant coronary stenosis (*O-VD*), one vessel disease (*1-VD*), two-vessel disease (*2-VD*) and three vessel disease (*3-VD*). (From [47] with permission)

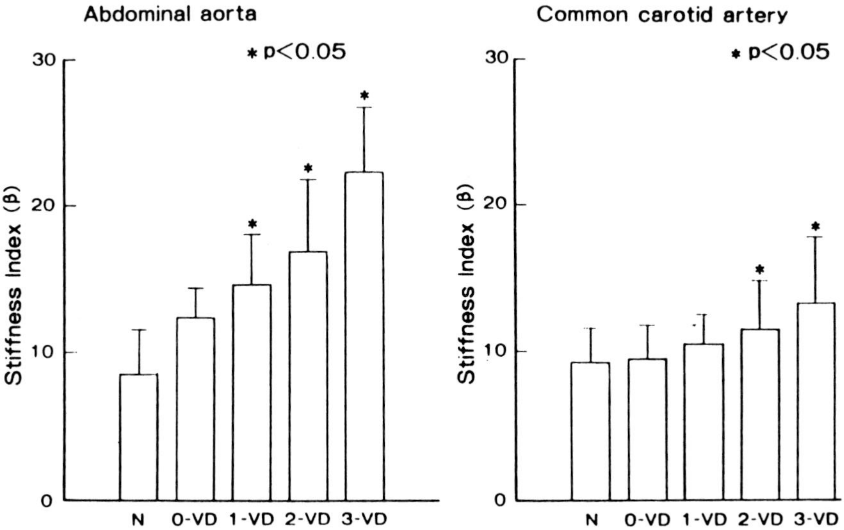

Fig. 18. Group mean values (±SD) of stiffness index β of abdominal aorta (*left*) and common carotid artery (*right*) in normal subjects (*N*), patients with myocardial infarction associated with no significant coronary stenosis (*O-VD*), one-(*1-VD*), two-(*2-VD*) and three-vessel disease (*3-VD*). *, significant difference from normal control ($P < 0.05$). (From [47] with permission)

infarction and compared to an age-matched control group (Fig. 17) [47]. β values were higher than the upper 95% confidence limits of the normal data in the common carotid artery of 28 patients ($P < 0.05$), and in the abdominal aorta and common carotid arteries, however, in patients with coronary artery in particular, had an arterial stiffness of the abdominal aorta higher than the 95% confidence limits of the normal data (Fig. 18). An average value of the stiffness index of the abdominal aorta was 8.58 ± 3.02 for the normal control, 12.25 ± 1.92 for patients with chest pain but no significant disease, 14.39 ± 3.62 for one-vessel disease, 16.63 ± 5.15 for two-vessel disease and 22.37 ± 4.29 for three-vessel disease.

In normal subjects, the β values were essentially the same in abdominal aorta and common carotid arteries, however, in patients with coronary artery disease, these values tended to be higher in the former than the latter in each group (Fig. 18). The proportion of subjects who exceed the nomogram in each group was increased with the extent of coronary artery disease.

Therefore, our observation of the higher prevalence of coronary artery sclerosis in those with more decreased distensibility of abdominal aorta supports the view that this artery is generally involved much earlier and more intensively in the atherosclerotic process than the other arteries. This is presumably related to the susceptibility of nutritional deficiency due to lack of penetrating vasa vasorum and its disposition for continuous exposure to unusual physical stress.

In summary, left ventriculo-arterial coupling is concerned with providing adequate cardiac output to peripheral perfusion and generation of adequate pressure in the ascending aorta. The coupling condition will be substantially modified by changes in arterial properties due to aging or arteriosclerosis in such a way that more pressure is elevated through an increase in arteriolar tone, or pulse pressure is increased through a decrease in aortic distensibility, an increase in arterial pulse wave velocity or creation of abnormal reflecting sites close to the heart. The appropriate treatment should be directed to reduce the disturbances which aggravate the optimal interaction between the ventricular and arterial properties.

References

1. Piene H, Sund T (1982) Does normal pulmonary impedance constitute the optimum load for the right ventricle? Am J Physiol 242:H154–H160
2. Elzinga G, Westerhof N (1973) Pressure and flow generated by the left ventricle against different impedances. Circ Res 32:178–186
3. Elzinga G, Piene H, de Jong J (1980) Left and right ventricular pump function and consequences of having two pumps in one heart. A Study on the isolated cat heart. Circ Res 46:564–574
4. van den Horn GJ, Westerhof N, Elzinga G (1985) Optimal power generation by the left ventricle. A study in the anesthetized open thorax cat. Circ Res 56:252–261
5. Sunagawa K, Maughan WL, Burkhoff D, Sagawa K (1983) Left ventricular interaction with arterial load studied in isolated canine ventricle. Am J Physiol 245: H773–H780
6. Sunagawa K, Maughan WL, Sagawa K (1985) Optimal arterial resistance for the maximal stroke work studied in isolated canine left ventricle. Circ Res 56:586–595
7. Asanoi H, Sasayama S, Kameyama T (1989) Ventriculo-arterial coupling in normal and failing heart in humans. Circ Res 65:483–493
8. Burkhoff D, Sagawa K (1986) Ventricular efficiency predicted by an analytical model. Am J Physiol 250:R1021–R1027
9. Suga H, Igarashi Y, Yamada O, Goto Y (1985) Mechanical efficiency of the left ventricle as a function of preload, afterload, and contractility. Heart Vessels 1:3–8
10. Elzinga G, Westerhof N (1980) Pump function of the feline left heart: changes with heart rate and its bearing on the energy balance. Cardiovasc Res 14:81–92
11. Suga H (1979) Total mechanical energy of a ventricle model and cardiac oxygen consumption. Am J Physiol 236:H498–H505
12. Suga H, Hayashi T, Shirahata M, Ninomiya I (1980) Critical evaluation of left ventricular systolic pressure volume area as a predictor of oxygen consumption rate. Jpn J Physiol 30:907–919
13. Teichholz LE, Kreulen T, Herman MV, Gorlin R (1976) Problems in echocardiographic volume determinations: echocardiographic-angiographic correlations in the presence and absence of asynergy. Am J Cardiol 37:7–11
14. Harris P (1987) Congestive cardiac failure: central role of the arterial blood pressure. Br Heart J 58:190–203
15. Asanoi H, Ishizaka S, Kameyama T, Miyagi K, Nozawa T, Sasayama S (1991) Neural modulation of optimal ventriculo-arterial coupling in conscious dogs. J Am Coll Cardiol 17(Suppl):374A

16. Sasayama S, Ohyagi A, Lee JD, Nonogi H, Sakurai T, Wakabayashi A, Fujita M, Kawai C (1982) Effect of the vasodilator therapy in regurgitant valvular disease. Jpn Circ J 46:433–441
17. Kameyama T, Asanoi H, Ishizaka S, Sasayama S (1991) Ventricular load optimization by unloading therapy in patients with heart failure. J Am Coll Cardiol 17: 199–207
18. Ishizaka S, Asanoi H, Kameyama T, Sasayama S (1991) Ventricular-load optimization by inotropic stimulation in patients with heart failure. Int J Cardiol 31: 51–58
19. Asanoi H, Sasayama S (1989) Relationship of plasma norepinephrine to ventricular-load coupling in patients with heart failure. Jpn Circ J 53:131–140
20. Sasayama S, Asanoi H (1989) Exercise hemodynamics in patients with heart failure. In: Hori M, Suga H, Baan J, Yellin EL (eds) Cardiac mechanics and function in the normal and diseased heart. Springer, Tokyo, pp 335–342
21. Shroff SG, Motz W, Janicki JS, Weber KT (1985) Importance of quantifying left ventricular systolic resistance in hypertrophy due to systemic hypertension. J Am Coll Cardiol 5:487
22. Cambell KB, Ringo JA, Neti C, Alexander JE (1984) Informational analysis of left ventricle/systemic arterial interaction. Ann Biomed Eng 12:209–231
23. Takahashi M, Sasayama S, Kawai C, Kotoura H (1980) Contractile performance of the hypertrophied ventricle in patients with systemic hypertension. Circulation 62:116–126
24. Gunther S, Grossman W (1979) Determinants of ventricular function in pressure-overload hypertrophy in man. Circulation 59:679–688
25. Wolinsky H, Glagov S (1964) Structural basis for the static mechanical properties of the aortic media. Circ Res 14:400–413
26. Roach MR, Burton AC (1959) The effect of age on the elasticity of human iliac arteries. Can J Biochem Physiol 35:681–690
27. Learoyd BM, Taylor MG (1966) Alterations with age in the viscoelastic properties of human arterial walls. Circ Res 18:278–292
28. Bader H (1967) Dependence of wall stress in the human thoracic aorta on age and pressure. Circ Res 20:354–361
29. Moritake K, Handa H, Okumura A, Hayashi K, Niimi H (1974) Stiffness of cerebral arteries: its role in the pathogenesis of cerebral aneurysms. Neurol Med Chir (Tokyo) 14:47–53
30. Hayashi K, Sato M, Handa H, Moritake K (1974) Biomechanical study of the constitutive laws of vascular walls. Exp Mech 14:440–444
31. Kawasaki T, Sasayama S, Yagi S, Asakawa T, Hirai T (1987) Non-invasive assessment of the age-related changes in stiffness of major branches of the human arteries. Cardiovasc Res 21:678–687
32. Hayashi K, Handa H, Nagasawa S, Okumura A, Moritake K (1980) Stiffness and elastic behavior of human intracranial and extracranial arteries. J Biomech 13: 175–184
33. Arndt JO, Stegall HF, Wicke HJ (1971) Mechanics of the aorta in vivo. Circ Res 28:693–704
34. Nichols WW, O'Rourke MF, Avolio AP, Yaginuma T, Murgo JP, Pepine CJ, Conti R (1987) Age-related changes in left ventricular/arterial coupling. In: Yin FCP (ed) Ventricular arterial coupling. Springer, New York, pp 79–114
35. Berry CL, Greenwald SE, Rivett JF (1975) Static mechanical properties of the developing and mature rat aorta. Cardiovasc Res 9:669–678

36. Wolinsky H (1972) Long-term effects of hypertension on the rat aortic wall and their relation to concurrent aging changes. Circ Res 3:301–309
37. Nagasawa S, Handa H, Okumura A, Naruo Y, Moritake K, Hayashi K (1979) Mechanical properties of human cerebral arteries. Part 1: effects of age and vascular smooth muscle activation. Surg Neurol 12:297–304
38. Yin FCP, Spurgeon HA, Kallman CH (1983) Age-associated alterations in viscoelastic properties of canine aortic strips. Circ Res 53:464–472
39. Yagi S, Kawaguchi Y, Nakayama K (1982) Ultrasonic thickness detection system for non-invasive evaluation of local young's modulus of living arterial wall. Proceedings of the Scientific Session of the Japanese Bio-rheology Society. Tokyo, pp 243–246
40. Farrar DJ, Bond MG, Sawyer JK, Green HD (1984) Pulse wave velocity and morphological changes associated with early atherosclerosis progression in the aortas of cynomolgus monkeys. Cardiovasc Res 18:107–118
41. Kawasaki T, Yagi S, Hirai T, Sasayama S (1989) Non-invasive measurement of Young's modulus of human common carotid arteries. J Jpn Coll Angiol 27:197–205
42. Nichols WW, O'Rourke MF, Avolio AP, Yaginuma T, Murgo JP, Pepine CJ, Conti CR (1985) Effects of age on ventricular-vascular coupling. Am J Cardiol 55: 1179–1184
43. Ross R (1986) The pathogenesis of atherosclerosis — an update. N Engl J Med 314:488–500
44. Roberts WC, Ferrans VJ, Levy RI, Fredrickson DS (1973) Cardiovascular pathology in hyperlipoproteinemia: anatomic observations in 42 necropsy patients with normal or abnormal serum lipoprotein patterns. Am J Cardiol 31:557–570
45. Sumner DS, Hokanson DE, Strandness DE Jr (1969) Arterial walls before and after endarterectomy. Arch Surg 99:606–611
46. Burton AC (1954) Relation of structure to function of the tissues of the wall of blood vessels. Physiol Rev 34:619–642
47. Hirai T, Sasayama S, Kawasaki T, Yagi S (1989) Stiffness of systemic arteries in patients with myocardial infarction. A noninvasive method to predict severity of coronary atherosclerosis. Circulation 80:78–86

9
Neurohumoral Mechanisms in Chronic Heart Failure

Masatsugu Hori[1], Toshifumi Kagiya[1], Hideyuki Sato[1], Hiroshi Sato[1], Akira Kitabatake[1], Masatake Fukunami[2], Noritake Hoki[2], Michitoshi Inoue[3]

Summary. In chronic heart failure, sympathetic nerve activity is stimulated mainly due to blunted cardiopulmonary and arterial baroreceptors. Neural reflex from the working skeletal muscles during exercise accelerates the activation of sympathetic activity. The renin-angiotensin-aldosterone system is also activated in heart failure and induces vasoconstriction and retension of sodium ions and water. In the early stage of heart failure, these neurohumoral activations may play a compensatory role in cardiac dysfunction. In advanced heart failure, however, these mechanisms exert detrimental effects on myocardial cells and circulatory hemodynamics: (1) sympathetic stimulation and elevated angiotensin II and vasopressin induce vasoconstriction and increase the cardiac afterload, (2) retension of sodium ions and water by aldosterone may cause pulmonary congestion and peripheral edema, (3) sustained sympathetic stimulation produces down-regulation of β-adrenoceptors, and thus, inotropic responsiveness of the heart is attenuated, and (4) myocardial cells are directly injured by excessive catecholamines and angiotensin II. Recent clinical reports on the treatment of chronic congestive heart failure suggest that angiotensin converting enzyme inhibitors are effective for improvement of cardiac function, exercise capacity and prognosis. Long-term β-blocker therapy is also effective, although administration of β-blockers more or less depresses cardiac function in the initial phase. Through these clinical experiences, we should reappraise our interpretation of previous reports on the pathophysiology of chronic heart failure and strategy for treatment of chronic heart failure.

Key words: Chronic heart failure — Neurohumoral abnormality — Sympathetic activity — Renin-angiotensin-aldosterone system — Neural reflex — Catecholamine-induced myocardial injury — β-adrenergic receptor — β-blocker therapy — Microtubule

[1] The First Department of Medicine Osaka University, Osaka, 553 Japan
[2] The Heart Center, Osaka Prefectural Hospital, Osaka, 558 Japan
[3] Department of Medical Information Science, Osaka University, Osaka, 553 Japan

Introduction

When cardiac pump function is depressed, a number of neurohumoral mechanisms are activated to maintain circulatory homeostasis by increasing peripheral vascular resistance and extracellular fluid volume [1, 2]. The contributions of sympathetic nerve activation and the renin-angiotensin-aldosterone system are prominent in this neurohumoral adjustment in congestive heart failure [3, 4]. Over the past few years, a beneficial compensatory role of neurohumoral activation has been reviewed. Recently, detrimental effects of this compensatory mechanism have been focused on. In this review, we discuss the role of neurohumoral activation in the progress of heart failure in view of the pathogenesis and treatment of this disease.

Neurohumoral Activation in Chronic Heart Failure

Sympathetic Nerve Activity and Neural Reflex

The baroreceptors located in artia and ventricles respond to changes in pressure and volume of the heart, relaying inhibitory signals to the central nervous system via the vagus nerve [5]. In the carotid sinus and aortic arch, there are mechanoreceptors which respond to local wall stretch and discharge inhibitory impulses to the central nervous system via the glossopharyngeal and vagus nerves [6]. Thus, these baroeceptors sensing the pressure and/or volume changes in the central cardiovascular system modulate the sympathetic outflow and vasopressin secretion from the hypophyseal section [7]. The vasomotor center in the hypothalamus discharges the sympathetic impulses by its excitation, but it is normally suppressed by the parasympathetic activity from the cardiopulmonary and arterial barorecptors [5, 6]. In congestive heart failure, the baroreflex is markedly impaired due to the decreased sensitivity of baroreceptors and consequently, inhibitory signals to the central nervous system are attenuated, leading to the sympathetic stimulation. A large amount of research has demonstrated the blunted baroreceptor function in heart failure although the precise mechanisms are still unclear [8, 9]. Left atrial receptors in experimental heart failure demonstrate attenuated responsiveness to changes in atrial pressure during volume expansion [8]. Dysfunction of baroreceptors in humans has also been enhanced during maneuvers which alter the central cardiac filling pressures, i.e., head-up tilt, application of lower body negative pressure or administration of vasodilator/vasoconstrictor agents [10, 11]. In normal subjects, sympathetic nervous and renin-angictensin systems are activated and vasopressin is released by lowering the filling pressure of the heart and sympathetic nervous activation can be assessed by increases in forearm vascular resistence and heart rate [10]. In patients with chronic heart failure, sympathetic tone is elevated, and changes in limb blood flow and plasma norepinephrine level are not clearly seen during the maneuvers which alter the cardiac filling pressure [10]. Baroreflex responsiveness is mostly impaired in patients with severe heart failure. It is important that arterial and cardiopulmonary baroreceptor dysfunction may precede the development of overt heart failure. Baroreceptor dysfunction is reversed, with improvement of pump function, by administration of digitalis [12] and angiotensin converting enzyme inhibitor, [8] and by heart transplantation [13]. Several lines of evidence have demonstrated that digitalis directly restores the baroreflex function by augmentation of the inhibitory influence of cardiac receptors with vagal afferent fibers [12]. Direct effects of ouabain on spontaneous firing of the isolated carotid sinus have also been demonstrated [14]. A possible mechanims that has been suggested for acute alteration of baroreceptors is activation of an electrogenic Na^+ pump during brief periods of pressure elevation since excitation of baroreceptors by mechanical stress is dependent on an increase in the Na^+ permeability of the receptor membrane which accumulates intracellular Na^+ and activates an electrogenic Na^+ pump [15]. The resultant hyperpolarization of the receptor membrane requires a greater degree of stretch which activates the baroreceptors. Ouabain blocks the increase in Na^+ pump activity and consequently membrane hyperpolarization is preserved. Lowering external K^+ by ouabain also blocks the electrogenic Na^+ pump in baroreceptors [16]. Thus, increased Na^+ pump activity may be involved in baroreceptor dysfunction in chronic heart failure. Angiotensin is also known to increase Na^+ influx [17] and the restoring effect of angiotensin converting enzyme inhibitor may be also attributed to attenuation of Na^+ pump activity with this agent.

It is well known that sympathetic activity is enhanced during exercise in normal subjects. In patients with chronic heart failure, it is more activated than normal subjects at the same level of the workload. Figure 1 shows the plasma norepinephrine levels during various workloads. In normal subjects, plasma norepinephrine levels are less than 700 pg/ml during the ordinary physical activity. In patients with congestive heart failure, plasma norepinephrine levels are increased with exercise of moderate intensity, and in severe heart failure plasma norepinephrine levels are more than 500 pg/ml, even at rest. Although the neural mechanisms responsible for the increased sympathetic activation during exercise are not fully clarified, two theories of neural control have been proposed; a direct action of the central command descending from the higher motor centers to the cardiovascular certral areas, and neural reflex from receptors in the skeletal work muscles. The central neural mechanism has been studied in humans as well as in animals. Involvement of the central neural mechanism has been documented by the observation that the heart rate and pressure responses to dynamic exercise are greater when partial neuromuscular blockers, e.g., decamethonium or tubocurarine, are administered [18] even though the workloads are not altered. Thus, the cardiovascular response may be related to greater motor command to achieve a given level of workload. As well as the central command, the reflex neural mechanism is also important in activation of sympathetic activity during exercise. In animal experiments, when the dorsal roots of L7 and S1, which carry the majority of the sensory input from the contracting hind limb to the spinal cord, are transected, increases in blood pressure, heart rate and left ventricular pressure during induced exercise

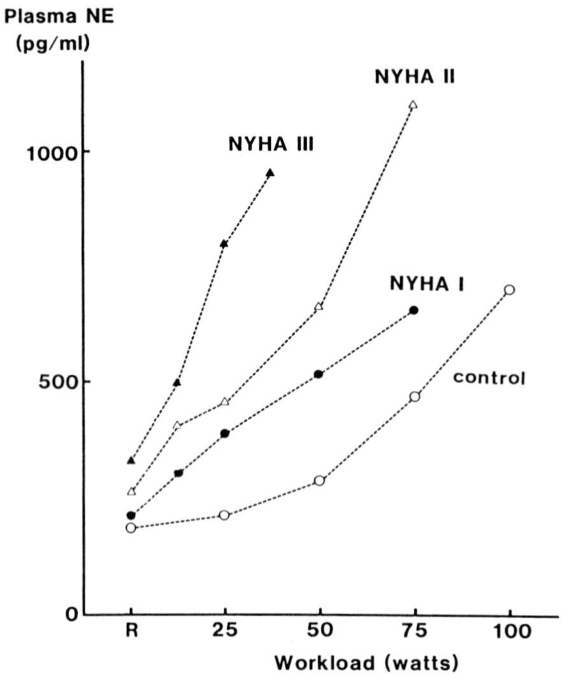

Fig. 1. Increase in plasma norepinephrine levels during exercise in normal subjects and patients with chronic heart failure. The data represent the mean values (5 normal subjects in control, 8 patients in NYHA I, 11 patients in NYHA II, 8 patients in NYHA III). Plasma norepinephrine levels at given workload are higher in advanced heart failure. *NE*, norepinephrine. (From [23])

of a hind limb by electrical stimulation are abolished [19]. This indicates that sensory endings on skeletal muscle traveling in the dorsal roots serve as the afferent limb of the reflex and regulate the sympathetic activity during exercise. The sensory fibers from skeletal muscle are classified into four groups according to anatomy and function. Group III and IV fibers may be mainly involved in the cardiovascular reflex response [20]. The receptors are generally classified into two types, ergoreceptors and nociceptors [21, 22]; ergoreceptors are activated by muscle contraction and nociceptors are stimulated by noxious stimuli.

In patients with cardiac dysfunction, and increase in cardiac output during exercise is disproportionate to the oxygen demand of the working skeletal muscle, and oxygen extraction by the muscle is increased as the workload increases. Resultant chemical changes, e.g., a decrease in oxygen concentration and pH and an increase in lactate in the venous blood, stimulate the nociceptors of the skeletal muscle, leading to sympathetic activation during exercise. The relationship between oxygen concentration in the mixed venous blood ($P\bar{v}O_2$) and plasma norepinephrine levels during exercise are depicted in Fig. 2 .The logarithmic plot clearly shows the linear relationship between these two parameters, indicating that sympathetic activity is stimulated by oxygen changes in the local blood during exercise by neural reflex [23]. In contrast to baroreceptors, however, the sensitivity of nociceptors is not altered in patients with chronic heart failure. Accordingly, in patients with severe heart failure, insufficient blood supply to the working muscle during exercise triggers sym-

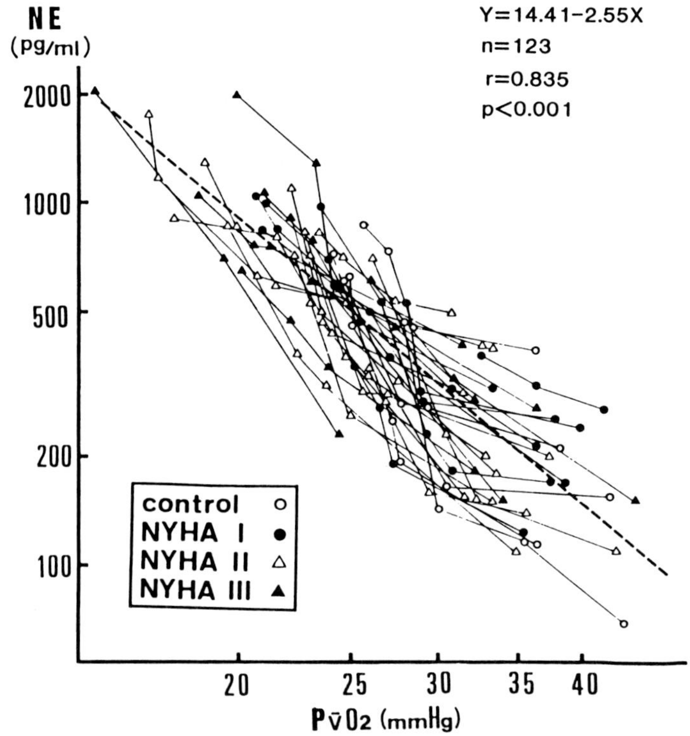

Fig. 2. Inverse correlation between venous PO_2 ($P\bar{v}O_2$) and plasma norepinephrine (*NE*) levels during exercise. Note that $P\bar{v}O_2$ and *NE* levels are depicted in a logarithmic plot. (From [23])

pathetic stimulation. This reflex mechanism may serve in concert with blunted baroreflex as a modulator of sympathetic activity in patients with chronic heart failure.

Activated Renin-angiotensin-aldosterone System and Arginine-vasopressin Secretion

Most patients with chronic heart failure demonstrate an excessive activation of the renin-angiotensin system at rest or during exercise, although the range of plasma levels are considerably large [24]. This is mainly due to the activated sympathetic activity since β-adrenergic stimulation enhances the release of renin from the juxtaglomerular cells [25]. The renin in the blood stream initiates the formation of angiotensin I which is transformed to angiotensin II by converting enzymes. Angiotensin II enhances the formation of aldosterone which increases the reabsorption of sodium by the renal tubules. In addition to the potent vasoconstrictor action, angiotensin II directly attenuates baroreceptor sensitivity and further activates sympathetic activity [26]. Angiotensin II also stimulates the release of vasopressin from the pituitary [26]. All of these hormones, i.e., norepinephrine, angiotensin II and vasopressin, are potent vasoconstrictors and increase vascular impedance. These processes make a vicious cycle in progression of the heart failure.

In acute heart failure, the renin-angiotensin system is markedly enhanced, serving for vasoconstriction and sodium retention. Extracellular fluid volume expansion occurs, resulting in restoration of blood pressure and return of plasma renin and aldosterone levels to normal. In this compensation phase, converting-enzyme inhibition has little or no effect in the reduction of blood pressure. In addition, the activation of the renin-angiotensin system is attenuated by the release of specific counter-regulatory hormones, e.g., prostaglandin E_2 and atrial natriuretic peptide [27, 28]. This may be a cause for the wide range of plasma renin levels in chronic heart failure. In patients with hyponatremic heart failure, however, plasma renin activity and prostagrandin E_2 are very high [29]. Increased prostaglandins (PGE_2 and PGI_2) further stimulates renin release [30]. Patients with hyponatremia are clinically decompensated and have poor prognosis. Thus hyponatremia of less than 133 meq/l observed in patients with moderate or severe heart failure usually indicates a high mortality rate. In such severe heart failure, administration of converting-enzyme inhibitors is effective to improve survival rate [31]. The rationale for converting-enzyme inhibitors for treatment of congestive heart failure may lie in the fact that angiotensin II exerts deleterious effects on ventricular function by increasing impedance of the cardiac output through its potent vasoconstriction and by exacerbation of loading conditions through retension of salt and water by the kidney. Converting-enzyme inhibitors may also preserve total body levels of potassium and reduce circulating levels of catecholamine [32, 33].

Vasopressin is a nonapeptide which is released from the supraoptic and paraventricular hypothalamic nuclei in response to osmotic and nonosmotic stimuli [34]. Arterial baroreceptors function in concert with the cardiopulmonary baroreceptors to increase vasopressin secretion in response to systemic hypotension [35]. Circulating levels of vasopressin are increased in patients with severe heart failure [36]. As well as norepinephrine and angiotensin II, vasopressin acts as a vasoconstrictor supporting systemic blood pressure in some patients with severe heart failure [37]. The levels of vasopressin has been reported to correlate with NYHA functional class: 50% of patients in NYHA class III and IV showed increased vasopressin concentration [38]. Vasopressin levels are high particularly in hyponatremic, hypo-osmolar patients with chronic heart failure [39]. However, the role of vasopressin in chronic heart failure is still unclear and further studies are necessary.

Role of Sympathetic Activity — Compensation or Exacerbation?

Despite the variety of etiologies of cardiac failure, cardiac compensatory mechanisms are usually common in the early stages of heart failure; an increase in the end-diastolic volume compensates for the reduced cardiac output causing the dilatation of the ventricle. However, the Frank-Starling mechanism is effective only in acute dysfunction of the heart and the resultant rise in left ventricular filling pressure may cause pulmonary congestion and lung edema.

Sustained stretch of ventricular muscle stimulates eccentric hypertrophy, i.e., dilation of the heart. In the dilated heart, muscle fibers bear the increased stress due to an enlargement of radius of curvature. As a result, moderate hypertrophy may occur to compensate for the increased stress even through systolic pressure remains unchanged. Enhanced sympathetic activity and the renin-angiotensin-aldosterone system may augment the cardiac hypertrophy [40, 41]. In mild heart failure, sympathetic activity is not activated at rest. However, during exercise sympathetic tone is markedly activated to compensate for the ventricular dysfunction, and heart rate is increased and myocardial contractility augmented. Compensatory mechanisms are inadequate to match the peripheral demand of blood supply especially during exercise and even at rest in advanced heart failure. Consequently, compensatory mechanisms are further activated; sympathetic tone is enhanced and the volume of the heart is further enlarged. Recent studies suggest that both α_1- and β-adrenergic activities contribute to the genesis of cardiac hypertrophy [42]. Thus, sympathetic activation, as well as mechanical load, should stimulate cardiac hypertrophy. Myocardial hypertrophy is frequently observed in failing hearts in which compensatory activation of sympathetic activity may serve as a detrimental factor for the myocardium because of a disturbance in myocardial energy utilization, abnormal Ca^{2+} handling and organic changes in intracellular organelles and receptors.

Cardiac Hypertrophy and Energy Metabolism

It has been speculated that myofibrillar growth involves the accumulation of myofilaments at the surface of existing bundles. The maintenance of myofibrillar size may be due to the existence of a critical perimitochondrial radius that is needed to supply ATP to the contractile proteins [43]. In volume-overloaded hypertrophy, a constant mitochondrial to myofibrillar volume ratio is maintained, but the capillary network may not increase in proportion to the muscle mass [44]. A relative deficiency in capillary luminal volume and surface in the ventricle is reported in a model of aortocaval fistula or intensive physical training [45]. Although a risk of blood supply may be higher in the pressure-overloaded heart (concentric hypertrophy), oxygen supply to the myocardium may be impaired in the volume-overloaded heart. Oxidative phosphorylation in mitochondria remains intact until very late in the course of failure [46]. Overall ATP and creatine phosphate concentrations remain normal although compensatory high phosphate energy source may play a key role. A defect of energy utilization at the electrical-contraction coupling may be more important in failing myocardium.

Role of Adrenergic Receptors in Chronic Heart Failure

It has long been demonstrated that inotropic effects of adrenergic stimulation are markedly reduced in animals with heart failure, whereas the blood pressure response appears to be unaltered. Recent development of the radioligand receptor binding assay technique has shown that reduced response to adrenergic stimulation is mainly attributed to desensitization of β-adrenoceptors and/or their down-regulation [47, 48]. Although a variety of biochemical changes associated with heart failure are documented, receptor changes may play a pivotal role in regulation of the contractile function of the heart. β-Adrenoceptors, which bind to agonists, stimulate the enzyme adenylate cyclase to form cyclic AMP which in turn promotes transmembrane Ca^{2+} influx and accerelates Ca^{2+} release from sarcoplasmic reticulum [49].

In normal hearts, β-adrenoceptors are not fully functioning. During exercise, however, sympathetic activity is markedly enhanced and thus, norepinephrine released from the nerve endings almost fully activates β-adrenoceptors located around the synapse. Therefore, abnormalities in the β-adrenoceptor pathway may cause the depressed cardiac function and clinical deterioration. Existence of desensitization of β-adrenoceptors has been speculated in view of the correlation of circulating catecholamine levels with the severity of heart failure [50]. This hypothesis is supported by pharmacologic studies which report that exposure of catecholamines results in down-regulation of β-adrenoceptors [51] and uncoupling of the receptors from adenylate cyclase [52]. In 1982, Bristow et al. first reported in human hearts that cardiac β-adrenoceptor density is markedly reduced in the failing hearts from cardiac transplant recipients or prospective donors [53]. Close correlations of the % reduction in maximal isoproterenol-mediated adenylate cyclase stimulation with that of β-adrenoceptor density indicates the functional coupling between β-adrenoceptors and subcellular signal transduction in failing hearts. Since their first report, several groups of investigators have confirmed that the β-adrenoceptor density is decreased in patients with chronic heart failure, regardless of etiology [54]. Mechanisms of desensitization of β-adrenoceptors are recently clarified by Lefkowitz and Caron [55]. They characterized an enzyme, β-adrenoceptor kinase, which phosphorylates the β-adrenoceptors when β-adrenoceptors are activated by an agonist. Thus, involvement of β-adrenoceptor kinase is the first step of desensitization. If the receptors were exposed to an agonist for a longer period, the receptors are sequest rated in the cytosolic space. Microfilaments may be involved in removal of β-adrenoceptors from the membrane surface toward the inner face [56], and further, microtubules may serve for internalization and degradation of the receptors [57].

Although β-adrenoceptor density appears to be correlated with the cardiac function and hence NYHA functional class (Fig. 3) [58], a change in receptor density is not the sole mechanism to explain the reduced responsiveness of the failing heart to adrenergic stimulation. Several lines of evidence demonstrate that GTP binding proteins which couple to β-adrenoceptors are altered in failing hearts though it is still controversial. Longabaugh et al. [59] reported a decrease in the stimulatory GTP binding proteins (Gs) in pressure-overloaded dogs. They observed that ADP ribosylation of Gs by chorela toxin is significantly decreased in the failing heart. They also reconstituted the solublized sarcolemma from failing ventricle into a fixed amount of cyc(-)membrane

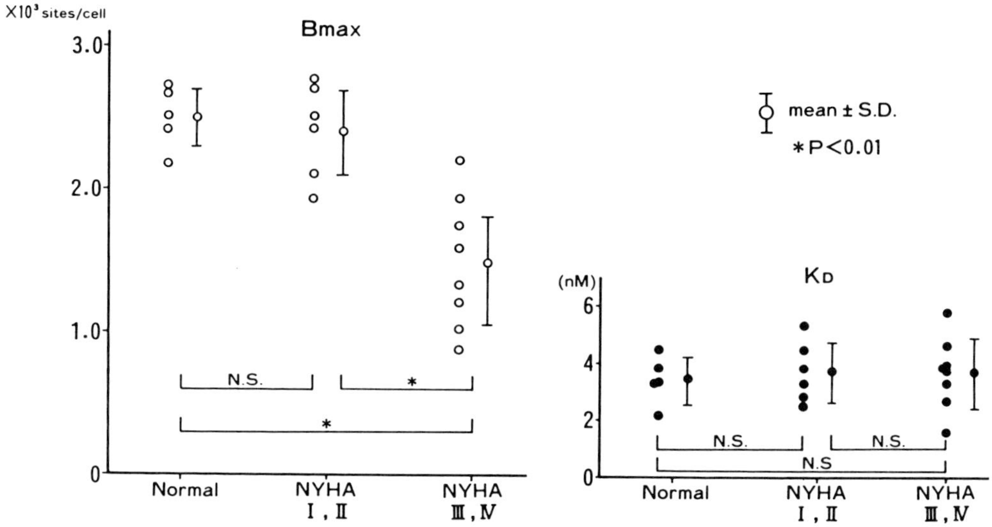

Fig. 3. β-Adrenoceptor number (B_{max}) and dissociation constant (K_d) of lymphocytes in patients with chronic heart failure. The hydrophilic β-adrenergic receptor ligand [^{3}H]CGP12177 was used to assess the cell-surface beta-receptor. In severe heart failure (NYHA III, IV), receptor number is significantly decreased. (From [58])

and observed a 50% reduction of adenylate cyclase activity when stimulated by NaF. Contrary to a decrease in Gs, Feldman et al. demonstrated that the activity of inhibitory GTP binding proteins ($G_{i\alpha}$) ($\alpha G_i 40$; 40 k mol pertussis toxin substrate) is increased by 36% in failing human hearts, whereas the stimulatory regulatory subunit (Gs_α) is not altered [60]. The increase in Gi and no change in Gs could explain a discrepancy in adenylate cyclase activities when stimulated by NaF and forskolin; forskolin-stimulated activity is decreased whereas NaF-stimulated adenylate cyclase activity is not altered. We also reported that forskolin-stimulated inotropic response (LV dP/dt max) is depressed, whereas isoproterenol-stimulated response appears normal in ischemic cardiomyopathy in dogs [61]. In this canine model with intracoronary microembolization, inotropic responses to isoproterenol and forskolin were both depressed in acute heart failure. A week after embolization, however, dogs recovered from ischemic insults with a compensatory increase in β-adrenoceptors. Despite restoration of the β-adrenoceptor-mediated inotropic response in this period, the responsiveness to forskolin stimulation was still depressed, suggesting that Gi may be increased, inhibiting the signal transduction of β-adrenoceptor stimulation (Fig. 4). Apparently the normal response to β-adrenoceptor stimulation in this model may be compensated for by the increased density of β-adrenoceptors.

The subpopulations of β_1 and β_2 subtypes is another point of interest in the study of the failing heart. Previous studies showed that human myocardium contains a relatively large proportion of β_2-adrenoceptors; 14%–40% in

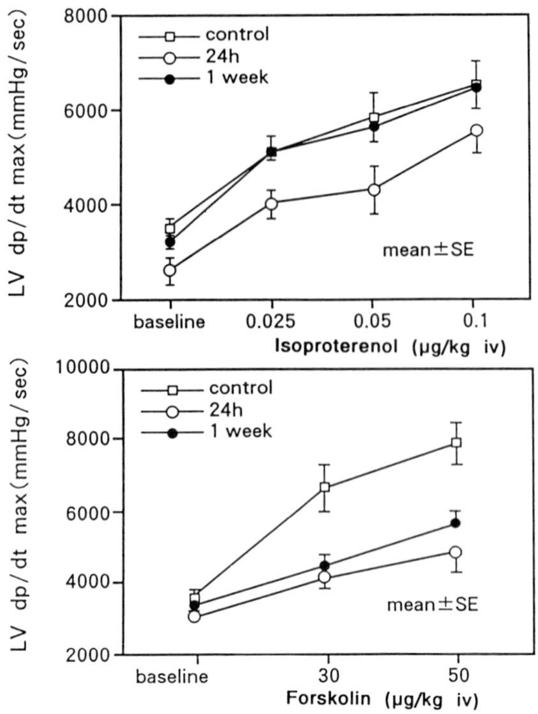

Fig. 4. Inotropic response to isoproterenol and forskolin in canine ischemic cardiomyopathy model. Hemodynamic studies were peformed in the conscious state before (*control*), and 24 h and 1 week after coronary embolization with 15 μm microspheres in dogs. Inotropic response to isoproterenol was recovered 1 week after embolization (*upper panel*) whereas inotropic response to forskolin remained depressed (*lower panel*). *LV*, left ventricle (Modified from [61])

ventricular muscle and 20%–55% in atrial tissues [62], whereas the population of β_2-adrenoceptors is very small in other species. Bristow et al. reported that in failing human left ventricles, the population of β_1-adrenoceptors is decreased [63]; the β_1:β_2 ratio was 60:38 due to selective down-regulation of β_1-adrenoceptors. This decrease in β_2-adrenoceptors and relative increase in β_2-adrenoceptors were in accordance with the reduced response to denopamine (β_1-agonist) and increased response to zinterol (β_2-agonist). Recently, differential pharmacological responses of β_1- and β_2-adrenoceptors have attracted our interest, especially in response to heart rate, since β_1-selective agonists, predominantly denopamine, increases the force of cardiac muscle, whereas chronotropic action is much less than isoproterenol. It follows that β_2-adrenoceptor stimulation preferentially increases heart rate. If this is the case, a relative increase in β_2-adrenoceptors in failing heart may serve as an accerelator of the heart rate in failing hearts.

In contrast to down-regulation of β-adrenoceptors, an increase in β-adrenoceptor density has been less extensively studied. However, previous studies reported several conditions in which β-adrenoceptors are increased, e.g., pressure-overloaded cardiac hypertrophy [64], myocardial ischemia [65], cardiac transplantation [66] and cardiomyopathic Syrian hamsters [67]. Under these conditions, β-adrenoceptors are more or less coupled with subcellular signal transduction and hence, an increase in β-adrenoceptors may play a compensatory role in intrinsic abnormalities in the heart. Therefore, excessive stimulation of sympathetic activity which may induce down-regulation of β-adrenoceptors could cause manifestation of overt heart failure. Tachyphylaxis of catecholamine therapy and acute exacerbation of heart failure after withdrawal of catecholamine may be attributed to down-regulation of β-adrenoceptors.

Catecholamine-induced Myocardial Injury

In cardiac failure, activated sympathetic activity serves as a compensatory mechanism for failing myocardium. However, sustained stimulation of adrenergic receptors deplete the cardiac norepinephrine stores. A reduction of tyrosine hydroxylase activity also contributes to a depletion of norepinephrine stores [68], although its physiological role in enhanced sympathetic activity in heart failure is still unclear. Despite desensitization of the heart to sympathetic stimulation, sustained exposure to catecholamines may injure the myocardium. It is well known that myocardial necrosis is induced by both exogenous and endogenous catecholamine in experimental animals [69]. Pathogenesis of catecholamine-induced myocardial necrosis is attributed to several factors. Of the mechanisms suggested, relative hypoxia is favored by many investigators [70]. It is thought that the oxygen supply is disproportionate to the increased oxygen demand due to β-adrenoceptor stimulation. Catecholamine is also known to enhance platelet aggregation, and platelet thrombi deposited in the coronary small vessels may play a role in precipitating the ischemic changes [71]. Recently, the role of free radicals in ischemic injury has been extensively discussed. Catecholamine injury can be explained in part by the formation of free radicals through a variety of the oxidation products of catecholamine [72]. Adrenochrome, an oxidation product of epinephrine, is thought to be a possible chemical which promotes lipid peroxidation leading to the cell membrane injury. It was demonstrated that adrenochrome depresses contractile activity in isolated perfused rat hearts [73].

In contrast to these cellular injuries derived from ischemia-related alterations of cellular membrane and organelles, myocardial Ca^{2+} overload is another key mechanism which may underlie the catecholamine-induced injury. This theory, which was originally presented by Fleckenstein [74], is in contrast to the previous idea that Ca^{2+} influx is secondary to increased permeability of sarcolemmal membrane. β-adrenoceptor stimulation increases the Ca^{2+} influx through voltage-dependent Ca^{2+} channels. An increase in the intracellular Ca^{2+} content results in myofilament overstimulation, increase of contractile force and oxygen requirement as well as excessive ATP breakdown. Thus, Ca^{2+} overload may be cardiotoxic. Recently, it has been suggested that myo-

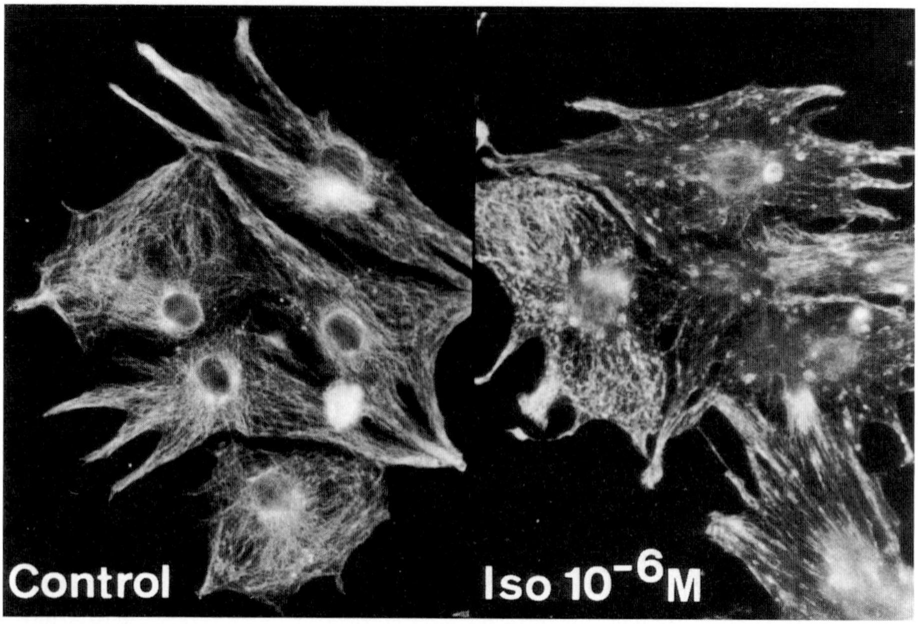

Fig. 5. Immunohistochemical studies of microtubules in cultured rat myocytes. The *left panel* shows the normal structure of microtubules, and the *right panel* depicts fragmentation and regional disruption of microtubules. (From [77])

cardial stunning is also caused by Ca^{2+} overload [75]. Reperfusion after transient ischemia enhances Ca^{2+} transport from extracellular space to intracellular space through Na^+/Ca^{2+} exchange [76]. The subcellular events caused by Ca^{2+} overload may be common in catecholamine-induced injury and reperfusion injury. Recently, we found that exposure of rat culture cardiomyocytes to isoproterenol causes depolymerization of microtubules (Fig. 5) [77]. The microtubule disruptions are inhibited by administration of Ca^{2+} channel blocker, diltiazem and low Ca^{2+} concentration of extracellular medium. Thus, sustained β-adrenoceptor stimulation could cause the cytoskeletal injury through Ca^{2+} overload. From these lines of evidence, one can assume that enhanced sympathetic activity in chronic heart failure may exert cardiotoxic action and produce a vicious cycle in heart failure.

Use of β-adrenoceptor Blockers for Treatment of Chronic Heart Failure

A challenge to the conventional therapy for congestive heart failure was first reported in 1975 by Waagstein et al. in Sweden [78]. These investigators treated several patients with chronic heart failure by β-adrenoceptor antagonists and found marked clinical improvement over a period of several months;

all patients had resting tachycardia and thus, β-blocker therapy significantly decreased the mean heart rate. Resolution of peripheral edema and ascites was observed with improvement of symptoms and exercise capacity. Noninvasive parameters of cardiac function, i.e., left ventricular ejection time and velocity of circumferential fiber shortening were increased. In 1979, these investigators also reported a prolongation of survival of 24 patients treated with β-blockers [79]. In the early 1980's, the same Swedish group extended the study to patients with dilated cardiomyopathy [80]. In this study, they reported the exacerbation of heart failure and cardiac function after withdrawal of β-blockers. Their experience of long-term treatment with β-blockers revealed that cardiac function and excessive capacity fall acutely with the initiation of β-blockade but long-term treatment improves the cardiac function and symptoms. However, these studies were not designed as a randomized controlled study, and not all patients were treated in the same fashion. In these studies, the dose of β-blockers was gradually and carefully increased from the initial dose of metoprolol of 5–10 mg/day. After this work, other investigators tested the beneficial effects of long-term treatment of chronic heart failure with β-blockers in randomized trials [81]. They also found that ventricular ejection increased and functional class improved. A study by Fowler et al. at Stanford [82] was most impressive; four of ten patients who tolerated metoprolol therapy were markedly improved and were removed from the transplant waiting list. We also studied 22 patients with dilated cardiomyopathy who were treated with metoprolol over a long-term period, and compared them with 22 patients with dilated cardiomyopathy treated with conventional drugs, e.g., digitalis, diuretics, and vasodilators. Three months after initiation of β-blocker treatment, the dimension of the left ventricle decreased and ejection fraction increased. Exercise tolerance fell initially but increased after a couple of months. Although favorable results for β-blocker therapy is accumulating, it has not been possible to identify specific subgroups of patients responsive to β-blocker treatment. Engelmeier et al. [83] suggested that patients with tachycardia are likely to respond to β-blocker therapy. Our experience suggests that β-blockers may preferably improve the cardiac function which has been progressively deteriorated and that β-blocker therapy may not be tolerated in patients with extremely advanced heart failure.

In contrast to the salutary effect of β-blockers, several reports are against the favorable effects of this drug. Ikram and Fitzpatrick [84] studied the effect of acebutorol, a β-blocker with intrinsic sympathetic activity, in 17 patients with chronic heart failure in a double-blind, randomized, crossover study over a period of one month. In this study, the beneficial effect of acebutorol was not observed in clinical symptoms, cardiac size and exercise capacity. Another study reported by Currie et al. [85] also demonstrated negative results in metoprolol therapy in a double-blind crossover study over four weeks. Unfavorable results were obtained in treatment for a relatively short period, and a longer period may be needed before clinical improvement. From these previous studies, β-blockers may be cardioprotective and the beneficial effect would appear after a long period, whereas the acute effect is deleterious.

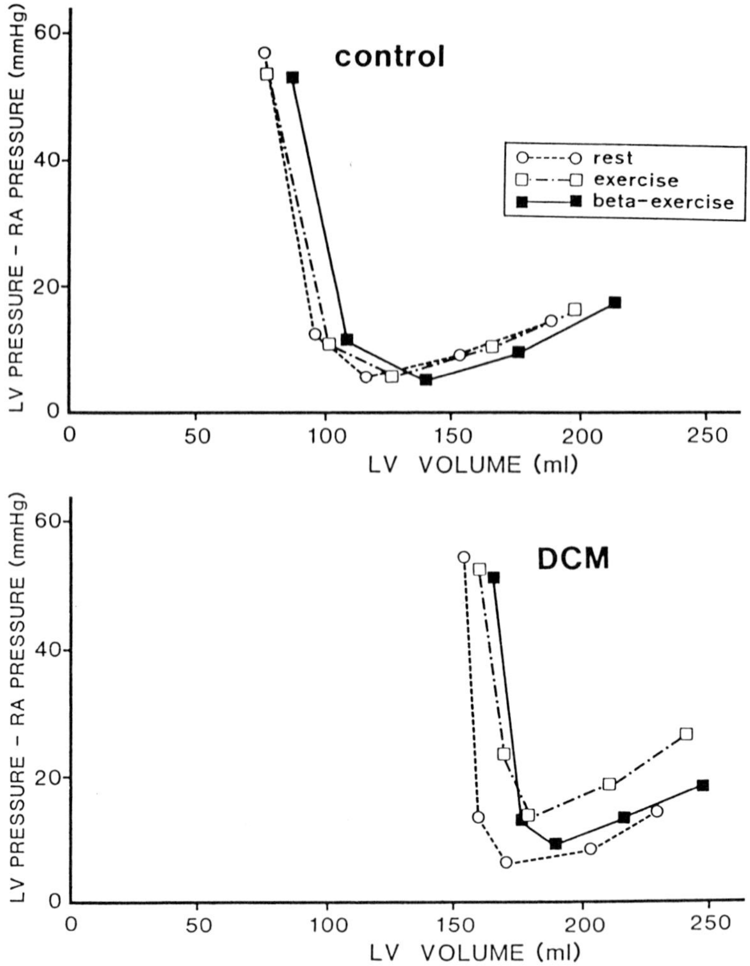

Fig. 6. Diastolic pressure-volume (P-V) relationship of the left ventricle in patients with dilated cardiomyopathy (*lower panel*) and in control subjects (*upper panel*). Immediately after exercise, the P-V relationship was shifted upward in patients with dilated cardiomyopathy. After administration of propranolol (0.1 mg/kg iv), this upward shift was markedly attenuated. In control subjects, the diastolic P-V relationship was not shifted. *LV*, left ventricle; *RA*, right atrium; *DCM*, dilated cardiomyopathy. (From [88])

A number of potential mechanisms for the beneficial effects of β-blocker treatment have been suggested [86]: (1) increased myocardial energy available for synthetic and reparative process, (2) improved diastolic relaxation, filling and compliance, (3) inhibition of sympathetically mediated vasoconstriction via prostaglandins and renin release, (4) protection against catecholamine-induced myocardial damage and necrosis, and (5) up-regulation of β-adrenoceptors. Grossman et al. [87] demonstrated impaired left ventricular relaxation and decreased diastolic chamber compliance. We studied the left ventricular chamber stiffness during exercise in patients with chronic heart failure. We observed that the left ventricular pressure-volume relationship was shifted upward during exercise and that this upward shift was significantly attenuated by administration of propranolol (Fig. 6) [88]. Attenuation of Ca^{2+} influx by β-blockade may be involved in improvement of myocardial distensibility during exercise. It is most likely that Ca^{2+} overload exists in the failing heart and this may cause myocardial injury. In dogs with heart failure produced by the intracoronary embolization of microspheres, we observed that the structures of microtubules, Ca^{2+}-sensitive cytoskelton, are severely disrupted. This histological abnormality may be attributed to the excessive sympathetic activity in dogs with heart failure since we observed that microtubules are sensitive to β-adrenoceptor stimulation which enhances Ca^{2+} influx, and that propranolol completely prevents the microtubule disruption induced by β-adrenoceptor stimulation. Up-regulation of β-adrenoceptors by administration of β-blockers may also play a role in restoration of inotropic reserve. We observed that lymphocyte β_2-adrenoceptors are up-regulated within a week after administration of metoprolol and down-regulated a few days after withdrawal in heart failure patients with dilated cardiomyopathy [89]. The relatively rapid response of β-adrenoceptors in not in accordance with the delayed improvement of exercise capacity and cardiac function that occurs usually more than three months after administration of β-blockers. This discrepancy may indicate that up-regulation of β-adrenoceptors does not play a crucial role in beneficial effect of β-blocker therapy. We also observed a decrease in heart rate and an increase in plasma renin activity during the metoprolol therapy. Thus, up-regulation of β-adrenoceptors contributes to the beneficial effects of β-blockers in heart failure in combination with other mechanisms, such as reduction of heart rate and inhibition of plasma renin release.

In conclusion, a subpopulation of patients whth chronic heart failure does respond to β-blocker therapy with symptomatic and functional improvement. Usually long-term treatment is necessary and clinical improvement is obtained after transient deterioration in acute period. The effective dose of β-blockers is rather low (60–120 mg/day of metoprolol) and a dose-response relationship could not be observed. However, the merit of this therapy is still controversial and large scale randomized, double-blind controlled trials will be necessary to reach a conclusive judgment.

References

1. Francis GS, Goldsmith SR, Olivari MT, Levine TB, Cohn JN (1984) The neurohormonal axis in congestive heart failure. Ann Intern Med 101:370–377
2. Watkins L, Burton JA, Haber E, Cant JR, Smith FW, Barger AC (1976) The renin-angiotensin system in congestive heart failure in conscious dogs. J Clin Invest 57:1606–1617
3. Thomas JA, Marks BH (1978) Plasma norepinephrine in congestive heart failure. Am J Cardiol 41:233–243

4. Curtiss L, Cohn JN, Vrobel T, Franciosa JA (1978) Role of the renin-angiotensin systemic vasoconstriction of chronic heart failure. Circulation 58:763–770
5. Ferguson DW, Abboud FM, Mark AL (1984) Selective impairment of baroreflex-mediated vasoconstrictor responses in patients with ventricular dysfunction. Circulation 69:451–460
6. Burch GE (1978) The role of the central nervous system in chronic congestive heart failure. Am Heart J 95:255–261
7. Cohn JN, Levine TB, Francis GS, Goldsmith S (1981) Neurohumoral control mechanisms in congestive heart failure. Am Heart J 102:509–514
8. Cody RJ, Franklin KW, Kluger J, Laragh JH (1982) Mechanisms governing the postural response and baroreceptor abnormalities in chronic congestive heart failure: effects of acute and long-term converting enzyme inhibition. Circulation 66: 135–142
9. Higgins CB, Vatner SF, Eckberg DL, Braunwald E (1972) Alterations in the baroreceptor reflex in conscious dogs with heart failure. J Clin Invest 51:715–724
10. Levine TB, Francis GS, Goldsmith SR, Cohn JN (1983) The neurohumoral and hemodynamic response to orthostatic tilt in patients with congestive heart failure. Circulation 67:1070–1075
11. Olivari MT, Levine TB, Cohn JN (1983) Abnormal neurohumoral response to nitroprusside infusion in congestive heart failure. J Am Coll Cardiol 2:411–417
12. Zucker IH, Peterson TV, Gilmore JP (1980) Ouabain increases left atrial stretch receptor discharge in the dog. J Pharmacol Exp Ther 212:320–324
13. Levine TB, Olivari MT, Carlyle P, Francis GS, Cohn JN (1982) Reversibility by heart transplantation of abnormal neurohumoral control mechanism in chronic congestive heart failure. Circulation 66(suppl II):II–192
14. Quest JA, Gillis RA (1974) Effect of digitalis on carotid sinus baroreceptor activity. Circ Res 35:247–255
15. Thomas RC (1972) Electrogenic sodium pump in nerve and muscle cells. Physiol Rev 52:563–594
16. Heesch CM, Abboud FM, Thames MD (1984) Acute resetting of carotid sinus baroreceptors. II. Possible involvement of electrogenic Na^+ pump. Am J Physiol 247:H833–H839
17. Berk BC, Aronow MS, Brock TA, Cragoe E, Gimbrone MA, Alexander RW (1987) Angiotensin II-stimulated Na^+/H^+ exchange in cultured vascular smooth muscle cells: evidence for protein kinase C-dependent and -independent pathways. J Biol Chem 262:5057–5064
18. Ochwadt B, Bücherl E, Kreuzer H, Loeschcke HH (1959) Beeinflussung der Atemsteigerung bei Muskelarbeit durch partillen neuromuskulären Block (Tubocurarin). Pflugers Arch 269:613–621
19. Mitchell JH, Reardon WC, McCloskey DI (1977) Reflex effects on circulation and respiration from contracting skeletal muscle. Am J Physiol 233:H374–H378
20. Waldrop TG, Rybicki KJ, Kaufman MP (1984) Chemical activation of group I and II muscle afferents has no cardiorespiratory effects. J Appl Physiol 56:1223–1228
21. Mitchell JH, Schmidt RF (1983) Cardiovascular reflex control by afferent fibers from skeletal muscle receptors. In: Shepherd JT, Abboud FM, Geiger SR (eds) Handbook of physiology — the cardiovascular system III. American Physiological Society, Bethesda, pp 623–658
22. Mitchell JH, Kaufman MP, Iwamoto GA (1983) The exercise pressor reflex: its cardiovascular effects, afferent mechanisms, and central pathways. Ann Rev Physiol 45:229–242

60. Feldman AM, Cates AE, Veazey WB, Hershberger RE, Bristow MR, Baughman KL, Baumgartner WA, Dop C (1988) Increase of the 40,000-MW pertussis toxin substrate (G protein) in the failing human heart. J Clin Invest 82:189–197
61. Hori M, Koretsune Y, Kagiya T, Watanabe Y, Iwakura K, Iwai K, Kitabatake A, Yoshida H, Inoue M, Kamada T (1989) A compensatory increase in beta-adrenoceptors for postischemic dysfunction following coronary microembolization in dogs. Cardiovasc Res 23:424–431
62. Heitz A, Schwartz J, Velly J (1983) β-Adrenoceptors of the human myocardium: determination of β_1 and β_2 subtypes by radioligand binding. Br J Pharmacol 80: 711–717
63. Bristow MR, Ginsburg R, Umans V, Fowler M, Minobe W, Rasmussen R, Zera P, Menlove R, Shah P, Jamieson S, Stinsom EB (1986) β_1- and β_2-Adrenergic receptor subtypes to muscle contraction and selective β^1-receptor down-regulation in heart failure. Circ Res 59:297–309
64. Tamai J, Hori M, Kagiya T, Iwakura K, Iwai K, Kitabatake A, Watanabe Y, Yoshida H, Inoue M, Kamada T (1989) Role of α_1-adrenoceptor activity in progression of cardiac hypertrophy in pressure-overloaded guinea pig hearts. Cardiovasc Res 23:315–322
65. Mukherjee A, Bush LR, McCoy KE, Duke RJ, Hagler H, Buja LM, Willerson JT (1982) Relationship between beta-adrenergic receptor numbers and physiological responses during experimental canine myocardial ischemia. Circ Res 50:735–741
66. Lurie KG, Bristow MR, Reitz BA (1983) Increased β-adrenergic receptor density in an experimental model of cardiac transplantation. J Thorac Cardiovasc Surg 86: 195–201
67. Kagiya T, Hori M, Iwakura K, Iwai K, Watanabe Y, Uchida S, Yoshida H, Kitabatake A, Inoue M, Kamada T (1991) Role of increased α_1-adrenergic activity in cardiomyopathic Syrian hamsters. Am J Physiol 260:H80–H88
68. Pool PE, Covell JW, Levitt M, Gibb J, Braunwald E (1967) Reduction of cardiac tyrosine hydroxylase activity in experimental congestive heart failure: its role in depletion of cardiac norepinephrine stores. Circ Res 20:349–353
69. Rona G, Chappel CI, Balazs T, Gaudry R (1959) An infarct-like myocardial lesion and other toxic manifestations produced by isoproterenol in the rat. Arch Pathol 67:443–455
70. Maling HM, Highman B (1958) Exaggerated ventricular arrhythmias and myocardial fatty changes after large doses of norepinephrine and epinephrine in unanesthetized dogs. Am J Physiol 194:590–596
71. Haft JI, Gershengorn K, Kranz PD, Oestreicher R (1972) Protection against epinephrine-induced myocardial necrosis by drugs that inhibit platelet aggregation. Am J Cardiol 30:838–843
72. Singal PK, Yates JC, Beamish RE, Dhalla NS (1981) Influence of reducing agents on adrenochrome-induced changes in the heart. Pathol Lab Med 105:664–669
73. Yates JC, Beamish RE, Dhalla NS (1981) Ventricular dysfunction and necrosis produced by adrenochrome metabolite of epinephrine: relation to pathogeneses of cardiomyopathy. Am Heart J 102:210–221
74. Fleckenstein A, Janke J, Doring HJ, Pachinger O (1973) Ca overload as the determinant factor in the production of catecholamine-induced myocardial lesions. In: Bajusz E et al. (Eds.) Recent advances in studies on cardiac structure and metabolism, cardiomyopathies. Vol 2 University Park Press, Baltimore, pp 455–466
75. Kusuoka H, Porterfield JK, Weisman HF, Weisfeldt ML, Marban E (1987) Pathophysiology and pathogenesis of stunned myocardium: depressed Ca^{2+} activation of

contraction as a consequence of reperfusion-induced cellular calcium overload in ferret hearts. J Clin Invest 79:950–961
76. Kitakaze M, Weisfeldt ML, Marban E (1988) Acidosis during early reperfusion prevents myocardial stunning in perfused hearts. J Clin Invest 82:920–927
77. Hori M, Sato H, Iwai K, Takashima S, Sato H, Inoue M, Kitabatake A, Kamada T (to be published) (1991) Disruption of microtubles in cultured neonatal rat cardiomyocytes during rapid contractions: protective effects of beta-adrenoceptor antagonist. Jpn Circ J
78. Waagstein F, Hjalmmarson A, Varnauskas E, Wallentin I (1975) Effect of chronic beta-adrenergic receptor blockade in congestive cardiomyopathy. Br Heart J 37: 1022–1036
79. Swedberg K, Waagstein F, Hjalmarson A, Wallentin I (1979) Prolongation of survival in congestive cardiomyopathy by beta receptor blockade. Lancet 1: 1374–1376
80. Swedberg K, Waagstein F, Hjalmarson A, Wallentin I (1980) Adverse effects of beta blockade withdrawal in patients with congestive cardiomyopathy. Br Heart J 44:134–142
81. Anderson JL, Lutz JR, Gilbert EM, Sorensen SG, Yanowitz FG, Melove RL, Bartholomew M (1985) A randomized trial of low-dose beta-blockade therapy for idiopathic dilated cardiomyopathy. Am J Cardiol 55:471–475
82. Fowler MB, Bristow MR, Laser JA, Ginsburg R, Scott LB, Schrowdwe JS (1984) Beta blocker therapy in severe heart failure: improvement related to $beta_1$-adrenergic receptor up regulation? Circulation 70(suppl II):II-112
83. Engelmeier RS, O'Conell JB, Walsh R, Rad N, Scanlon PJ, Gunnar RM (1985) Improvement in symptoms and exercise tolerance by metoprolol in patients with dilated cardiomyopathy: a double-blind, randomized, placebo-controlled trial. Circulation 72:536–546
84. Ikram H, Fitzpatrick D (1981) Double-blind trial of chronic oral beta-blockade in congestive cardiomyopathy. Lancet 2:490–493
85. Currie PJ, Kelly MJ, McKenzie A, Harper RW, Lim YL, Federman J, Anderson ST, Pitt A (1984) Oral beta-adrenergic blockade with metoprolol in chronic severe dilated cardiomyopathy. J Am Coll Cardiol 3:203–209
86. Alderman J, Grossman W (1985) Are β-adrenergic-blocking drugs useful in the treatment of dilated cardiomyopathy? Circulation 71:854–857
87. Grossmann W, McLaurin LP, Rolett EL (1979) Alterations in left ventricular relaxation and diastolic compliance in congestive cardiomyopathy. Cardiovasc Res 13:514–522
88. Ozaki H, Sato H, Matsuyama, T, Yokoyama H, Hori M, Kitabatake A, Kamada T, Takeda H, Inoue M (1989) Acute effects of β-blocker on left ventricular diastolic pressure-volume relation during exercise in patients with dilated cardiomyopathy. Shinzo 21(suppl 2):40–44
89. Kagiya T, Hori M, Fukunami M, Hoki N, Iwakura K, Kurihara T, Watanabe Y, Kamada T (1987) Role of beta-adrenergic receptors in beta-blocker therapy for chronic heart failure in patients with dilated cardiomyopathy. Circulation 76(suppl IV):IV-308

10

Effects of Rapid Pacing Stress on Ventricular Function of Hypertrophied Human Heart

Yasuyuki Nakamura[1], Takashi Konishi[2], Toshiaki Kumada[2], Chuichi Kawai[2]

Summary. Rapid pacing stress has been used to study hemodynamics, ventricular function and metabolism in ischemic heart disease. This method was applied to patients with left ventricular hypertrophy but without coronary artery disease in order to gain an insight into the mechanism responsible for the transition from compensation to failure in cardiac hypertrophy. Seven patients with LV hypertrophy (H) (three patients with aortic stenosis and four patients with hypertrophic non-obstructive cardiomyopathy) and six controls with chest pain syndrome (C) were studied. The coronary arteriograms were normal and no LV dysfunction was present on pre-pacing LV grams in all the cases. Although the pre-pacing LV ejection fractions (EF) were not different in the two groups, the post-pacing EF diminished in H (68.2 ± 7.8 to 63.5 ± 12.8%, $P < 0.05$), but not in C. The pre-pacing LV end-diastolic pressure (EDP) was slightly higher in H (H, 14.4 ± 6.5; C, 9.0 ± 2.2 mmHg, $P < 0.05$), and EDP increased markedly after pacing only in H (30.0 ± 7.4 mmHg, $P < 0.01$), while the LV end-diastolic volume index in H increased slightly (80.3 ± 29.7 to 86.4 ± 25.3 ml/M^2, n.s.), indicating a decrease in LV chamber compliance with pacing in H. Thus, LV systolic function and chamber compliance deteriorate with pacing in hypertrophied hearts with normal LV contraction before pacing. Susceptibility to pacing stress may suggest a role of the diminished coronary reserve in the development of ultimate failure in hypertrophy.

Key words: Coronary reserve — Heart failure — Hypertrophy — Pacing stress

[1] First Department of Medicine, Shiga University of Medical Science, Shiga, 520–21 Japan
[2] Third Division, Department of Internal Medicine, Faculty of Medicine, Kyoto University, Japan

Introduction

Cardiac hypertrophy is one of the adaptive mechanisms of the heart against abnormal loading conditions. Interest in the function of the hypertrophied heart has spawned a number of studies of hypertrophy models and of patients with hypertrophy of various etiologies. Work has included isolated cardiac muscle studies [1, 2], intact heart studies in animals with opened chests [3], and studies of conscious animals [4–6] as well as of humans [7, 8]. The results have been varied depending on the models used and the stages of hypertrophy studied. According to serial observation studies, initial normal function in the adaptation stage and the transition to pump failure in the late stage has been demonstrated [3, 6]. The findings have been well accepted by clinical cardiologists who observe different stages of the patients with hypertrophy.

The question then arises about the mechanism for the transition from adaptation to failure, and there have been a number of hypotheses. In order to gain an insight into the mechanism, we studied left ventricular function in patients with hypertrophy before and after intervention with rapid pacing stress.

Pacing Stress Testing

Rapid Pacing as a Method for Ischemic Intervention

In order to study hemodynamics, ventricular function and metabolism during ischemia in patients with coronary artery disease, several intervention methods have been utilized at the time of cardiac catheterization, thallium myocardial scintigraphy and echocardiography. These include dynamic exercise tests [9, 10], isometric exercise tests [11], infusion of catecholamines such as dobutamine [12], and the chronotropic stress test with pacing tachycardia [13–15]. Atrial pacing was first introduced by Sowton et al. as a stress test during cardiac catheterization to evaluate patients with ischemic heart disease [13]. Of these stress tests, pacing tachycardia is one of the most frequently used methods because of its easy applicability, good reproducibility, reliability and safety.

Hemodynamic Effects of Rapid Pacing

The mechanism for induction of ischemia by rapid pacing has been attributed to an increase in myocardial oxygen consumption secondary to the increased heart rate and to an increase in myocardial contractility because of the Treppe effect [16]. Compared with dynamic exercise, however, a rise in rate-pressure product (heart rate × peak systolic pressure), an estimate of myocardial oxygen consumption, is minimal [17]. Furthermore, the minute stroke work with rapid pacing does not increase significantly enough to account for ischemia in patients with coronary artery disease, since the stroke work per beat during rapid pacing falls substantially due to a drop in the stroke volume which inversely correlates with the heart rate, and there is no change or even a decrease in the aortic pressure. However, ischemia does occur with rapid pacing in patients with coronary artery disease. Parker et al. measured arterial and coronary sinus blood lactate concentration before, during and after rapid pacing and demonstrated the shift from lactate extraction to lactate production with pacing [18]. More recently, Heller et al. demonstrated myocardial ischemia on thallium myocardial scans during rapid pacing in the patients with coronary artery disease [19]. The area of hypoperfusion on the thallium scans during pacing refilled on the delay images.

Since ischemia is definitely induced easily with rapid pacing in patients with coronary artery disease despite a minimal increase in myocardial oxygen demand, a more important mechanism for ischemia with this intervention has to be substantiated. With rapid pacing, the diastolic filling period shortens inversely with the heart rate. Initially, the isovolumic relaxation rate may not change, in contrast to tachycardia induced by exercise or catecholamine infusion when it accelerates. Shortening of the diastole and no change in the relaxation rate during rapid pacing may not cause any deleterious effects on coronary circulation in normal subjects, but this condition can limit coronary supply in patients with coronary artery disease whose coronary reserve is diminished, and hence it may result in ischemia. Ischemia causes impaired relaxation and a decrease in left ventricular compliance. These two changes may further deteriorate coronary circulation in patients with ischemic heart disease, and thus a vicious circle may be established. Therefore, one of the important mechanisms for ischemia with rapid pacing in patients with diminished coronary reserve appears to be the generation of the vicious circle in coronary circulation as described above.

Pacing Induced Changes in Hemodynamics and Ventricular Function in Coronary Artery Disease

Before discussing the effects of rapid pacing in hypertrophy, it would be worth looking at the changes induced by rapid pacing in patients with coronary artery disease [15].

The effect of pacing was studied in 11 patients with coronary artery disease. All of the 11 patients with coronary artery disease developed typical anginal pain during pacing tachycardia, and the hemodynamics and the ventricular functions were examined in the post-pacing beat. Figure 1 shows the results. As seen in Figure 1a, the heart rate and the peak left ventricular pressure did not change significantly. The left ventricular end-diastolic pressure rose significantly with ischemic intervention. Impairment of ventricular ejection is indicated by decreases in the ejection fraction and the percent shortening (%L) of the ischemic segment. The relaxation time constant increased significantly, implying impairment of relaxation with ischemia. The %L of the control segment did not change in post-pacing beats. The peak rate of early left ventricular filling (LVPF), the LVPF/stroke volume (SV), and the LVPF/end-

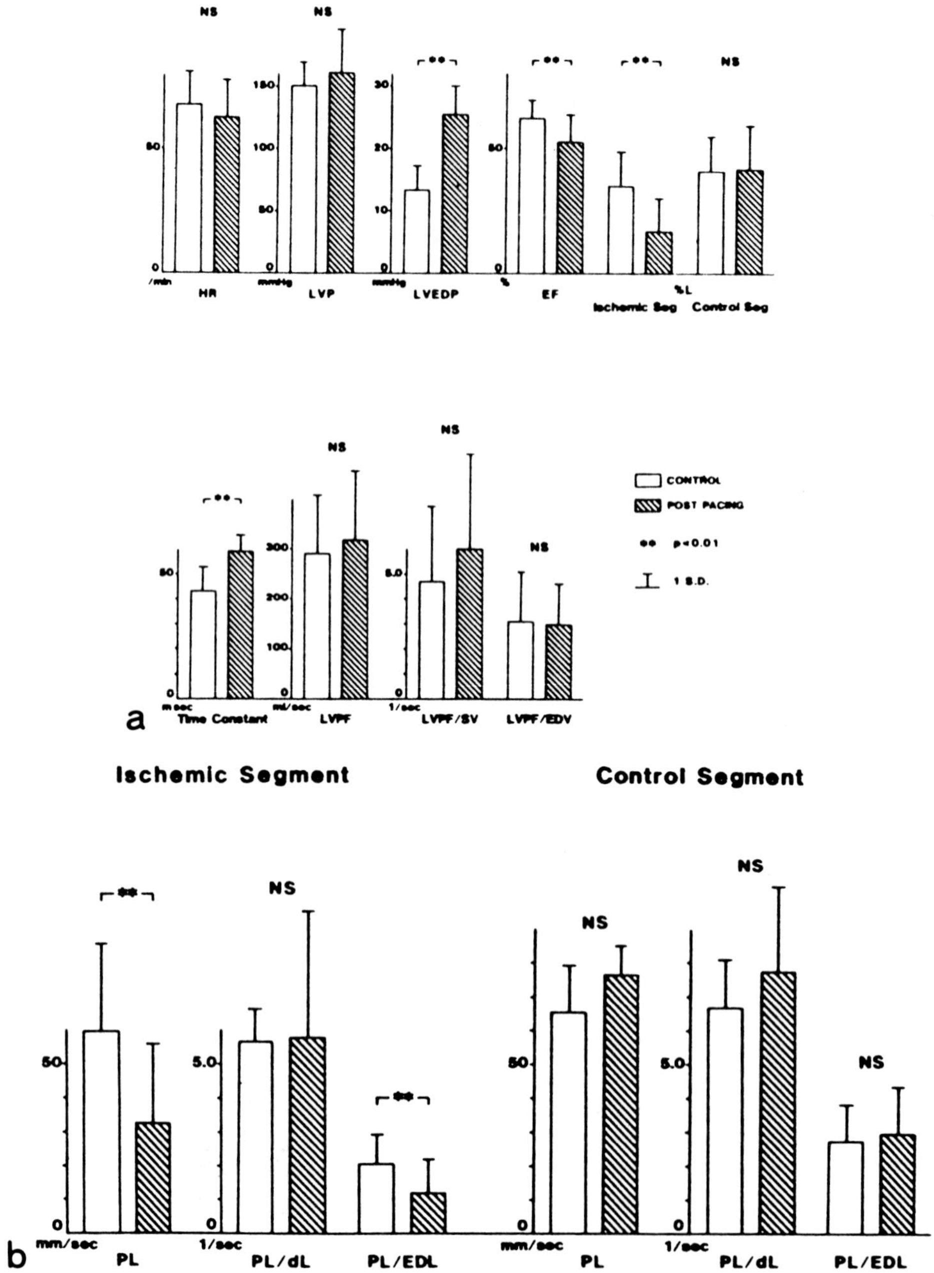

Fig. 1. a Effects of pacing induce ischemia on hemodynamics and ventricular function. The heart rate (*HR*) and peak left ventricular pressure (*LVP*) did not change significantly. The left ventricular end-diastolic pressure (*LVEDP*) rose significantly with ischemic intervention. Impairment of ventricular ejection is indicated by decreases in

diastolic volume (EDV) did not change significantly. Figure 1b shows the effects of pacing induced ischemia on regional myocardial lengthening. In the ischemic segment, the peak rate of lengthening (PL) decreased with pacing induced ischemia, as did the PL/end-diastolic segment length (EDL). However, the PL/extent of shortening (dL) did not change with ischemic intervention. Analysis of the control segment showed a tendency to increase in these three variables in post pacing beats. In short, substantial deterioration in global ejection, segment shortening, and relaxation occurred during pacing-induced ischemia in the patients with coronary artery disease. The early diastolic global filling rate did not change, probably because of an increase in left atrial pressure with ischemia.

Chronotropic Stress in Cardiac Hypertrophy

Ischemic intervention with rapid pacing, as used in studies of heart function in patients with coronary artery disease, was used in the present study of the hypertrophied heart in order to test the following hypothesis: diminished coronary reserve is an important factor for transition from compensation to ultimate pump failure in cardiac hypertrophy.

Study Patients and Methods

We studied seven patients with left ventricular hypertrophy, three with aortic stenosis and four with hypertrophic non-obstructive cardiomyopathy whose coronary arteriogram and resting left ventriculogram were normal. The patients, two women and five men, had a mean age of 55 years. Six patients with chest pain but normal coronary arteriograms and left ventriculograms served as the

←

the ejection fraction (*EF*) and the percent shortening (*%L*) of the ischemic segment. The relaxation time constant (*Time Constant*) increased significantly, implying impairment of relaxation with ischemia. The *%L* of the control segment did not change in post-pacing beats. The peak rate of early left ventricular filling (*LVPF*), the LVPF/stroke volume (*SV*), and the LVPF/end-diastolic volume (*EDV*) did not change significantly. Control data, *open bars*; post-pacing data, *shaded bars*. $^{**}P < 0.01$, N.S. = not statistically significant. n = 11 except for *Time Constant*, where n = 7. **b** Effects of pacing-induced ischemia on regional myocardial dynamics. In the ischemic segment, the peak rate of lengthening (*PL*) decreased with pacing induced ischemia, as did the PL/end-diastolic segment length (*EDL*). However, the PL/extent of shortening (*dL*) did not change with ischemic intervention. Analysis of the control segment showed a tendency to increase in these three variables in post-pacing beats. (From [15] with permission)

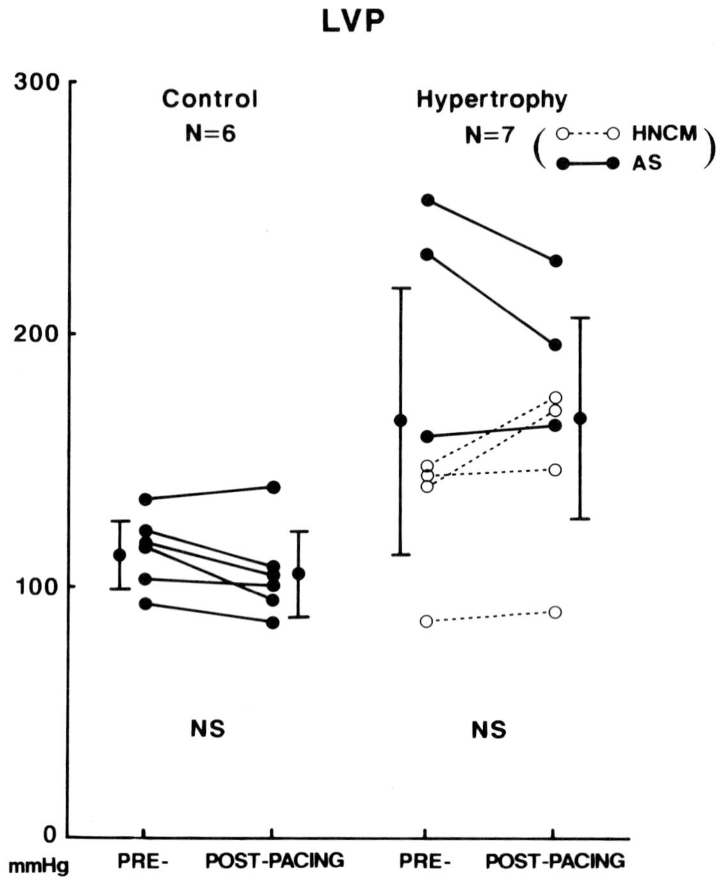

Fig. 2. Changes in left ventricular pressure (*LVP*) before and after rapid right ventricular pacing. No significant changes were seen in the both groups. *HNCH*, hypertrophic non-obstructive cardiomyopathy; *AS*, aortic stenosis; N.S., not statistically significant

control (mean age, 46 years). After a routine left ventriculogram, we waited until the left ventricular pressure returned to the baseline, and right ventricular pacing was started at a rate of $150\,min^{-1}$. The pacing duration was 6 min for all patients but one with hypertrophic cardiomyopathy who discontinued pacing at 5 min due to angina-like chest pain. Chest pain was induced in another patient with aortic stenosis. No chest pain was induced in the control patients. The second left ventriculogram was obtained immediately after pacing was stopped.

Changes Induced by Rapid Pacing in Patients with Left Ventricular Hypertrophy

Figure 2 shows left ventricular pressure before and after rapid right ventricular pacing. No significant changes were seen in both groups. In addition, the heart

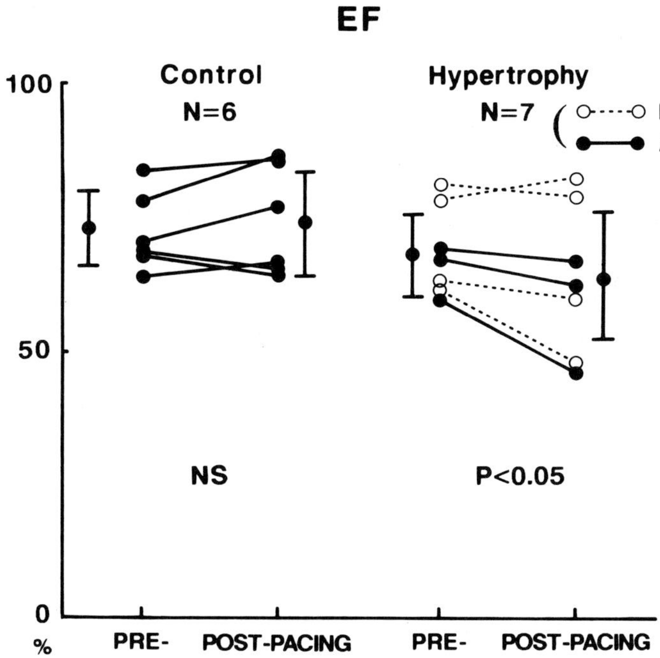

Fig. 3. Changes in the left ventricular ejection fraction (*EF*). No changes in the ejection fraction were noted in the controls (from 72.3 ± 6.7 to 74.3 ± 9.6%, n.s.). However, there was a slight but significant decline in the ejection fraction in the hypertrophy group with ischemic intervention (from 68.2 ± 7.8 to 63.5 ± 12.8%, $P < 0.05$). *HNCM*, hypertrophic non-obstructive cardiomyopathy; *AS*, aortic stenosis; N.S., not statistically significant

rate did not change (not shown). Figure 3 shows changes in the left ventricular ejection fraction. No changes were noted in the controls (from 72.3 ± 6.7 to 74.3 ± 9.6%, n.s.), but there was a slight but significant decline in the ejection fraction in the hypertrophy group with ischemic intervention (from 68.2 ± 7.8 to 63.5 ± 12.8%, $P < 0.05$). Therefore, rapid pacing provoked left ventricular contraction abnormality in hypertrophied hearts whose resting contraction was well preserved.

As seen in Fig. 4, the isovolumic relaxation time constant (Tau) was higher in the hypertrophy group than in the controls, even prior to ischemic intervention ($P < 0.05$). The post-pacing Tau increased further in the hypertrophy, but no change was found in the controls (control patients: 36.4 ± 3.9 vs. 37.4 ± 6/0 msec, n.s.; hypertrophy patients: 54.6 ± 9.1 vs. 68.4 ± 12.1 msec, $P < 0.01$). Thus, myocardial relaxation was impaired in the hypertrophied heart with preserved systolic function. The impairment in relaxation became worse in the post-pacing beats.

The most prominent change was seen in the left ventricular end-diastolic pressure in the hypertrophy group as seen in Fig. 5. It rose from 14 ± 6 to 30.0

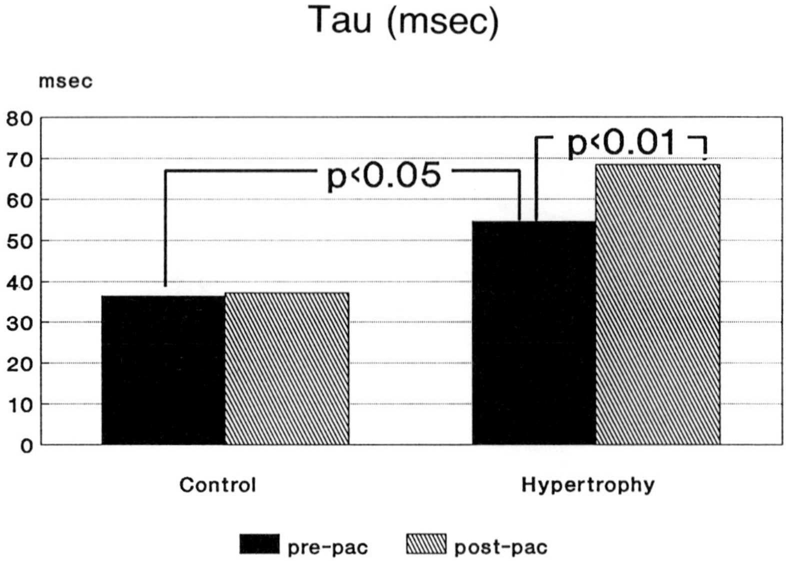

Fig. 4. Changes in isovolumic relaxation time constant (*Tau*). The isovolumic relaxation time constant (*Tau*) was increased in the hypertrophy group compared to the controls even prior to ischemic intervention ($P < 0.05$). Post-pacing *Tau* increased further in the hypertrophy group, but no change was found in the controls (controls: 36.4 ± 3.9 vs. 37.4 ± 6/0 msec, n.s.; hypertrophy group: 54.6 ± 9.1 vs. 68.4 ± 12.1 msec, $P < 0.01$)

± 7 mmHg ($P < 0.01$) with pacing, on average. The change in the controls was not significant. In contrast to the change in the left ventricular end-diastolic pressure, the left ventricular end-diastolic volume index showed virtually no change in both groups, as shown in Fig. 6. The prominent rise in the left ventricular end-diastolic pressure without significant change in the left ventricular volume may indicate significant reduction in chamber compliance in the hypertrophy patients with ischemic intervention.

Figure 7 shows the diastolic pressure-volume relations in patients with aortic stenosis. The results from patient KAN may indicate a significant increase in the chamber stiffness constant, whereas in the other two patients, the upward shift of pressure-volume relations may account for the rise in left ventricular end-diastolic pressure. Figure 8 shows the diastolic pressure-volume relations in the patients with hypertrophic non-obstructive cardiomyopathy. In the results from patient INA, an increase in chamber stiffness was seen, and in those from patient TAK, an upward shift of the relation was seen. In the results from patient HAY, an upward shift of the relation and also an increase in the end-diastolic volume were observed. In short, the mechanisms for a reduction in chamber compliance with ischemic intervention in hypertrophy may not be uniform, rather more than one mechanism may be operating.

Fig. 5. Changes in left ventricular end-diastolic pressure (*LVEDP*). *LVEDP* rose from 14 ± 6 to 30.0 ± 7 mmHg ($P < 0.01$) with pacing, on average. The change in the controls was not significant. *HNCM*, hypertrophic non-obstructive cardiomyopathy; *AS*, aortic stenosis; n.s., not statistically significant

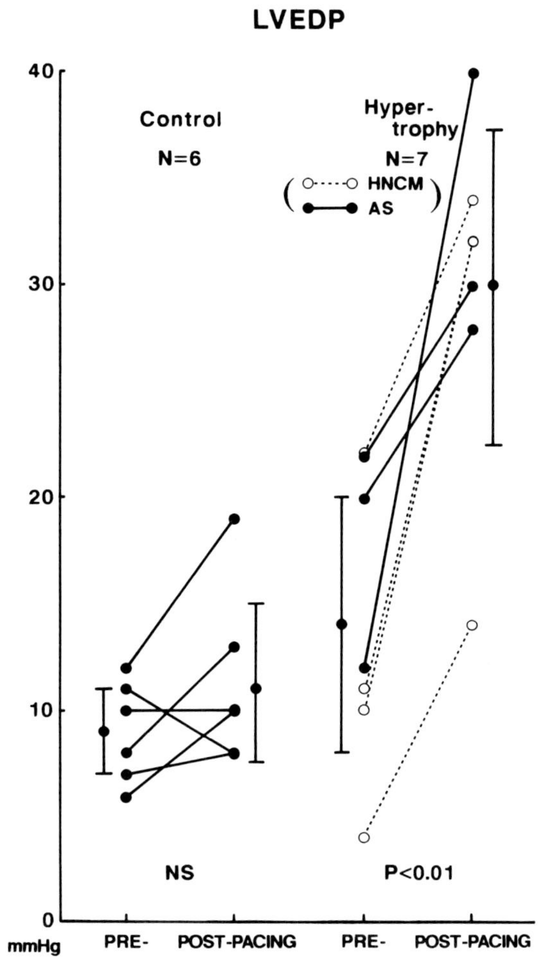

Quest for the Mechanisms for the Transition from Compensation to Failure in Cardiac Hypertrophy

There have been a number of investigations into the mechanisms for the transition from compensation to pump failure in cardiac hypertrophy. The following may only described some of the mechanisms so far postulated, but they seem to be important and are directly or indirectly related to interpretation of our present study.

Cardiac Myosin Isozyme Redistribution

In small animals, cardiac hypertrophy causes a shift of heavy chain myosin isozymes, and an isozyme of a lower ATPase activity (V_3 or β-type) predominates [20]. This shift has been paralleled with a decrease in maximal speed

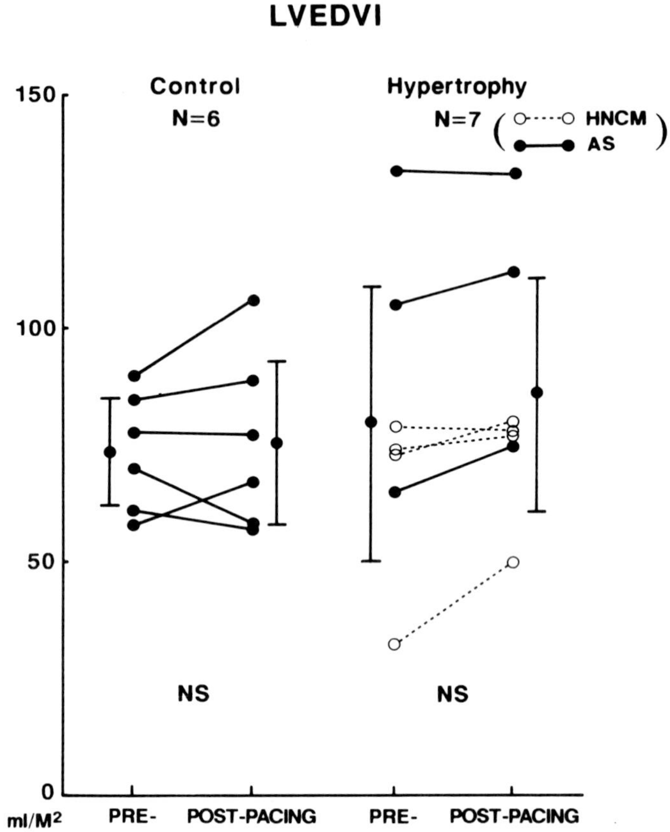

Fig. 6. Changes in left ventricular end-diastolic volume index (*LVEDVI*). In contrast to the change in the LVEDP, the LVEDVI shows virtually no change in the both groups. *HNCM*, hypertrophic non-obstructive cardiomyopathy; *AS*, aortic stenosis; N.S., not statistically significant

of muscle shortening (V_{max}) and an increase in myothermal economy [21]. A similar change has been reported to occur in hypothyroid rat myocardium [22]. However, many studies, including our own, have shown that the overall myocardial energy efficiency is reduced in the hypertrophied heart [23, 24] (see Chapter 6). Furthermore, myosin isozyme redistribution in larger animals or humans has been reported to play only a minor role since β-myosin is the major component of ventricular myocardium even in the normal heart [25, 26].

Abnormal Calcium Handling in Cardiac Hypertrophy

Mitochondrial calcium metabolism in cardiac hypertrophy has been controversial [27, 28]. However, calcium uptake and calcium ATPase of sarcoplasmic reticulum (SR) of the hypertrophied heart have been uniformly found to be depressed [28, 29]. Recently, Komuro et al. [30] found that the mRNA levels

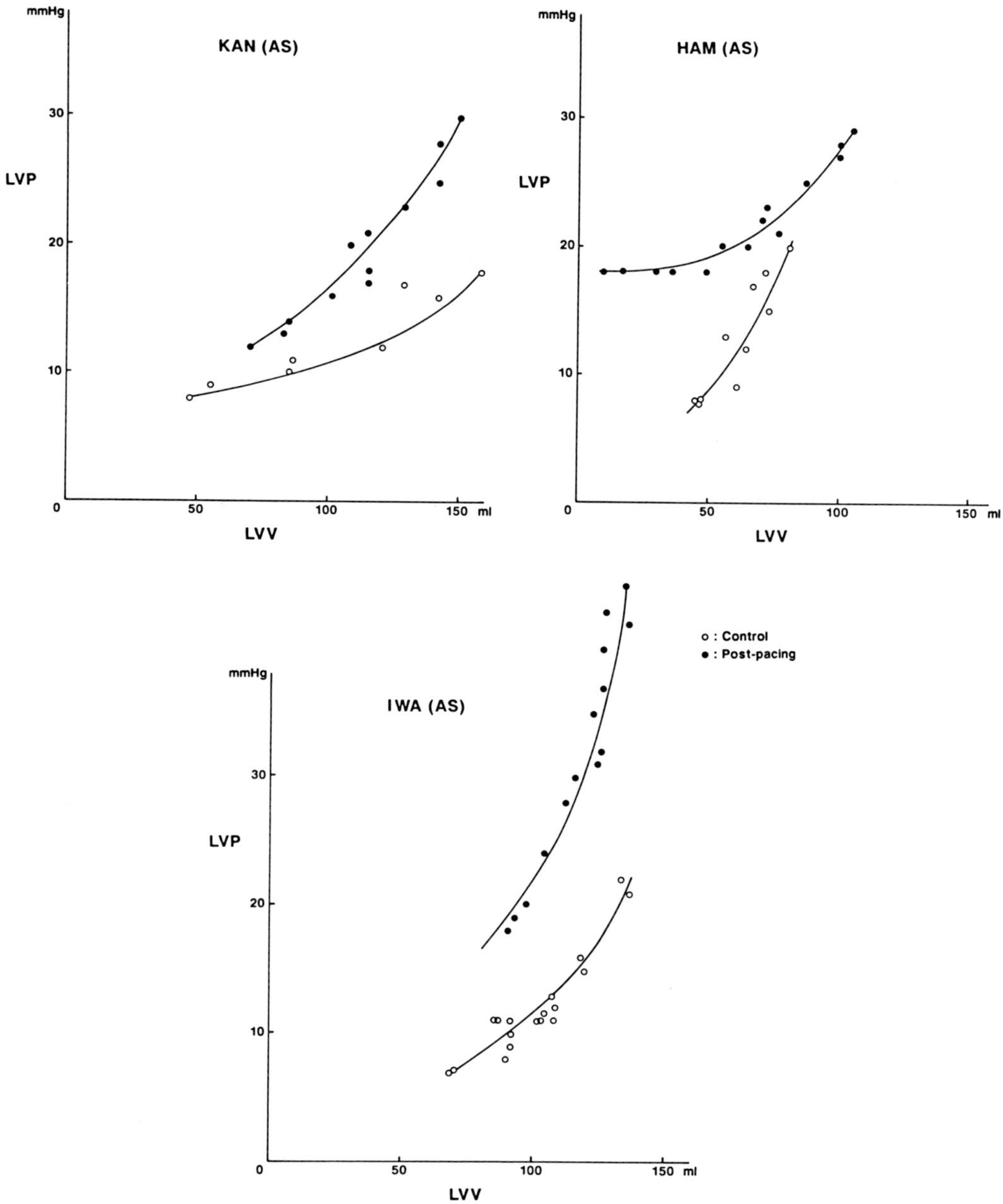

Fig. 7. Diastolic pressure-volume relations in patients with aortic stenosis. The results from patient KAN may indicate a significant increase in chamber stiffness constant, whereas in the other two patients, the upward shift of the pressure-volume relations may account for the rise in left ventricular end-diastolic pressure. *LVV*, left ventricular volume; *LVP*, left ventricular pressure; *AS*, aortic stenosis

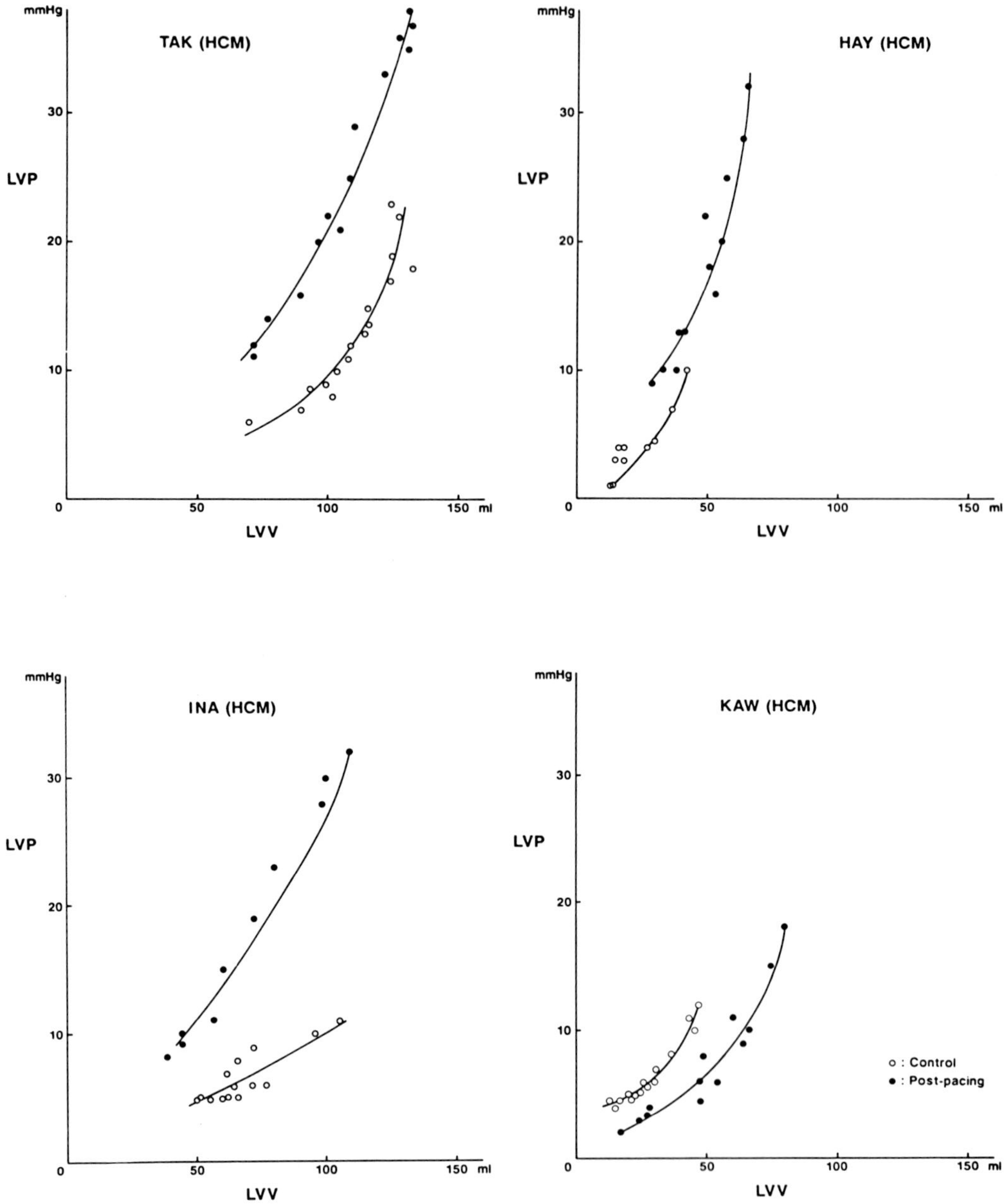

Fig. 8. Diastolic pressure-volume relations in the patients with hypertrophic non-obstructive cardiomyopathy. In patient INA, an increase in chamber stiffness was seen and in patient TAK, an upward shift of the relation was seen. In patient HAY, an upward shift of the relation and also an increase in the end-diastolic volume were observed. *LVV*, left ventricular volume; *LVP*, left ventricular pressure; *HCM*, hypertrophic (non-obstructive) cardiomyopathy

of calcium ATPase in SR of the pressure overloaded heart were decreased and that the expression of cardiac calcium-ATPase in SR is regulated by pressure overload. This change in SR calcium-ATPase may well be in concert with the results of the present study as well as other mechanical studies of hypertrophied myocardium and heart, where impairment of relaxation has been found universally even when the contractile function is found to be normal.

Diminished Coronary Reserve in Hypertrophy

Linzbach [31] proposed the hypothesis that heart failure in hypertrophy is caused by relative ischemia due to inadequate capillary growth compared with the hypertrophy of the muscle fiber. According to Henquell et al. [32] who measured intercapillary distance in hypertrophied rat hearts beating in situ, the capillary reserve in hypertrophy was fully utilized and the mean functional intercapillary distance was greater than normal. They thought this was responsible for the focal necrosis and fibrosis observed in hypertrophy and for the development of circulatory failure. Our study has demonstrated that this mechanism indeed is operating in human hypertrophied hearts of patients with aortic stenosis and hypertrophic non-obstructive cardiomyopathy, as ischemic intervention with rapid pacing resulted in systolic dysfunction and deterioration in diastolic functions.

Afterload Excess

Stress-shortening analyses in whole hearts of experimental models and humans have shown that the difference in shortening between compensated hypertrophied hearts and failing hypertrophied hearts are due to differences in afterload [6, 8, 33]. Afterload excess or afterload mismatch has been observed in hypertrophy with depressed contractile function, and changes in the inotropic state were not seen in the majority of the cases. It is not surprising to see that a study of isolated cardiac muscle from an aged SHR showed a normal shortening speed and a normal peak-developed tension even though an SHR of the same age exhibited depressed pump function in an in-situ whole heart study [3, 34]. This is because in isolated cardiac muscle studies, all mechanical indices are normalized by cross-sectional area, and the data expressed after excluding the effect of different afterloads. Therefore, the indices do not become depressed until very late.

Gaasch et al. [6] recently proposed the following mechanism for transition to pump failure in hypertrophy: intermittent ischemia due to limited coronary reserve in hypertrophy may result in impaired myocardial protein synthesis, and thus left ventricular wall thickness does not increase in proportion to the product of systolic pressure and radius. Therefore, hypertrophic hearts with pump failure exhibit afterload excess. There appears to be a firm cause and effect relation, and our present observations also seem to support the hypothesis.

References

1. Spann JF Jr, Buccino RA, Sonnenblick EH, Braunwald E (1967) Contractile state of cardiac muscle obtained from cats with experimentally produced ventricular hypertrophy and heart failure. Circ Res 21:341–354
2. Bing OHL, Matsushita S, Fanburg BL, Levine HJ (1971) Mechanical properties of rat cardiac muscle during experimental hypertrophy. Circ Res 28:234–245
3. Pfeffer MA, Pfeffer JM, Frohlich ED (1976) Pumping ability of the hypertrophying left ventricle of the spontaneously hypertensive rat. Circ Res 38:423–429
4. Sasayama S, Ross J Jr, Franklin D, Bloor CM, Bishop S, Dilley RB (1976) Adaptation of the left ventricle to chronic pressure overload. Circ Res 38:172–178
5. Morioka S, Simon G (1982) Echocardiographic evidence for early left ventricular hypertrophy in dogs with renal hypertension. Am J Cardiol 49:1891–1898
6. Gaasch WH, Zile MR, Hoshino PK, Apstein CS, Blaustein AS (1989) Stress-shortening relations and myocardial blood flow in compensated and failing canine hearts with pressure-overloaded hypertrophy. Circulation 79:872–883
7. Hood WP Jr, Rackley CE, Rolett EL (1968) Wall stress in the normal and hypertrophied human left ventricle. Am J Cardiol 22:550–558
8. Gunther S, Grossman W (1979) Determinants of ventricular function in pressure-overloaded hypertrophy in man. Circulation 59:679–688
9. Thadani U, West RO, Mathew TM, Parker JO (1977) Hemodynamics at rest and during supine and sitting bicycle exercise in patients with coronary artery disease. Am J Cardiol 39:776–783
10. Carroll JD, Hess OM, Hirzel HO, Krayenbuehl HP (1983) Dynamics of left ventricular filling at rest and during exercise. Circulation 68:59–67
11. Helfant RH, DeVilla MA, Meister SG (1971) Effect of sustained isometric handgrip exercise on left ventricular performance. Circulation 44:982–993
12. Mannering D, Cripps T, Leech G, Mehta N, Valentine H, Gilmour S, Bennett ED (1988) The dobutamine stress test as an alternative to exercise testing after acute myocardial infarction. Br Heart J 59:521–526
13. Sowton GE, Balcon R, Cross D, Frick MH (1967) Measurement of the angina threshold using atrial pacing. Cardiovasc Res 1:301–307
14. Fujita M, Sasayama S, Kawai C, Eiho S, Kuwahara M (1981) Automatic processing of cineventriculograms for analysis of regional myocardial function. Circulation 63:1065–1074
15. Nakamura Y, Sasayama S, Nonogi H, Miyazaki S, Fujita M, Kihara Y, Konishi T, Kawai C (1987) Effects of pacing-induced ischemia on early left ventricular filling and regional myocardial dynamics and their modification by nifedipine. Circulation 76:1232–1244
16. Ricci D, Orlick A, Alderman E (1979) Role of tachycardia as an inotropic stimulus in man. J Clin Invest 63:695–703
17. McKay RG, Grossman W (1986) Hemodynamic stress testing during pacing tachycardia. In: Grossman W (ed) Cardiac catheterization and angiography, 3rd edn. Lea & Febiger, Philadelphia pp 267–281
18. Parker JO, Chiong MA, West RO, Case RB (1969) Sequential alterations in myocardial lactate metabolism, S-T segments, and left ventricular functions during angina induced by atrial pacing. Circulation 40:113–131
19. Heller GV, Aroesry JM, Parker JA, McKay RG, Silverman KJ, Als AV, Come PC, Kolodny GM (1984) The pacing stress test: thallium-201 myocardial imaging after atrial pacing. Diagnostic value in detecting coronary artery disease compared with exercise testing. J Am Coll Cardiol 3:1197–1204

20. Lompre AM, Schwartz K, d'Albis A, Lacombe G, Thiem NV, Swynghedauw B (1979) Myosin isozyme redistribution in chronic heart overload. Nature 282: 105–107
21. Alpert NR, Mulieri LA (1982) Increased myothermal economy of isometric force generation in compensated cardiac hypertrophy induced by pulmonary artery constriction in the rabbit. A characterization of heat liberation in normal and hypertrophied right ventricular papillary muscles. Circ Res 50:491–500
22. Holubarsch Ch, Goulette RP, Litten RZ, Martin BJ, Mulieri LA, Alpert NR (1985) The economy of isometric force development, myosin isoenzyme pattern and myofibrillar ATPase activity in normal and hypothyroid rat myocardium. Circ Res 56:78–86
23. Gunning JF, Coleman HN (1973) Myocardial oxygen consumption during experimental hypertrophy and congestive heart failure. J Mol Cell Cardiol 5:25–38
24. Cooper G IV, Satava RM Jr, Harrison CE, Coleman HN III (1973) Mechanism for the abnormal energetics of pressure-induced hypertrophy of cat myocardium. Circ Res 33:213–223
25. Gorza L, Mercadier JJ, Schwartz K, Thornell LE, Sartore S, Schiffino S (1984) Myosin types in the human heart. An immunofluorescence study of normal and hypertrophied atrial and ventricular myocardium. Circ Res 54:694–702
26. Wisenbaugh T, Allen P, Cooper GIV, Holzgrefe H, Beller G, Carabello B (1983) Contractile function, myosin ATPase activity and isozymes in the hypertrophied pig left ventricle after a chronic progressive pressure overload. Circ Res 53:332–341
27. Sobel BE, Spann JF Jr, Pool PE, Sonnenblick EH, Braunwald E (1967) Normal oxidative phosphorylation in mitochondria from the failing heart. Circ Res 21: 355–363
28. Sordahl LA, McCollum WB, Wood WG, Schwartz A (1973) Mitochondria and sarcoplasmic reticulum function in cardiac hypertrophy and failure. Am J Physiol 224:497–502
29. Ito Y, Suko J, Chidsey CA (1974) Intracellular calcium and myocardial contractility. V. Calcium uptake of sarcoplasmic reticulum fractions in hypertrophied and failing rabbit hearts. J Mol Cell Cardiol 6:237–247
30. Komuro I, Kurabayashi M, Shibazaki Y, Takaku F, Yazaki Y (1989) Molecular cloning and characterization of a Ca^{2+}+Mg^{2+}-dependent adenosine triphsophatase from rat cardiac sarcoplasmic reticulum. Regulation of its expression by pressure overload and developmental stage. J Clin Invest 1102–1108
31. Linzbach AJ (1960) Heart failure from the point of view of quantitative anatomy. Am J Cardiol 5:370–382
32. Henquell L, Odoroff CL, Honig CR (1976) Intercapillary distance and capillary reserve in hypertrophied rat hearts beating in situ. Circ Res 41:400–408
33. Sasayama S, Franklin D, Ross J Jr (1977) Hyperfunction with normal inotropic state of the hypertrophied left ventricle. Am J Physiol 232:H418–H425
34. Cohen ME, Bing OHL (1987) Performance of papillary muscles from the aging spontaneously hypertensive rat: Temporal changes in isometric contraction parameters. Proc Societ Exp Biol Med 185:318–324

11

Regional Work of the Left Ventricle and Contractility Index Independent of Ventricular Size

Motoaki Sugawara[1], Kiyoharu Nakano[1], Masatoshi Kawana[1], Jun Umemura[1], Shigetake Sasayama[2], Blase A. Carabello[3]

Summary. We describe here a new method of defining regional work and regional contractility of the myocardium of the ventricular wall using the relationship between mean wall stress (σ) and the natural logarithm of reciprocal of wall thickness (ln(1/H)). Regional work of the ventricle normalized to a unit volume of myocardium is equal to the area surrounded by the loop described by the σ-ln(1/H) relation during a cardiac cycle. The constant k_{SM} of the end systolic σ-ln(1/H) relation, $\sigma = C\exp(k_{SM} \ln(1/H))$, corresponds to the myocardial elastic stiffness constant, which is sensitive to changes in contractile state, insensitive to changes in loading conditions and independent of ventricular size.

Key words: Cardiac function — Work — Contractility — Wall stress — Wall thickness

Introduction

Various attempts have been made to analyze regional myocardial function of the ventricle. The set of variables which describe the working condition of a small region of the ventricular wall in the greatest detail will be the stress and strain tensors in that region. Unfortunately, there are as yet no reliable methods to measure directly each component of stress tensor in the ventricular wall. Several authors have reported mathematical estimations of the stress tensor components under various assumptions on the ventricular geometry and

[1] The Heart Institute of Japan, Tokyo Women's Medical College, Shinjuku-ku, Tokyo, 162 Japan
[2] The Second Department of Internal Medicine, Faculty of Medicine, Toyama Medical and Pharmaceutical University, Toyama, 930-01 Japan
[3] Division of Cardiology, Department of Medicine, Medical University of South Carolina, Charleston, SC 29425-2221, U.S.A.

constitutive relations. However, there are quantitative and qualitative discrepancies between the stress distributions calculated for the various ventricular models [1, 2], and there is no agreement about which is the most realistic representation of the actual stress distribution across the ventricular wall. Therefore, detailed analyses based on stress and strain tensors are, at present, of little practical utility.

We have proposed the use of the relationship between the mean wall tension (T) and the area (A) of a region of interest of the ventricular wall to analyze regional myocardial function [3]. We showed that regional ventricular work can be calculated by the T-A relationship and that the regional myocardial function can be satisfactorily investigated on the basis of the T-A diagram. The validity of this method was also confirmed by Goto et al. [4] and the applications are described in Chap. 5.

Although the method based on the T-A relationship is still useful in analyzing regional myocardial function, it has two shortcomings:

1. Investigators can choose the size of area arbitrarily, and the wall thickness of the selected region in each experiment differs from those in every other experiment. Therefore, the results derived from the T-A relationships in different experiments cannot be compared quantitatively.
2. Measurement of the regional area A is difficult in clinical cases, which means that application of the method is limited to animal experiments only.

We have improved the method to overcome these shortcomings [5–7]. The first step was to normalize the results derived from the T-A relationship to unit volume of myocardium, which makes it possible to compare the results obtained from hearts with different area sizes and wall thicknesses. This step led us to the use of a new relationship between mean wall stress (σ) and the natural logarithm of A (area strain). The next step was to substitute the regional area A by a variable which can be easily measured in clinical cases too. On the assumption that the myocardium is incompressible throughout one cardiac cycle, the reciprocal of wall thickness (1/H) is proportional to the regional area. Since wall thickness is readily measured by several methods, we used 1/H in place of A.

The relation between σ and 1/H gives a new index of myocardial contractility as well. Suga et al. [8] and Sagawa [9] designated the slope of the end-systolic pressure-volume relationship as the maximum elastance of the ventricle, E_{max}, and various studies have shown that E_{max} is useful in evaluating the contractile state of the ventricle. However, E_{max} depends not only on myocardial contractility but also on heart size. In this respect, E_{max} is not normalized, i.e., the values of E_{max} of hearts of differing size cannot be compared. On the other hand, the index derived from the relation between σ and 1/H does not include the effects of ventricular geometry as a parameter [10, 11].

We shall now describe our new methods and survey the results of animal experiments and clinical applications.

Regional Work Normalized to Unit Volume of Myocardium

Calculation of Regional Work

The mechanical work done by a region of interest of the ventricular wall is given by

$$RW = -\int T dA \tag{1}$$

where RW is regional work, T is the mean wall tension, A is the area of a regional midwall layer of the ventricle, and the integral is taken over a cardiac cycle [3]. The integration value is equal to the area surrounded by the loop described by the T-A relation during a cardiac cycle. (See Chap. 5)

Normalization of Regional Work

Figure 1 shows a schematic illustration of an imaginary section of myocardium that has a midwall layer area A and a wall thickness H. The volume Vm of the section is given by

$$Vm = A \times H \tag{2}$$

Since the myocardium is incompressible, Vm is constant. If we wish to examine RWM, the regional work per unit volume of myocardium, we divide RW by Vm. Division of Eq. (1) by Vm (=AH) yields

$$\begin{aligned} RWM = RW/Vm &= -(1/AH)\int T dA \\ &= -\int (T/H)(dA/A) \end{aligned} \tag{3}$$

Here, since AH is constant, it can be moved into the integral sign. The mean wall stress σ is defined as T/H. Using this definition and the relation dA/A = d(ln A), we obtain

$$RWM = -\int \sigma d(\ln A) \tag{4}$$

Meaning of the Natural Logarithm of Regional Area and Definition of Area Strain

Since d(ln A), or dA/A, expresses a relative change in area, we define dε, the "incremental area strain," by dε = d(ln A). Thus, the total area strain is given by

$$\varepsilon = \int_{Ao}^{A} d\varepsilon = \int_{Ao}^{A} d(\ln A) = \ln A - \ln Ao = \ln(A/Ao)$$

where Ao is the unstressed area, i.e., the area corresponding to a state of zero stress. To obtain a stress-strain ($\sigma - \varepsilon$) relation, Ao is required. However, in the calculation of regional work (Eq. (4)), and in the analysis of the stiffness-stress ($d\sigma/d\varepsilon - \sigma$) relation (see pp. 271–278), Ao is not required [11]. In fact, the unstressed area Ao is difficult to measure or define in the working heart, and the stiffness-stress relation is more suitable than the stress-strain relation to

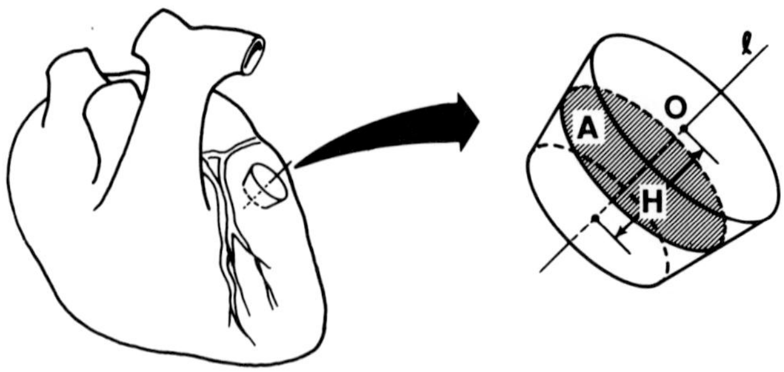

Fig. 1. Schematic illustration of the imaginary frustum of myocardium that has a volume of Vm. *A*, area of the midwall layer of the frustum; *H*, wall thickness measured along *l*; *l*, a straight line perpendicular to the epicardial surface and passing through a selected point *O*. Vm = *A* × *H*. (From [7] with permission of the American College of Cardiology)

characterize the properties of nonlinearly elastic materials such as the myocardium. Therefore, omitting Ao, we newly define the area strain by

$$\varepsilon = \ln A \tag{5}$$

Use of Reciprocal of Wall Thickness in Place of Regional Area

Taking logarithms of Eq. (2) and rearranging yield

$$\ln A = \ln \mathrm{Vm} + \ln(1/H)$$

Differentiation of the above equation on the assumption that Vm is constant yields

$$d(\ln A) = d(\ln(1/H)) \tag{6}$$

Substitution of d(ln(1/H)) for d(ln A) in Eq. (4) gives

$$\mathrm{RWM} = -\int \sigma d(\ln(1/H)) \tag{7}$$

Changes in the area A are difficult to measure in clinical cases. On the other hand, changes in the wall thickness H can be easily measured using conventional echocardiography or cineangiography. Therefore, substitution of wall thickness for regional area has increased the applicability of the method.

Regional Work of the Human Ventricle

Regional work of the interventricular septum and of the posterior wall of the left ventricle was calculated from the measured pressure and dimension data in normal subjects and in patients with heart disease.

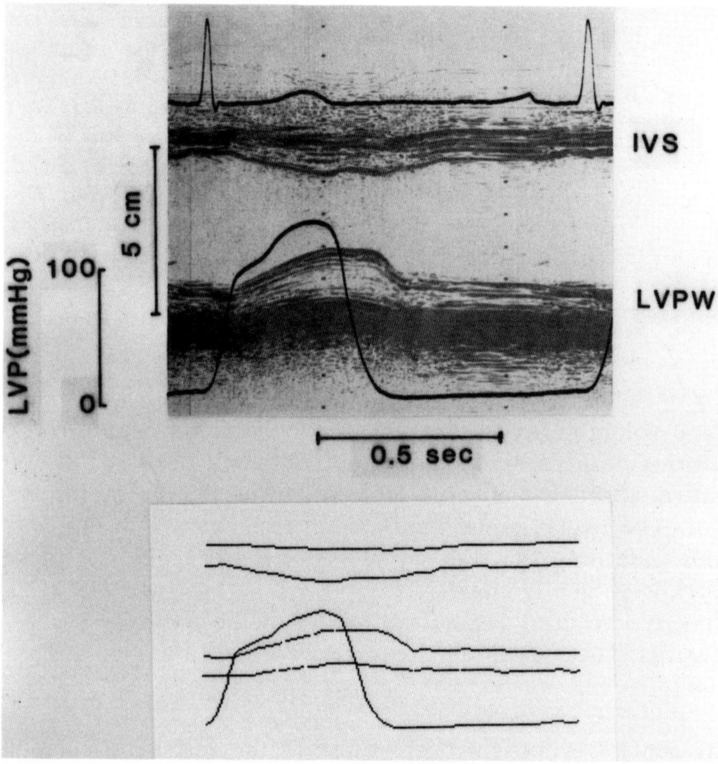

Fig. 2. Original recordings of the left ventricular pressure (*LVP*) and M-mode echocardiogram from a normal subject (*top*) and the tracings digitized with a hand-controlled cursor (*bottom*). *IVS*, interventricular septum; *LVPW*, left ventricular posterior wall. (From [7] with permission of the American College of Cardiology)

Methods of Clinical Measurements

A micromanometer-tipped catheter was inserted into the left ventricle, and echocardiography was performed using a phased-array scanner (Toshiba Sonolayer SSH60A) with a 2.25 MHz transducer. The transducer was placed in the third or fourth intercostal space at the left sternal edge, and a short-axis view of the left ventricle at the level of the papillary muscles or the mitral valve was obtained. The M-mode cursor was positioned centrally in the two-dimensional image of the short-axis cross section of the left ventricle, and the derived M-mode image was recorded. Left ventricular pressure was recorded simultaneously with the M-mode echocardiogram at a paper speed of 100 mm/s (Fig. 2). The left ventricular pressure and echocardiographic recordings were digitized over one cardiac cycle with the use of a hand-controlled cursor (Fig. 2). The data were fed into a computer system, and σ-ln(1/H) relations for the ventricle were delineated with a digital plotter (Fig. 3). The area that is surrounded by the σ-ln(1/H) loop during a cardiac cycle is equal to regional

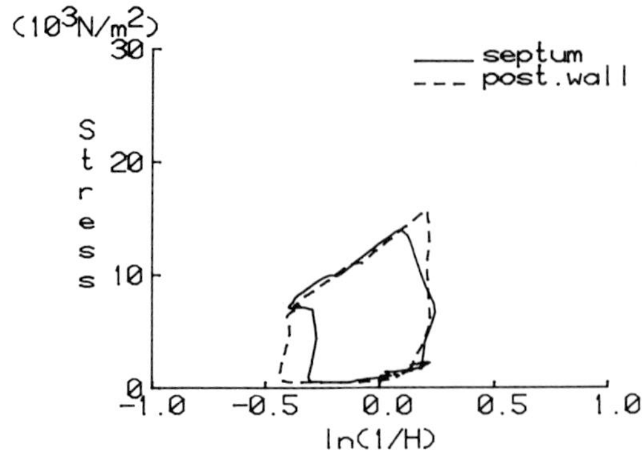

Fig. 3. The mean wall stress-natural logarithm of the reciprocal of wall thickness (σ-*ln(1/H)*) loops of the ventricular septum (*solid line*) and the posterior (*post.*) wall of the left ventricle (*dotted line*) obtained from the data in Fig. 2. (From [7] with permission of the American College of Cardiology)

work per unit volme of myocardium. If the loop rotates counterclockwise, the region performs positive work. If the loop rotates clockwise, the region performs negative work; that is, work is done on that region by the surrounding myocardium. The two regional loops (counterclockwise) in Fig. 3 show similar behavior indicating that the septal regional work and the posterior wall regional work were nearly equal.

For simplicity, we used a spherical model of the left ventricle to calculate mean wall stress. The mean wall stress σ was defined by

$$\sigma = P \times D/4H \tag{8}$$

where P is the left ventricular pressure, D the left ventricular short axis diameter, and H the wall thickness. Since the left ventricle is generally considered to be a prolate ellipse and not a sphere, some error is introduced by the assumption of a spherical shape. The mean wall stress calculated on this assumption is 27% underestimated compared with the mean wall stress calculated for an ellipsoid model in which the ratio of the minor and major axes is 0.5 [7]. Therefore, a spherical model underestimates actual regional work by about 27%. However, this underestimation is consistent in the model, and causes no practical problem, if we keep it in mind each time we calculate regional work (see p. 265).

Regional Left Ventricular Work in Patients with Anteroseptal Infarction

Study Patients. Sixteen patients were selected for this study from the Heart Institute of Japan, Tokyo Women's Medical College, and the Second Department of Internal Medicine, Toyama Medical and Pharmaceutical University [7]. Eight patients were referred to the catheterization laboratory because of a chest pain syndrome but subsequently demonstrated normal ejection fraction, and had no significant coronary disease and no regional wall motion abnormality. Two additional patients showed 75% and 90% stenosis of the luminal diameter in the left anterior descending coronary artery but had no ventriculographic regional wall motion abnormalities. These two patients were included in the normal wall motion group.

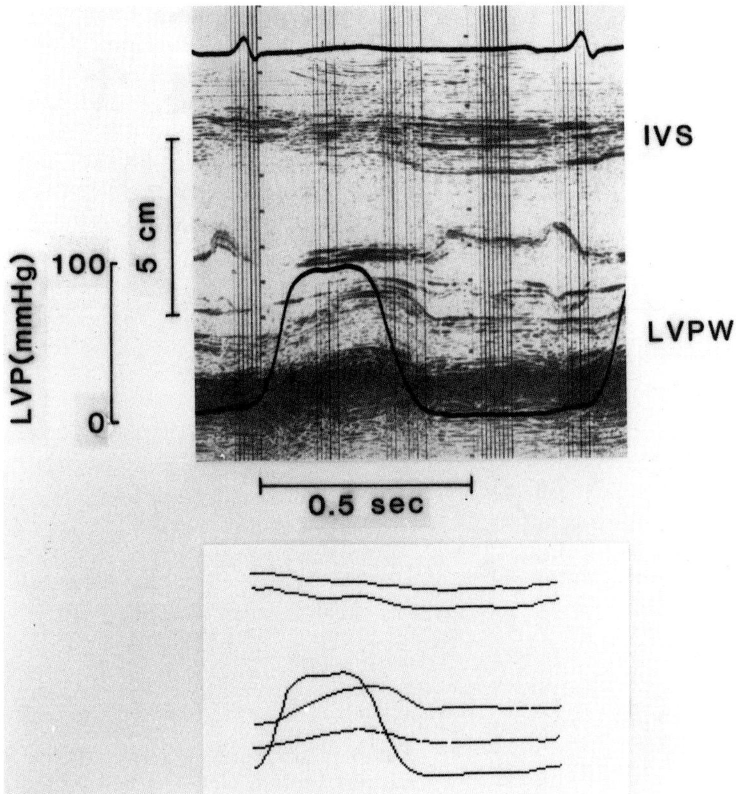

Fig. 4. Original recordings of the left ventricular pressure and M-mode echocardiogram from a patient with anteroseptal infarction (*top*) and the tracings digitized with a hand-controlled cursor (*bottom*). *IVS*, interventricular septum; *LVPW*, left ventricular posterior work; *LVP*, left ventricular pressure

Six patients had previous anteroseptal myocardial infarction established by at least two of the following criteria: (1) history of characteristic chest pain, (2) electrocardiographic (ECG) changes with evolution of Q waves in the anterior chest leads, and (3) elevation of serum creatine kinase. The studies were performed more than one month after the infarction. In all six cases, biplane ventriculography demonstrated anteroapical and septal wall motion abnormalities. Although four of these six patients had coronary lesions in addition to those in the left anterior descending artery, none had abnormalities of left ventricular wall motion in areas supplied by the other coronary arteries. These six patients represent the anteroseptal infarct group.

Statistics. The data in this and the following sections are expressed as mean ± SD. Comparisons between regional septal wall work and regional left ventricular posterior wall work in the same patients in each group were made using a

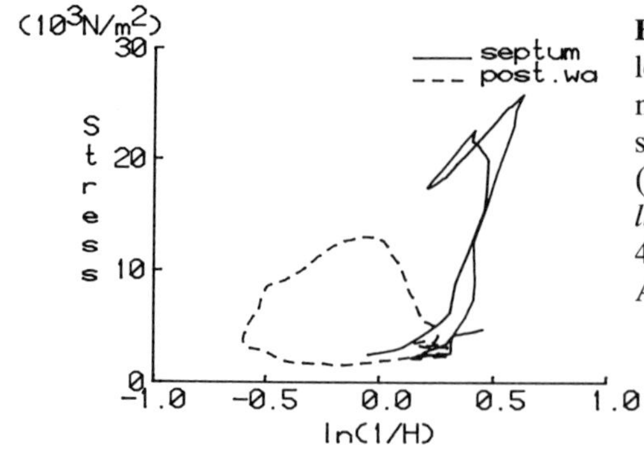

Fig. 5. The mean wall stress-natural logarithm of the reciprocal of wall thickness (*σ-ln(1/H)*) loops of the ventricular septum (*solid line*) and the posterior (*post.*) wall of the left ventricle (*dotted line*) obtained from the data in Fig. 4. (From [7] with permission of the American College of Cardiology)

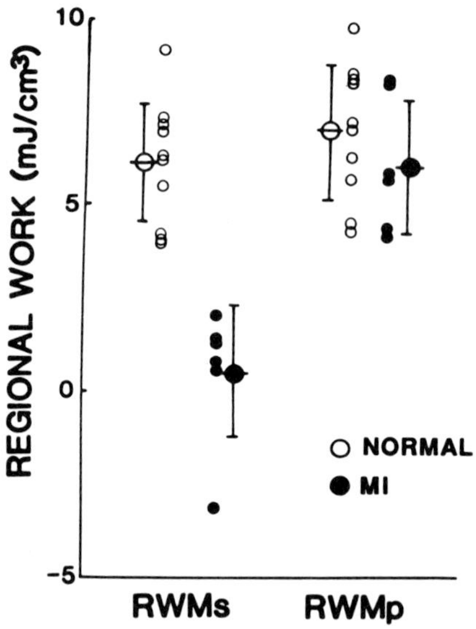

Fig. 6. The regional work of the interventricular septum (*RWMs*) and of the posterior wall of the left ventricle (*RWMp*) in the normal group (*open circle*) (n = 10) and the anteroseptal myocardial infarct (*MI*) group (*closed circle*) (n = 6). (From [7] with permission of the American College of Cardiology)

paired Student's t test. When regional work in different groups was compared, an unpaired t test was performed.

Results. Figure 4 reproduces representative original recordings of the left ventricular pressure and the M-mode echocardiogram obtained from a patient with anteroseptal infarction and the tracings digitized with the hand-controlled cursor. Figure 5 shows the regional work (σ-ln(1/H)) loops of the ventricular septum and the posterior wall obtained from the same patient in Fig. 4. Both σ and ln(1/H) of the septum increased during systole and decreased during diastole. In contrast, the posterior wall shows the normal pattern. The septal regional work was 1.5 mJ/cm^3, whereas the posterior wall regional work was 4.2 mJ/cm^3.

Figure 6 shows the regional work of the interventricular septum and of the posterior wall of the left ventricle in the normal group and the anteroseptal infarct group. In the normal group, septal regional work was slightly lower than posterior wall regional work (6.1 ± 1.7 versus 7.0 ± 1.8 mJ/cm^3; $P <$ 0.005). However, the difference was small. In the anteroseptal infarct group, the septal regional work was remarkably reduced compared with posterior wall regional work (0.6 ± 1.9 versus 6.1 ± 1.8 mJ/cm^3; $P < 0.001$). In one case, the σ-ln(1/H) loop rotated clockwise and the septal regional work was negative.

Validation of the Regional Work Estimated by the Present Method

Since the regional work of the ventricular wall has not yet been calculated in man, the value of the regional work obtained here cannot be validated directly. However, according to the law of conservation of energy, the total regional work accumulated over the myocardial volume of the left ventricle must correspond to the total mechanical work performed by the entire left ventricle. If a unit volume of myocardium in every part of the left ventricle performs the same amount of regional work, the regional work per unit volume of myocardium multiplied by the left ventriclar myocardial volume must be equal to the total work performed by the entire left ventricle, which is obtained from the pressure-volume curve. This is obviously not the case in the anteroseptal myocardial infarction group. There is a considerable difference in regional work between the septum and posterior wall in this group. However, in the normal group, the regional difference is small. Therefore, we take the average of the septal regional work and the posterior regional work in each case in the normal group, and multiply it by the left ventricular myocardial volume. Figure 7 shows the relation between the average regional work per unit volume, RWM, multiplied by the left ventricular myocardial volume, LVM, and the total work, TW. Although the (RWM × LVM) is linearly correlated with TW, the value of (RWM × LVM) was slightly smaller than the value of TW.

The accuracy of our method is limited by the accuracy in determining the mean wall stress. For simplicity, we used a spherical model. In this case, the mean wall stress is, as previously mentioned, underestimated by about 27% compared with an ellipsoidal model. The dotted line shows a prediction line corresponding to the case that (RWM × LVM) is 27% smaller than TW. This line falls within the 95% confidence band of the regression relation between TW and RWMxLVM and coincides well with the linear regression line, which is denoted by the solid line. This suggests the validity of our methods of calculating the regional work.

Regional Left Ventricular Work in Patients with Hypertrophic Cardiomyopathy

All the data which we shall use here were obtained at the Heart Institute of Japan, Tokyo Women's Medical College. Figure 8 reproduces representative original recordings of the left ventricular pressure and the M-mode echocardiogram obtained from a patient with hypertrophic cardiomyopathy (HCM), and the tracings for computer feeding obtained from the same original

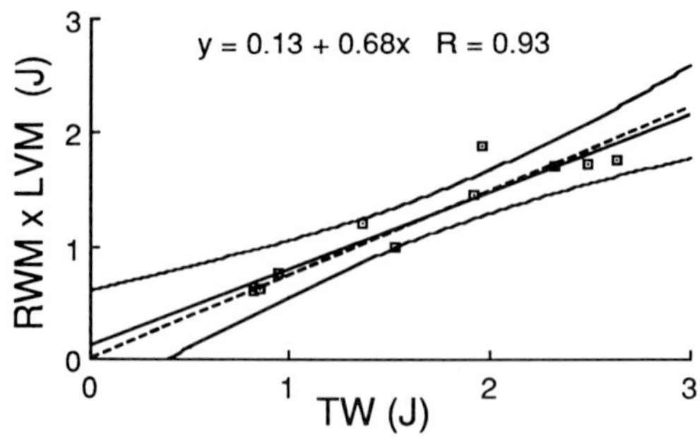

Fig. 7. Relation between the average regional work per unit volume multiplied by the left ventricular myocardial volume (*RWM* × *LVM*) and total work (*TW*) in the normal group (n = 10). The *solid line* is the linear regression line. The *dotted line* is the *RWM* × *LVM* versus *TW* relation predicted if spherical wall stress underestimates ellipsoid stress by 27%. The *curved lines* are the edges of the 95% confidence band for the actual *RWM* × *LVM* versus *TW* relation. *LVM*, left ventricular myocardium volume; *RWM*, average of regional work of interventricular septum (*RWMs*) and posterior wall of the left ventricle (*RWMp*); *TW*, total work performed by the entire left ventricle. (From [7] with permission of the American College of Cardiology)

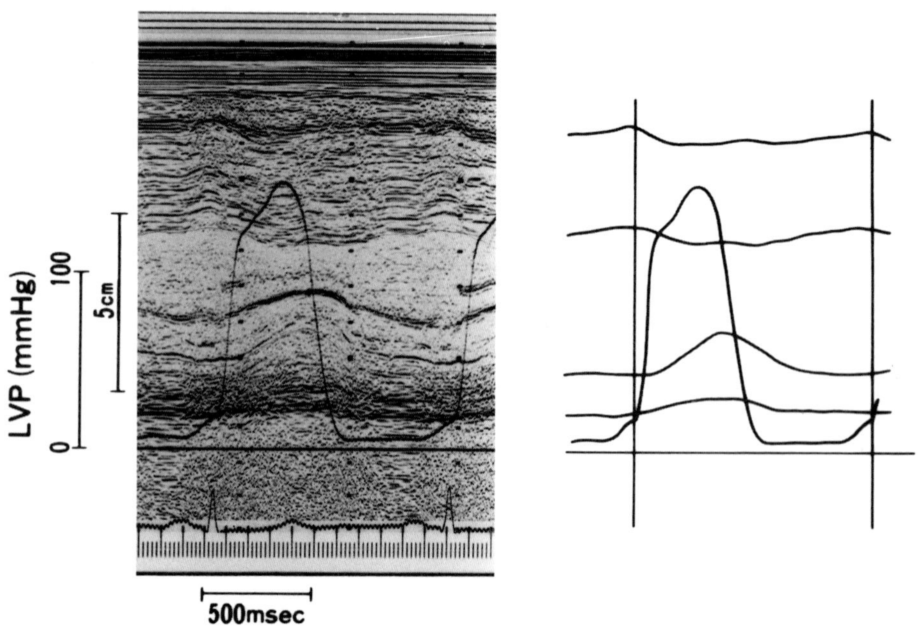

Fig. 8. Original recordings of the left ventricular pressure (*LVP*) and M-mode echocardiogram from a patient with hypertrophic cardiomyopathy (*left*) and the tracings for computer feeding (*right*)

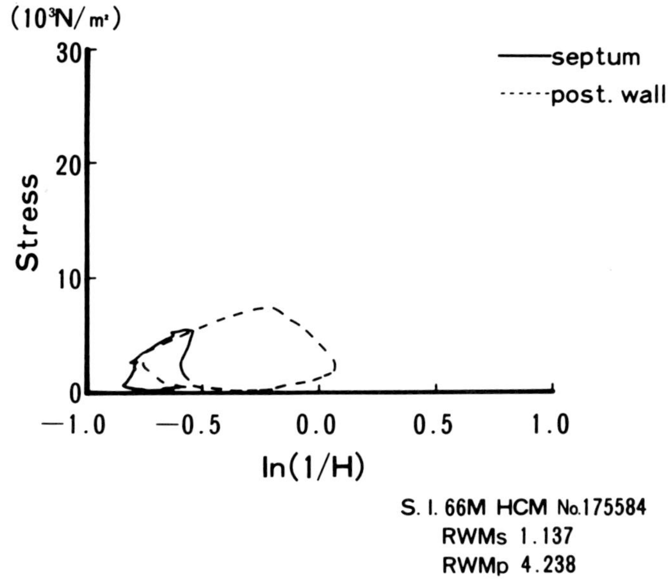

Fig. 9. The mean wall stress-natural logarithm of the reciprocal of wall thickness (σ-*ln(1/H)*) loops of the ventricular septum (*solid line*) and the posterior (*post.*) wall of the left ventricle (*dotted line*) obtained from the data in Fig. 8. *RWMs*, regional work of the interventricular septum; *RWMp*, regional work of the posterior wall of the left ventricle

recordings. Asymmetric septal hypertrophy is obvious. Figure 9 shows the σ-ln(1/H) loops obtained from the tracing in Fig. 8. The septal regional work was remarkably reduced compared with the posterior wall regional work (1.1 versus 4.2 mJ/cm^3). We compared the data obtained from seven normal cases and six patients with HCM. In the normal group, the septal wall thickness was 10.0 ± 1.7 mm and the posterior wall thickness was 10.6 ± 1.8 mm. In the HCM group, the septal wall thickness was 20.5 ± 5.1 mm and the posterior wall thickness was 15.0 ± 0.9 mm. There were no significant differences in the peak dP/dt and the ejection fraction of the left ventricle between the normal and the HCM groups (1680 ± 410 versus 1750 ± 330 mmHg/s; 65 ± 6 versus 71 ± 6%). However, in the HCM group, the septal regional work was markedly reduced compared with the posterior wall regional work (0.5 ± 0.6 versus 3.8 ± 1.4 mJ/cm^3) (Fig. 10). The posterior wall regional work was also reduced significantly as compared with that of the septum (6.1 ± 1.7 mJ/cm^3) and the posterior wall (7.0 ± 2.0 mJ/cm^3) in the normal group (Fig. 10).

Changes in Left Ventricular Regional Work During Coronary Angioplasty

We examined nine patients with angina pectoris during percutaneous transluminal coronary angioplasty (PTCA) of the left anterior descending artery using echocardiography and micromanometry at the Heart Institute of Japan,

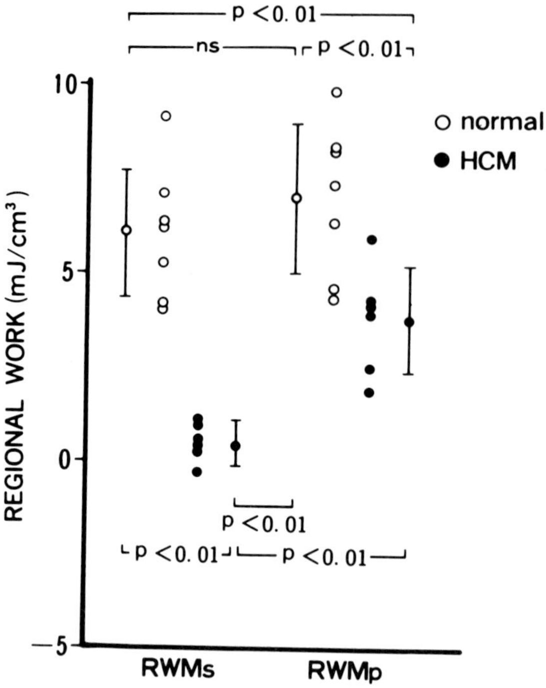

Fig. 10. The regional work of the interventricular septum (*RWMs*) and of the posterior wall of the left ventricle (*RWMp*) in the normal group (*open circle*) (n = 7) and the hypertrophic cardiomyopathy group (*closed circle*) (n = 6)

Tokyo Women's Medical College. The top left panel of Fig. 11 reproduces original recordings obtained before inflation of the balloon. The bottom left panel shows the tracings for computer feeding. The right panels are those obtained during inflation of the balloon. Figure 12 shows the pressure-volume curves and the σ-ln(1/H) loops obtained from the tracings in Fig. 11. The regional work of the septum, the ischemic region, was reduced markedly, whereas that of the posterior wall, the non-ischemic region, increased significantly. The total work, however, remained unchanged.

Figure 13 shows representative changes in the σ-ln(1/H) loops before and during inflation and after deflation of the balloon. The typical changes can be described as follows. During inflation of the balloon, the septal regional work decreased with time to nearly zero or negative at about 100 s after the onset of inflation of the balloon. During this period, the end-systolic and end-diastolic points of the septal σ-ln(1/H) loop moved together towards the right, i.e., the σ-ln(1/H) loop as a whole moved towards the right. On the other hand, the posterior wall regional work nearly doubled during the same period. The end-systolic point of the posterior wall σ-ln(1/H) loop moved towards the left and the end-diastolic point moved towards the right, but the loop as a whole stayed at nearly the same position. Within 20 s after deflation of the balloon, the septal σ-ln(1/H) loop moved back to nearly the same position as before inflation, and the septal regional work increased and became slightly larger

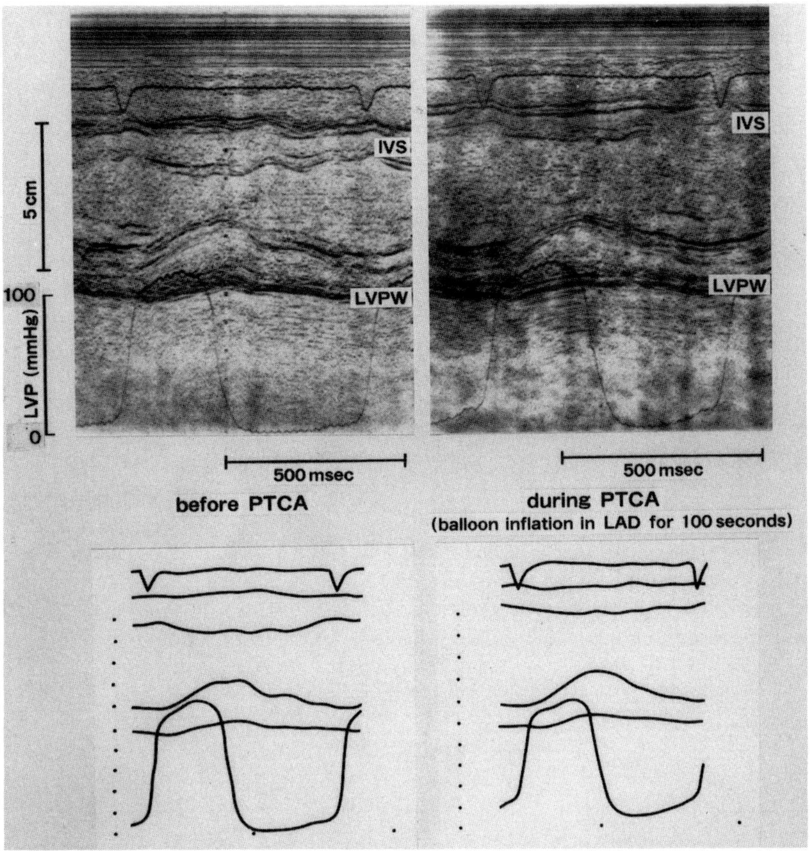

Fig. 11. Original recordings of the left ventricular pressure (*LVP*) and M-mode echocardiogram before (*top left*) and during (*top right*) percutaneous transluminal coronary angioplasty (*PTCA*) of the left anterior descending artery (*LAD*) and the tracings for computer feeding (*bottom*). *IVS*, interventricular septum; *LVPW*, left ventricular posterior wall

than that before inflation. The posterior wall σ-ln(1/H) loop shrank but the posterior wall regional work still remained slightly greater than that before inflation.

The changes in regional work before and about 100 s after the onset of balloon inflation in nine patients were as follows. The septal regional work decreased from 3.6 ± 0.9 to −1.9 ± 4.0 mJ/cm^3 ($P < 0.01$). On the other hand, the posterior wall regional work increased from 4.9 ± 1.1 to 8.6 ± 0.9 mJ/cm^3 ($P < 0.01$). The total left ventricular work was not changed significantly by the balloon inflation. Before the inflation, the septal regional work was significantly smaller than the posterior wall regional work ($P < 0.01$). It is not clear whether this is an effect of the presence of the catheter in the left anterior descending coronary artery. The catheter might have increased the resistance of the artery and reduced blood flow even before inflation of the

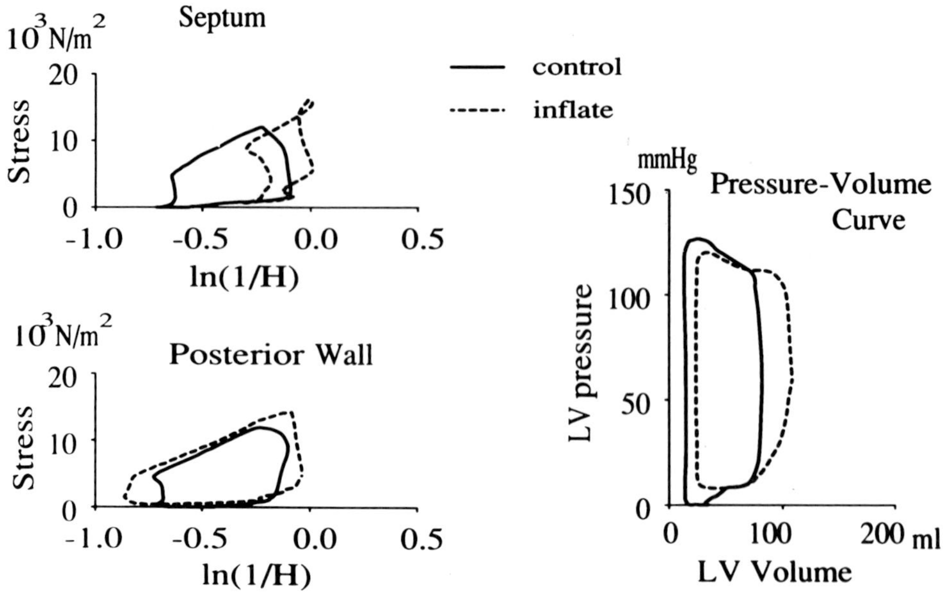

Fig. 12. The pressure-volume curves (*right*) and the mean wall stress-natural logarithm of the reciprocal of wall thickness (σ-*ln(1/H)*) loops of the ventricular septum (*left top*) and the posterior wall of the left ventricle (*left bottom*) before (*solid line*) and during (*dotted line*) percutaneous transluminal coronary angioplasty obtained from the data in Fig. 11

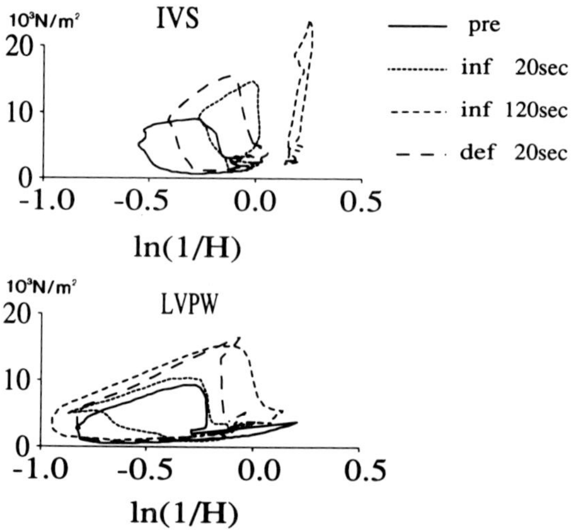

Fig. 13. Representative changes in the mean wall stress-natural logarithm of the reciprocal of wall thickness (σ-*ln(1/H)*) loops before and during inflation and after deflation of the balloon. *IVS* (*top*), loops of the interventricular septum; *LVPW* (*bottom*), loops of the posterior wall of the left ventricle; *pre*, before the onset of inflation of the balloon; *inf 20 sec*, 20 seconds after the onset of inflation of the balloon; *inf 120 sec*, 120 seconds after the onset of inflation of the balloon; *def 20 sec*, 20 seconds after deflation of the balloon

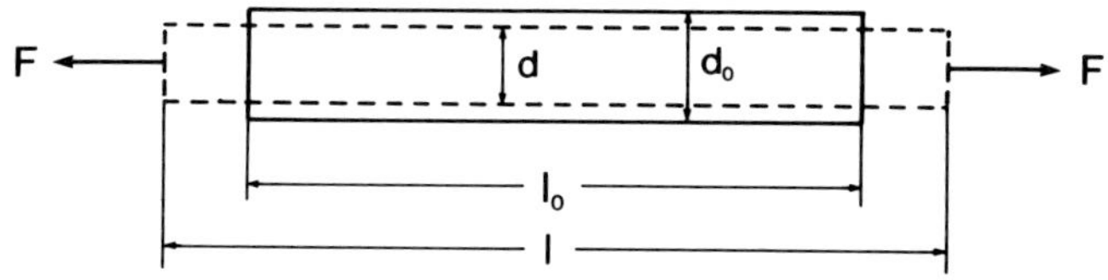

Fig. 14. Longitudinal and transverse strains caused by a longitudinal stress. *F*, force; *d*, diameter; d_o, diameter at zero force; *l*, length; l_o, length at zero force

balloon. The detailed mechanism of the changes in regional work during PTCA is still unknown at present.

Contractility Index Independent of Ventricular Size

All the experimental data which we shall use in this section, except Fig. 16, were obtained in the experimental catheterization laboratory at the Medical University of South Carolina [11].

Meaning of the Slope of the Relation Between Wall Stress and The Natural Logarithm of the Reciprocal of Wall Thickness

The analogy of an incompressible Hookean material enables a clear understanding of the meaning of the slope of the σ-ln(1/H) relationship. Let us consider a fiber with cross-sectional area C, diameter d ($C = \pi d^2/4$) and length 1, on each end of which a force F is applied (Fig. 14). The longitudinal stress across any cross section of the fiber, σ_1, is given by $\sigma_l = F/C$. The ratio of extension along the fiber, i.e., the longitudinal strain ε_l is defined by $\varepsilon_l = \ln(l/l_o)$, where l_o is the length of the fiber when $F = 0$. In an ordinary elastic material (Hookean material), it turns out that the ratio of σ_l to ε_l is a constant of the material, i.e., it is independent of F, C and l as long as F is not excessive [12]. This ratio is denoted by E and known as Young's modulus:

$$E = \sigma_l/\varepsilon_l \tag{9}$$

where E has the same dimension (force/area) as σ_l since ε_l is dimensionless.

Elongation of the fiber is always accompanied by a contraction of its cross section. The ratio of contraction is expressed by the transverse strain ε_d:$\varepsilon_d = \ln(d/d_o)$, where d_o is the diameter when $F = 0$. In elongation, ε_d is a negative number. The quantity ν, defined by

$$\nu = -\varepsilon_d/\varepsilon_l \tag{10}$$

is also a constant of the material, which is called Poisson's ratio of transverse contraction to longitudinal extension. In case of incompressible materials such as the myocardium, $\nu = \frac{1}{2}$. From Eqs. (9) and (10) we obtain

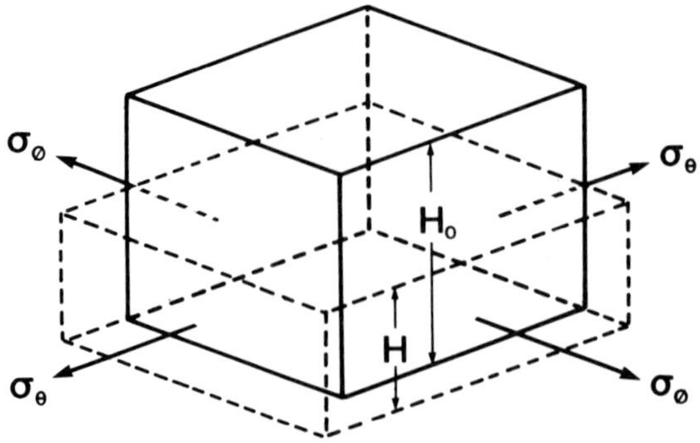

Fig. 15. Deformation of an incompressible body. The rectangular solid delineated by a *solid line* shows the body before deformation, and that delineated by a *broken line* shows the body after deformation. *H*, thickness; H_o, thickness at zero stress; σ_θ, stress; σ_ϕ, stress

$$\varepsilon_d = -(\nu/E)\sigma_l \tag{11}$$

Let us consider a rectangular solid body with thickness H, which is subjected to stresses σ_θ and σ_ϕ (Fig. 15). It is assumed that the stresses are uniformly distributed over the cross sections. The extension along σ_θ is accompanied by a reduction of thickness (thinning) of the solid body, the ratio of which is obtained from Eq. (11):

$$\varepsilon_{H1} = -(\nu/E)\sigma_\theta$$

where ε_{H1} is the strain in the direction of thickness. The extension along σ_ϕ is also accompanied by a thinning which is given by

$$\varepsilon_{H2} = -(\nu/E)\sigma_\phi$$

The total thinning caused by σ_θ and σ_ϕ is expressed by a superposition of these two strains:

$$\varepsilon_H = \varepsilon_{H1} + \varepsilon_{H2} = -(\nu/E)(\sigma_\theta + \sigma_\phi) \tag{12}$$

ε_H is the strain given by

$$\varepsilon_H = \ln(H/H_o) \tag{13}$$

where H_o is the thickness corresponding to a state of zero stress. Rearrangement of Eq. (12) and the assumption that $\nu = ½$ (incompressible) yield

$$(\sigma_\theta + \sigma_\phi)/2 = -E\varepsilon_H \tag{14}$$

If we imagine that the solid body in Fig. 15 is a region of the left ventricular wall and σ_θ and σ_ϕ are circumferential and meridional stresses, the left hand side of Eq. (14), $(\sigma_\theta + \sigma_\phi)/2$, is equal to the mean wall stress σ which is used in our $\sigma - \ln(1/H)$ relations:

$$\sigma = (\sigma_\theta + \sigma_\phi)/2 \tag{15}$$

Substitution of Eq. (15) into Eq. (14) yields

$$\sigma = -E\varepsilon_H \tag{16}$$

Differentiation of Eq. (13) yields

$$d\varepsilon_H = d\ln H = -d\ln(1/H) \tag{17}$$

Note that H_o does not appear in this differential relation since it is constant. Differentiation of Eq. (16) and use of Eq. (17) yield

$$d\sigma/d\ln(1/H) = E \tag{18}$$

As previously mentioned, ln(1/H) is a substitution for the area strain lnA. Equation (18) shows that the slope of the σ-ln(1/H) relation gives Young's modulus E for a linearly elastic (Hookean) material as might be expected from a stress-strain relationship.

The myocardium does not necessarily exhibit a linear relation between stress (σ) and strain (ln(1/H)). If the stress-strain relation is curvilinear, Young's modulus is replaced by the term "tangent modulus" or "elastic stiffness," which defines the slope at any point of a stress-strain curve. In such a case, the stiffness-stress relations express elastic properties of a material. If the stress-strain relation is of the exponential form, as is often the case in biological materials:

$$\sigma = C\exp(k\ln(1/H)) + B \tag{19}$$

the elastic stiffness is

$$\begin{aligned} d\sigma/d\ln(1/H) &= kC\exp(k\ln(1/H)) \\ &= k\sigma - kB \end{aligned} \tag{20}$$

The elastic stiffness in this case is a linear function of the stress σ and k is called the "stiffness constant" which is also an index related to the elastic property of a material.

New Contractility Index Relating End-Systolic Stress and the Natural Logarithm of Reciprocal of Wall Thickness

Figure 16 shows representative changes in the σ-ln(1/H) loop during volume unloading and pressure loading in a dog. Volume unloading was accomplished by decreasing venous return through slow inflation of a catheter-mounted balloon in the inferior vena cava. Pressure loading was accomplished by increasing the aortic resistance through slow inflation of another catheter-mounted balloon in the descending aorta. The end-systolic σ-ln(1/H) data point moved on the same single line (not necessarily rectilinear) during both loadings. The analogy from the end-systolic pressure-volume relation (E_{max}) which moves on a rectilinear line in the pressure-volume plane gives the idea that the end-systolic σ-ln(1/H) relation may also be useful in assessing changes in contractile state. We shall show that this is the case.

First, let us see the detailed functional relation between the end-systolic σ and ln(1/H). In Fig. 16, the relation appears to be linear. In fact, the linear fit to the end-systolic σ-ln(1/H) data points always achieves a very good correlation coefficient (r) usually greater than 0.95. However, the exponential fit achieves a higher value of r than the linear fit [11]. Figure 17 (left panel) shows a representative exponential fit to the end-systolic σ-ln(1/H) data points during

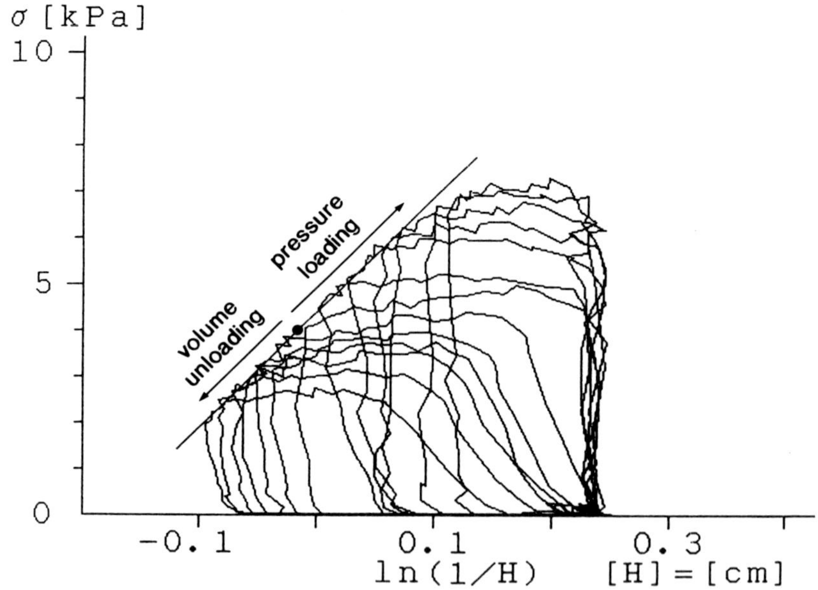

Fig. 16. Representative changes in the mean wall stress-natural logarithm of the reciprocal of wall thickness (σ-*ln(1/H)*) loop during *volume unloading* and *pressure loading* from a dog. kPa = $10^3\,N/m^2$. σ, mean wall stress

volume unloading in a dog. (In the figures hereafter, stress is expressed in kdynes/cm^2, whereas it is expressed in $10^3\,N/m^2$ in the previous figures. 10 kdynes/cm^2 = $10^3\,N/m^2$.) The most general form of the exponential curve equation is Eq. (19). However, as shown in Fig. 17, the fitting of end-systolic σ-ln(1/H) to a simple exponential curve expressed as $\sigma = C\exp(k\ln(1/H))$ does not differ significantly from that to Eq. (19). (Theoretical reasoning for this will be shown later.) The end-systolic stiffness-stress relation is also shown in Fig. 17 (right panel), the slope of which, k, can be termed the end-systolic stiffness constant of the myocardium (k_{SM}) [11]. k_{SM} = 3.3 in this case. Note that the rectilinear stiffness-stress relation coincides with the origin of the stiffness-stress co-ordinate system, since the constant B in Eq. (19) or (20) was taken as zero in this approximation.

Figure 18 demonstrates the effect of changes in inotropic state on k_{SM} from a representative dog [11]. k_{SM} was examined during β-blockade, during β-blockade plus isoflurane anesthesia (a negative inotropic agent), and after reversal of β-blockade plus infusion of dobutamine (a positive inotropic agent). Isoflurane (ISO) decreased k_{SM} from 3.3 to 2.7 and dobutamine (DOB) increased k_{SM} to 4.7. It is clearly seen that k_{SM} is sensitive to changes in inotropic state.

We shall now consider the reason why the fitting of end-systolic σ-ln(1/H) to $\sigma = C\exp(k_{SM}\ln(1/H))$ applies well. We assume that the fitting to Eq. (19) is correct. Then, let us examine the order of magnitude of the error caused by omitting B from Eq. (19).

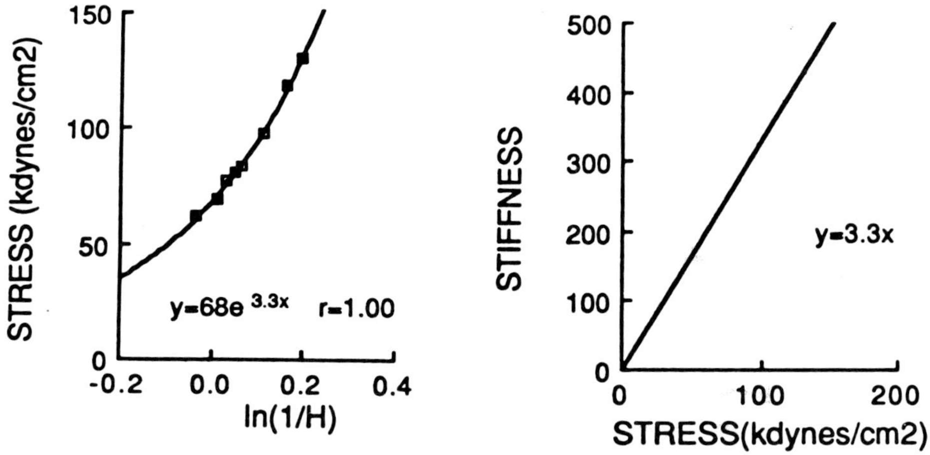

Fig. 17. Exponential fit to the end-systolic stress-strain (mean wall stress-natural logarithm of the reciprocal of wall thickness) data points (*left*) and stiffness-stress relation (*right*) during volume unloading from a representative dog. Note that stress is expressed in kdynes/cm^2 (10 kdynes/cm^2 = 10^3 N/m^2). (From [11] with permission of the American Heart Association)

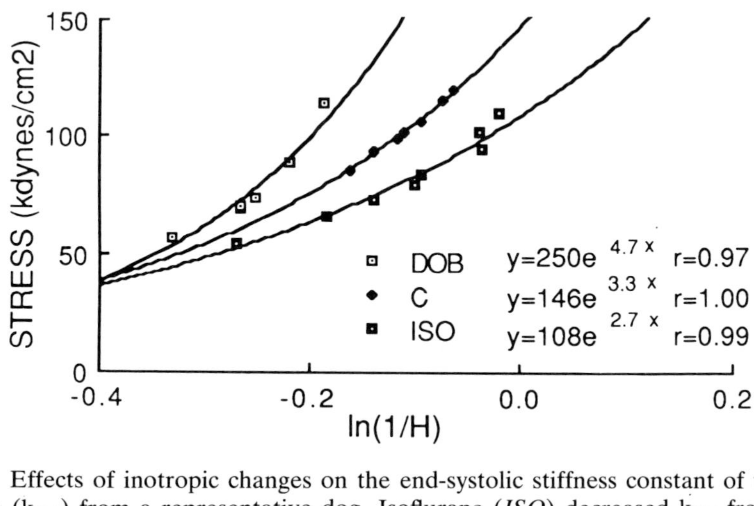

Fig. 18. Effects of inotropic changes on the end-systolic stiffness constant of the myocardium (k_{SM}) from a representative dog. Isoflurane (*ISO*) decreased k_{SM} from 3.3 to 2.7 and dobutamine (*DOB*) increased k_{SM} to 4.7. *C*, control state under β-blockade. Note that stress is expressed in kdynes/cm^2 (10 kdynes/cm^2 = 10^3 N/m^2). (From [11] with permission of the American Heart Assoication)

Division of Eq. (19) by C gives

$$\sigma/C = \exp(k\ln(1/H)) + B/C \tag{21}$$

If we assume that the end-systolic wall thickness reaches a value H_d when the end-systolic stress becomes zero, we obtain from Eq. (21)

$$0 = \exp(k\ln(1/H_d)) + B/C$$

Therefore,

$$B/C = -\exp(k\ln(1/H_d)) \tag{22}$$

We do not know whether a constant value of H_d exists or not. However, we may consider that H_d takes a value near to that of the wall thickness corresponding to the dead volume V_d at which the end-systolic pressure volume relation line intercepts with the volume axis. We did not actually measure H_d, but it is likely that H_d takes a value greater than 2 cm in a normal dog (say 20 kg in weight). Therefore, $\ln(1/H_d)$ is likely to be less than −0.7. Since the smaller value of k gives the greater value of $\exp(k\ln(1/H_d))$, we choose $k = k_{SM} = 2.7$ from Fig. 18. Substituting $\ln(1/H_d) = -0.7$ and $k = 2.7$ into Eq. (22) gives

$$\begin{aligned} B/C &= -\exp(2.7 \times (-0.7)) \\ &= -0.15 \end{aligned}$$

If we put $H_d = 2.5$ cm, and $k_{SM} = 4.7$ (enhanced contractile state in Fig. 18), then

$$B/C = -0.01$$

Giving a physiological value of 1 cm to H yields

$$\exp(k\ln(1/H)) = 1$$

Since B/C is small compared with 1, B/C can be omitted from Eq. (21) with sufficient accuracy for the physiological range of wall stress. Therefore, the fitting of end-systolic σ-$\ln(1/H)$ to a simple exponential curve $\sigma = C\exp(k_{SM}\ln(1/H))$ is a good approximation.

Independency of the End-Systolic Stiffness Constant of the Myocardium from Ventricular Size

Figure 19 demonstrates the relation between k_{SM} and end-diastolic volume during β-blockade (to stabilize inotropic state) in normal dogs [11]. Eight puppies, 6–8 weeks old and weighing 6.4 ± 2.5 kg and 17 adult dogs, weighing 22.3 ± 5.0 kg, were studied. End-diastolic volume ranged from 14 to 30 ml in puppies and from 33 to 82 ml in adult dogs. Despite this wide range of ventricular volumes, k_{SM} was nearly constant with a narrow distribution, 3.6 ± 0.4, and was independent of left ventricular size.

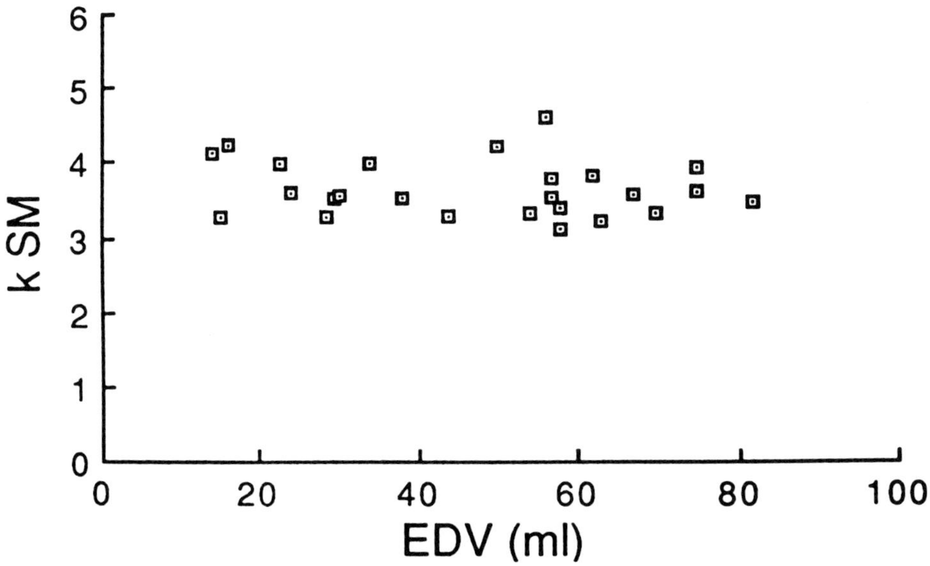

Fig. 19. Relation between the end-systolic elastic stiffness constant of the myocardium (k_{SM}) and end-diastolic volume (*EDV*) in 25 β-blockaded dogs. (From [11] with permission of the American Heart Association)

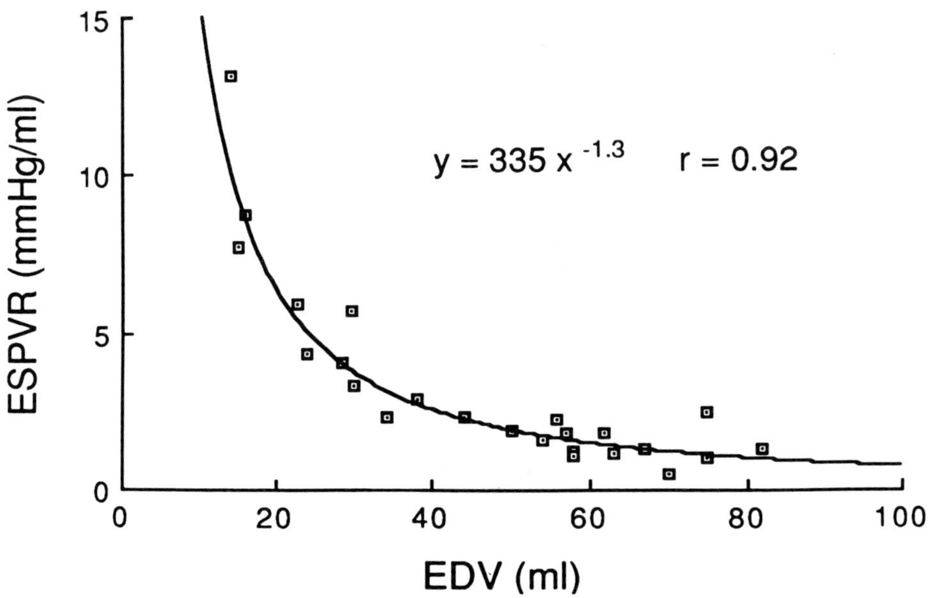

Fig. 20. Relation between E_{max}, the slope of end-systolic pressure-volume relation (*ESPVR*) and end-diastolic volume (*EDV*) in all dogs during *B*-blockade. (From [11] with permission of the American Heart Association)

Figure 20 shows the relation between E_{max} and end-diastolic volume in the same β-blockaded dogs as in Fig. 19. Contrary to k_{SM}, E_{max} was closely related to left ventricular size by a logarithmic function ($r = 0.92$) [11].

Conclusions

We have introduced a new method of estimating regional work of the left ventricle using the relation between mean wall stress (σ) and the natural logarithm of reciprocal of wall thickness ($\ln(1/H)$). Regional work is easily calculated from readily available clinical parameters. We have applied the method to patients with heart disease. Using the end-systolic σ-$\ln(1/H)$ relation, we have defined the end-systolic stiffness constant of the myocardium, k_{SM}, which is sensitive to changes in contractile state, insensitive to changes in loading condition and independent of cardiac size. k_{SM} should be useful for the comparison of myocardial contractility among ventricles with differing size and between different pathological states in the same ventricle.

With its ability to estimate regional work and myocardial contractility, the method based on the σ-$\ln(1/H)$ relation should be valuable in assessing regional myocardial function quantitatively.

Acknowledgments. This work was partly supported by a research grant for cardiovascular diseases (lA-l) from the Ministry of Health and Welfare of Japan.

References

1. Huisman RM, Sipkema P, Westerhof N, Elzinga G (1980) Comparison of models used to calculate left ventricular wall force. Med Biol Eng Comput 18:133–144
2. Yin FCP (1981) Ventricular wall stress. Circ Res 49:829–842
3. Sugawara M, Tamiya K, Nakano K (1985) Regional work of the ventricle: wall tension-area relation. Heart Vessels 1:133–144
4. Goto Y, Suga H, Yamada O, Igarashi Y, Saito M, Hiramori K (1986) Left ventricular regional work from wall tension-area loop in canine heart. Am J Physiol 250 (Heart Circ Physiol 19):H151–H158
5. Nakano K, Sugawara M, Tamiya K, Satomi G, Koyanagi H (1986) A new approach to defining regional work of the ventricle and evaluating regional cardiac function: mean wall stress-natural logarithm of reciprocal of wall thickness relationship. Heart Vessels 2:74–80
6. Sugawara M, Nakano K (1987) A method of analyzing regional myocardial function: mean wall stress-area strain relationship. Jpn Circ J 51:120–124
7. Nakano K, Sugawara M, Kato T, Sasayama S, Carabello BA, Asanoi H, Umemura J, Koyanagi H (1988) Regional work of the human left ventricle calculated by wall stress and the natural logarithm of reciprocal of wall thickness. J Am Coll Cardiol 12:1442–1448
8. Suga H, Sagawa K, Shoukas AA (1973) Load independence of the instantaneous pressure-volume ratio of the canine left ventricle and effects of epinephrine and heart rate on the ratio. Circ Res 32:314–322.

9. Sagawa K (1981) The end-systolic pressure-volume relation of the ventricle: definition, modifications and clinical use. Circulation 63:1223–1227
10. Sugawara M, Nakano K (1989) A new method of analyzing regional myocardial function of the ventricle. In: Hori M, Suga H, Baan J, Yellin EL (eds) Cardiac mechanics and function in the normal and diseased heart. Springer, Tokyo, pp 249–256
11. Nakano K, Sugawara M, Ishihara K, Kanazawa S, Corin WJ, Denslow S, Biederman RWW, Carabello BA (1990) Myocardial stiffness derived from end-systolic wall stress and logarithm of reciprocal of wall thickness: contractility index independent of ventricular size. Circulation 82:1352–1361
12. Sommerfeld A (1964) Mechanics of deformable bodies. Academic Press, New York

12

Selective Stimulation of High-Affinity β_1-Receptors: Its Implication in the Treatment of Mild Heart Failure

Teruyuki Yanagisawa[1], Kuniaki Ishii[1], Hitoshi Yokoyama[1], Hideo Kurosawa[1], Norio Taira[1]

Summary. In this article, we focus on the different natures of the subtypes of β-receptors and β-receptor pathways in cardiac function. We have demonstrated the possible existence of three subtypes of β-receptors, i.e., β_2-receptors, high-affinity β_1-receptors (the so-called β_1-receptors), and low-affinity β_1-receptors (akin to β_3-receptors) in cardiac muscle, which are coupled with increases in myocardial cyclic AMP content and positive inotropic effects. Although the increase in cyclic AMP produced via β_2-receptors is proportional to their fraction of total β-receptor density, the cyclic AMP produced by stimulation of β_2-receptors may not couple well to the positive inotropic effect. Cyclic AMP generated by the activation of high-affinity β_1-receptors seems to be coupled with the positive inotropic effect much more effectively than that via low-affinity β_1-receptors. Since a large increase in cyclic AMP may result in phosphorylation of β-receptors by cyclic AMP-dependent protein kinase, stimulation of β_2-receptors or the low affinity state of β_1-receptors is causally related to the development of tolerance and to the adverse effects of nonselective β-full agonists. It is conceivable that with denopamine, unlike with isoproterenol, tolerance can hardly develop, and there are no adverse effects resulting from its partial agonistic property and its selectivity for high-affinity β_1-receptors. The selective stimulation of high-affinity β_1-receptors would be beneficial for the management of congestive mild heart failure. In contrast, stimulation of low-affinity β_1-receptors by endogenous catecholamines or nonselective β-agonists will contribute to deteriorating hemodynamic, symptomatic and prognostic consequences in patients with congestive heart failure.

Key words: Subtypes of β-adrenergic receptors — Cyclic AMP — Cardiac muscle — Denopamine — Congestive heart failure

---

[1] Department of Pharmacology, Tohoku University School of Medicine, Sendai, 980 Japan

Introduction

The cardiac β-adrenergic mechanism has been one of the most intensively investigated biological mechanisms. Adrenergic mechanisms are thought to be involved to various degrees in cardiovascular diseases or syndromes, such as myocardial infarction, angina pectoris, pheochromocytoma, orthostatic hypotension, some subgroups of essential hypertension, and certain arrhythmias [1]. However, recognition of a potential role of the adrenergic mechanisms in the pathophysiology and consequently the concepts about treatment of heart failure have been controversial and confused [2].

It is well-known that the sympathetic nervous system is activated at rest or during exercise in most patients with heart failure. Is activation of the sympathetic nervous system beneficial or detrimental to the patient with chronic heart failure? On one hand, the increase in sympathetic nerve activity might be favorable if the released catecholamines act to increase cardiac output and to lower left ventricular filling pressure. Withdrawal of such beneficial actions might explain why agents interfering with the sympathetic nervous system adversely affect the hemodynamic and clinical status of patients with heart failure. In patients with severe heart failure, treatment with xamoterol, a β_1-selective partial agonist (Fig. 1), was associated with an increase in mortality [3]. Thus, even a β_1 partial agonist may not be beneficial in patients with severe heart failure because of its antagonistic property for β-receptors. On the other hand, generalized adrenergic activation produces peripheral vasoconstriction, and salt and water retention. Furthermore, it fosters the release of other vasoconstricting humoral factors, e.g., renin, angiotensins, endothelin, etc., and may exert direct deleterious effects on the myocardial cell [1]. These adverse effects could have important deteriorating hemodynamic, symptomatic and prognostic consequences.

In facing these markedly divergent possibilities, which is beneficial for patients with chronic heart failure to enhance or to diminish the effects of sympathetic nervous system? In Chapter 9, Hori and Inoue outline the therapeutic implication of β-blockers, and we would like to focus on the different natures of the subtypes of β-receptors and β-receptor pathways concerning cardiac functions. Furthermore, we would like to discuss the mechanisms of the beneficial effects of selective stimulation of high-affinity β_1-receptors for the treatment of mild heart failure.

Drawbacks of Nonselective β-full Agonists in the Treatment of Heart Failure

Isoproterenol and adrenaline are nonselective β-full agonists commonly employed for the management of acute cardiogenic shock. Long-term therapy with them as inotropic agents has met with only limited success in treatment of congestive heart failure. Such limitation has been explained by the following drawbacks:

Fig. 1. The chemical structures of β_1-selective agonists.

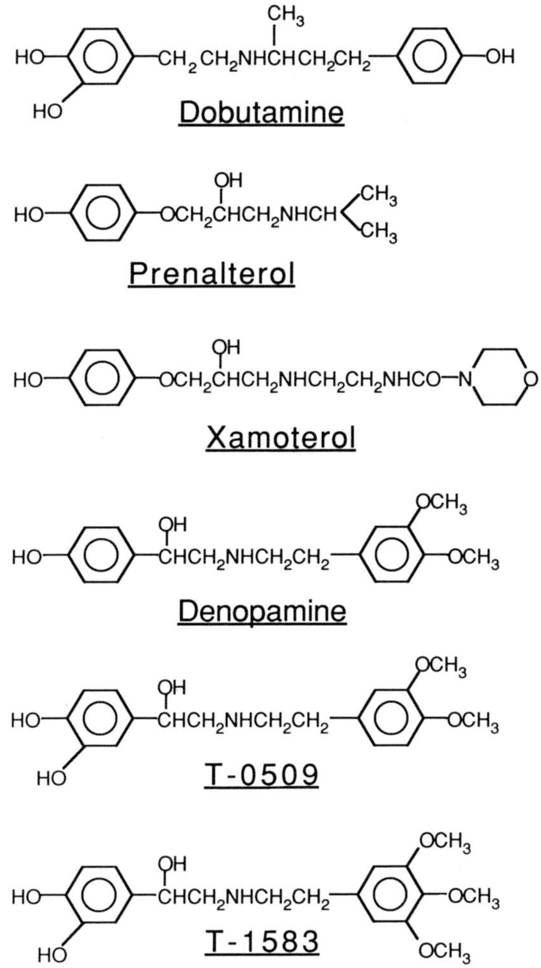

1. Production of marked tachycardia,
2. Induction of arrhythmias,
3. Increased oxygen consumption in the myocardium,
4. Induction of tolerance due to desensitization and downregulation of β-receptors,
5. Possible adverse metabolic effects, e.g., increased concentrations of glucose, lactate and free fatty acids and a decreased K^+ concentration in the plasma,
6. Possible ventricular hypertrophy,
7. Inconsistent bioavailabilities via enteral administration.

Other catecholamines with nonselective β-full agonistic activity seem to share more or less the same drawbacks mentioned above. Such unfavorable effects of nonselective β-full agonists may be due to their full-agonistic stimulation of both β_1- and β_2-receptors [4]. Although noradrenaline is a relatively selective β_1-agonist, it has α_1- and α_2-agonistic activities which contribute to some other drawbacks, i.e., an increase in blood pressure. Even dobutamine, a so-called β_1-selective full agonist, has some β_2- and α_1-agonistic activity [5].

To What Extent Are β_2-Receptors Involved in the Action of Nonselective β-Agonists?

Previous studies using radioligand binding techniques have shown that myocardial tissue of various species contains various proportions of β_2-receptors [6]. In human left ventricular and canine ventricular myocardial membranes, the proportions of β_2-receptors have been reported to be about 25% and 15% of total β-receptors, respectively [6–9]. All of the β-receptors, i.e., β_1- and β_2-receptors, are thought to be closely coupled to adenylate cyclase in human and canine right atria [8, 9]. However, in general, the positive inotropic effect of catecholamines is thought to be related to β_1-receptors in ventricular muscles, in spite of the evidence for the coexistence of β_1- and β_2-receptors in ventricular muscles. One reason for such discrepancy between the positive inotropic effects mediated by β-receptors and the results obtained from radioligand binding studies or studies of adenylate cyclase activity in cardiac muscles might be due to the unavailability of agonists highly selective for β_1- or β_2-receptors, and likewise selective antagonists.

Recently, some highly selective β_1- and β_2-agonists and antagonists have been made available, so that it has become possible to undertake a systematic analysis of the positive inotropic effects mediated by β_1- and β_2-receptors [10]. In the canine isolated right ventricular muscle, isoproterenol, T-1583 or T-0509 (β_1-selective agonists), and procaterol (a β_2-selective agonist) produced positive inotropic effects accompanied by a concomitant increase in cyclic AMP content of the tissue, via binding to β_1- and/or β_2-receptors, respectively. Interestingly, the concentration-response curves for procaterol became biphasic due to its different affinities for β_1- and β_2-receptors (Fig. 2, left). The biphasic curves were modified by atenolol (β_1-antagonists) or ICI 118,551 (β_2-antagonists) as predicted, and computer-simulated from the affinities of each β-antagonist for and the fractions of β_1- and β_2-receptors (Fig. 2, right). The fraction of β_2-receptors in total β-receptors was about 15% as has been reported [6], the increases in cyclic AMP produced by procaterol was 15%–20% above the baseline and the maximum positive inotropic effect due to their stimulation was about 10% of Ca-max [10].

Liang and Molinoff [9] have reported the close coupling of β_1- and β_2-receptors to adenylate cyclase in canine atria. Such close coupling seems to also exist in canine ventricular muscles. Although a significant correlation was found between the positive inotropic effect and an increased cyclic AMP content produced by procaterol, the slope was significantly different from those of isoproterenol and T-1583 (Fig. 3). Selective stimulation of β_2-receptors by procaterol and that of β_1-receptors by T-1583 produced an increase in cyclic

AMP content to almost the same extent. However, the positive inotropic effect was much smaller with procaterol than with T-1583. Thus, the cyclic AMP produced by stimulation of β_2-receptors may not couple well to the positive inotropic effect.

Even in human ventricular myocardium, cyclic AMP produced via the β_2-receptor-enzyme pathway seems to be less efficiently used by cellular effectors involved in contractility than that produced via the β_1-receptor-enzyme pathway [11–13]. When the cardiac muscles are exposed to isoproterenol, β_2-receptors are stimulated and an increase in cyclic AMP content occurs. The positive inotropic effect mediated, however, through β_2-receptors may be so marginal that the effect seems not to be detected in the concentration-response curves. Indeed, the curves were shifted to the right by atenolol, a β_1-selective antagonist, and were not modified by ICI 118,551 ($<10^{-7}$ M), a β_2-selective antagonist. Thus, the positive inotropic effect of nonselective β-agonists is due mainly to stimulation of β_1-receptors, and cyclic AMP produced by stimulation of β_2-receptors seems not to be coupled well to the positive inotropic effect [10].

How Different Are the Cardiac Effects of Denopamine, a β_1-Selective Partial Agonist, from Those of Isoproterenol?

Denopamine is an orally-active, β_1-selective cardiotonic drug which has been used to treat patients with congestive heart failure in Japan for nearly two years. According to basic pharmacological studies, denopamine produces less increase in heart rate [14] and myocardial oxygen consumption [15] or arrhythmias [16, 17] than the nonselective β-agonist isoproterenol. Moreover, with denopamine, unlike isoproterenol, scarcely self- or cross-tolerance develops [18]. These properties seem favorable for the treatment of mild heart failure. The less positive chronotropic effect of denopamine than isoproterenol has been ascribed to its β_1-selectivity [14], because both β_1- and β_2-receptors are thought to be involved in positive chronotropy [19]. The smaller increase in myocardial oxygen consumption with denopamine than with isoproterenol has partly been attributed to the β_1 selectivity [15], because the heart rate, one of the major determinants of myocardial oxygen consumption, is increased less by selective β_1 than by nonselective β stimulation. However, the smaller activation of adenylate cyclase by denopamine and the resultant smaller increase in cyclic AMP in myocardial cells than by isoproterenol are thought to be responsible for the smaller increase in myocardial oxygen consumption with denopamine than with isoproterenol [20, 21]. The reduced arrhythmogenic action of denopamine compared to isoproterenol has also been explained in similar terms [16, 17, 21]. Such properties of denopamine are thought to be derived from its partial agonistic property as well as its high β_1 selectivity [20, 21]. The lower tolerance produced by denopamine than by isoproterenol is presumed to be entirely due to its partial agonistic property [18]. Thus, the question arises about which property of denopamine, the β_1 selectivity or

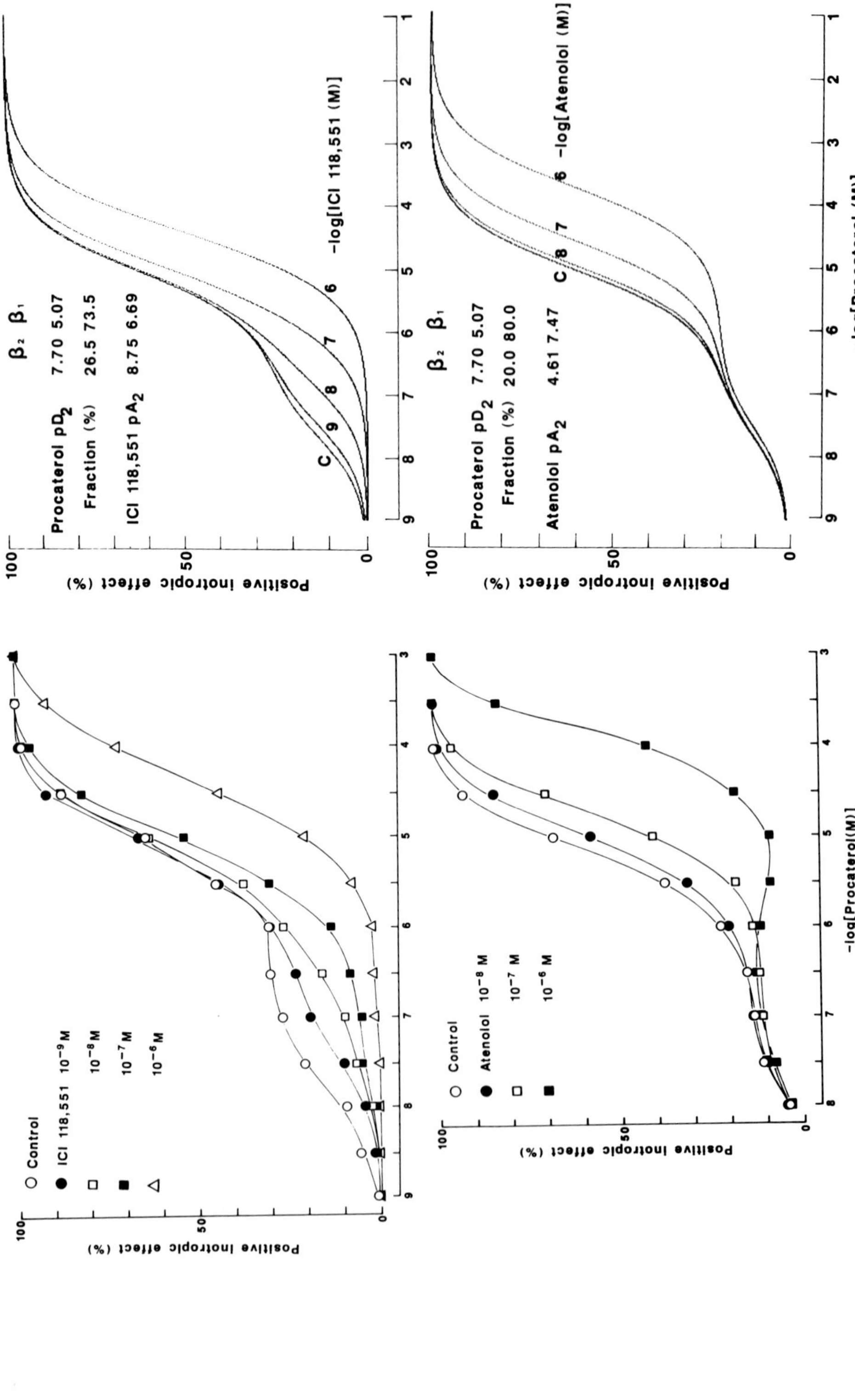
Control
ICI 118,551 10⁻⁹ M
10⁻⁸ M
10⁻⁷ M
10⁻⁶ M
Positive inotropic effect (%)
Control
Atenolol 10⁻⁸ M
10⁻⁷ M
10⁻⁶ M
-log[Procaterol(M)]
β2 β1
Procaterol pD2 7.70 5.07
Fraction (%) 26.5 73.5
ICI 118,551 pA2 8.75 6.69
-log[ICI 118,551 (M)]
β2 β1
Procaterol pD2 7.70 5.07
Fraction (%) 20.0 80.0
Atenolol pA2 4.61 7.47
-log[Atenolol (M)]
-log[Procaterol (M)]

Fig. 2. Positive inotropic effect of procaterol and selective antagonism of ICI 118,551 or atenolol in the canine right ventricular muscle. *Left* Cumulative concentration-response curves for the positive inotropic effect of procaterol became biphasic because its pD_2 values of positive inotropic effects via β_2- and β_1-receptors were 7.93 ± 0.12 (n = 18) and 5.12 ± 0.05 (n = 25), respectively. The maximum positive inotropic effect of procaterol was about 50% that of isoproterenol or Ca-max. Thus, the maximum positive inotropic effect via β_2-receptors stimulated by procaterol was about 10% that of isoproterenol or Ca-max. ICI 118,551 (10^{-9}–10^{-7} M) selectively antagonized the positive inotropic effect of procaterol at lower concentrations, whereas atenolol (10^{-8}–10^{-6} M) did at higher concentrations (from [10]). *Right* The biphasic concentration-response curves of procaterol and their selective modification by ICI 118,551 or atenolol were computer-simulated by the following logistic equation:

$$E = E_{max(\beta 2)} \times \frac{A}{A + K_{a(\beta 2)}} + (1 - E_{max(\beta 2)}) \times \frac{A}{A + K_{a(\beta 1)}}$$

where E and $E_{max(\beta 2)}$ are the normalized positive inotropic effect and maximum effect via β_2-receptors (fraction), respectively; A is procaterol concentration; $K_{a(\beta 2)}$ and $K_{a(\beta 1)}$ are EC_{50} values of procaterol for positive inotropic effects via β_2- and β_1-receptors, respectively. In the presence of ICI 118,551 or atenolol, $K_{a(\beta 2)}$ and $K_{a(\beta 1)}$ should be $K_{a(\beta 2)} \times (1 + B/K_{b(\beta 2)})$ and $K_{a(\beta 1)} \times (1 + B/K_{b(\beta 1)})$, respectively. Where B is antagonist concentration, $K_{b(\beta 2)}$ and $K_{b(\beta 1)}$ are binding constants (derived from pA_2 values) of each antagonist for β_2- and β_1-receptors, respectively

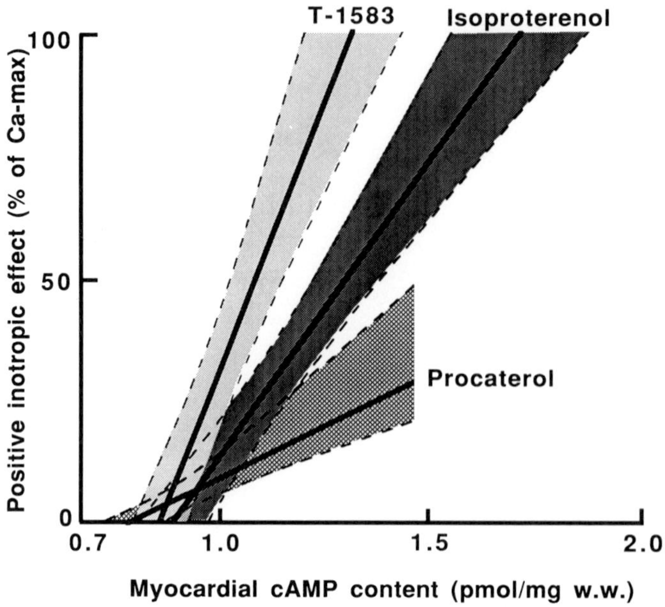

Fig. 3. Relationship between myolcardial cyclic AMP contents and positive inotropic effect in the presence and absence of T-1583, isoproterenol, and procaterol in canine right ventricular muscle. *Solid lines* are regression lines calculated from control values and those in the presence of T-1583 (10^{-8} and 10^{-7} M), isoproterenol (10^{-8} – 10^{-6} M), and procaterol (10^{-8} and 10^{-7} M), respectively. Dashed lines are 95% confidential intervals of each regression line. X intercepts, the control cyclic AMP content, are not different from each other. (Modified from [10] with permission)

the partial agonistic property, determines the characteristics favorable for the treatment of heart failure. To settle this question, it is urgent to obtain details on how selective and how partially agonistic denopamine is for β_1-receptors. In the next section, we describe the results obtained from our recent studies [22, 23].

Denopamine Behaves as a Full Agonist in the Single-concentration Regimen, but as a Partial Agonist in the Cumulative-concentration Regimen

In isolated canine ventricular muscles (trabecular muscles from the right ventricle) when single concentrations of denopamine (10^{-7}–3×10^{-4} M) were applied to single muscles (single-concentration regimen), a sigmoid concentration-positive inotropic curve was produced that attained a maximum at about 10^{-5} M, which was about 97.3% of the maximum with isoproterenol

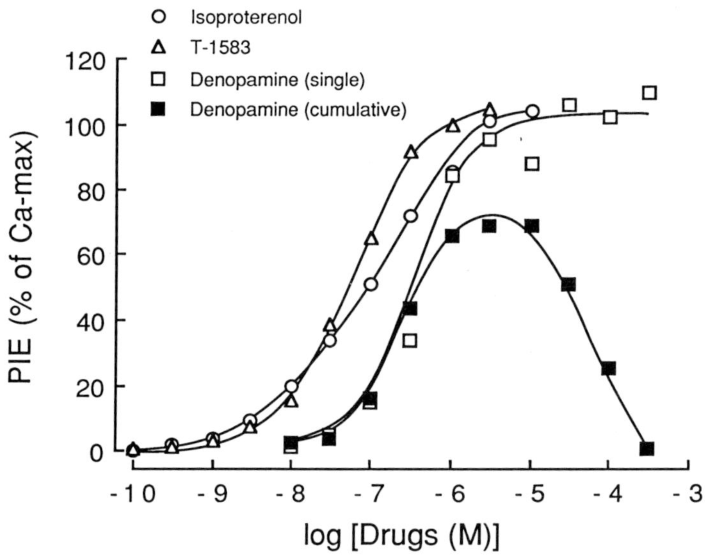

Fig. 4. Concentration-positive inotropic effect curves of denopamine as compared with that of isoproterenol in canine ventricular muscle. The sigmoid curve for denopamine was obtained with administration of single concentrations to single muscles, whereas the bell-shaped curve was obtained with cumulative administration at 30-min intervals. The sigmoid curve for isoproterenol was obtained with cumulative administration at 5-min intervals. The effects are expressed as percentages of the maximum effect obtained with 12.5 mM $CaCl_2$ (Ca-max) which was nearly equal to isoproterenol maximum. Data points are means ± SE (n = 6–12). (Modified from [10, 22] with permission)

(Fig. 4) [22]. The pD_2 ($-\log EC_{50}$) value of denopamine was determined to be 6.26 ± 0.11 (mean ± SE; n = 6–12) by computer-fitting the concentration-effect curve to a logistic equation:

$$E = M \times \frac{A^p}{A^p + K^p}$$

where E is normalized effect, M is maximum effect, A is agonist concentration, K is EC_{50} value of agonist and p is slope factor. Isoproterenol, whether applied in the single- or cumulative-concentration regimen, produced essentially the same sigmoid concentration-effect curve. Computer-fitting of the curve to the logistic equation yielded a pD_2 value of 7.05 ± 0.14 for isoproterenol [22]. Thus, in the single-concentration regimen, denopamine behaved as a nearly full agonist and seemed different only in potency; denopamine was about three times less potent than isoproterenol. Careful inspection of the concentration-effect curves for both agonists, however, revealed that the curve of denopamine was steeper than that of isoproterenol (Fig. 4); the slope factor was nearly unity (1.14 ± 0.41) for denopamine as against 0.77 ± 0.03 for isoproterenol [10]. Denopamine, when applied cumulatively (cumulative-concentration regimen) to canine ventricular muscles at about 30-min intervals, produced a bell-shaped concentration-positive inotropic curve. The curve ascended at 10^{-7} to 10^{-6} M to about 75.3% of that attained with the single concentration-regimen, and descended at higher concentrations nearly leading to abolition of the positive inotropic effect (Fig. 4). The pD_2 value of denopamine determined at the ascending limb of the curve was 6.64 ± 0.06 and the slope factor of the curve 1.32 ± 0.07. Thus, even with the cumulative-concentration regimen, denopamine was about one-third as potent as isoproterenol.

Denopamine is Selective for β_1-Receptors

In the presence of the β_1-selective antagonist atenolol, bell-shaped concentration-positive inotropic effect curves of denopamine were shifted to the right in a parallel way. Schild analysis of the antagonism by atenolol of the ascending limb of the curves yielded a pA_2 value of 7.66 ± 0.03 (n = 6) for atenolol [22]. The curves of denopamine were not affected by the concentrations of ICI 118,551 which antagonize β_2-receptors but were shifted to the right in a parallel way by the high concentrations which antagonize β_1-receptors. Its pA_2 value was 7.22 ± 0.23 (n = 6) with denopamine, which is the same as that of a β_1-antagonist [22]. Thus, it can be concluded that denopamine produced a positive inotropic effect by stimulating β_1-receptors exclusively in canine ventricular muscle.

Denopamine Antagonizes the Positive Inotropic Effects of Isoproterenol in Two Different Affinity States or Subtypes of β_1-Receptors

In the presence of cumulative concentrations of denopamine (3×10^{-5}–3×10^{-4} M) attained by addition at 30-min intervals, cumulative concentration-positive inotropic effect curves of isoproterenol determined with administration at 5-min intervals shifted to the right (Fig. 5a). The rightward shift of the curves became obvious when the concentration-effect curves of isoproterenol in the presence of cumulative concentrations of denopamine were normalized by expressing them as percentages of their maxima subtracted by the effects which had already been produced by denopamine (Fig. 5b). Another feature which became obvious by this normalization is that the concentration-effect curves of isoproterenol became steeper as the cumulative concentrations of denopamine were raised; the slope factor was 0.87 ± 0.12 in the absence of denopamine (control) and 1.05 ± 0.10 in the presence 3×10^{-4} M denopamine [23]. In other words, denopamine antagonized more effectively the lower concentration part than the higher concentration part of the curves for isoproterenol. This implies that isoproterenol produced a positive inotropic effect by stimulating non-homogeneous states or subtypes of β_1-receptors, e.g., the high- and low-affinity (states or subtypes of) β_1-receptors, and also that denopamine antagonized more effectively high- than low-affinity β_1-receptors.

Fig. 5. a Concentration-positive inotropic effect curves of isoproterenol obtained in the presence and absence (control) of cumulative concentrations of denopamine in canine ventricular muscles. Data points are means ±SE (n = 6). **b** The normalized curves of those shown in **a**. (From [23] with permission)

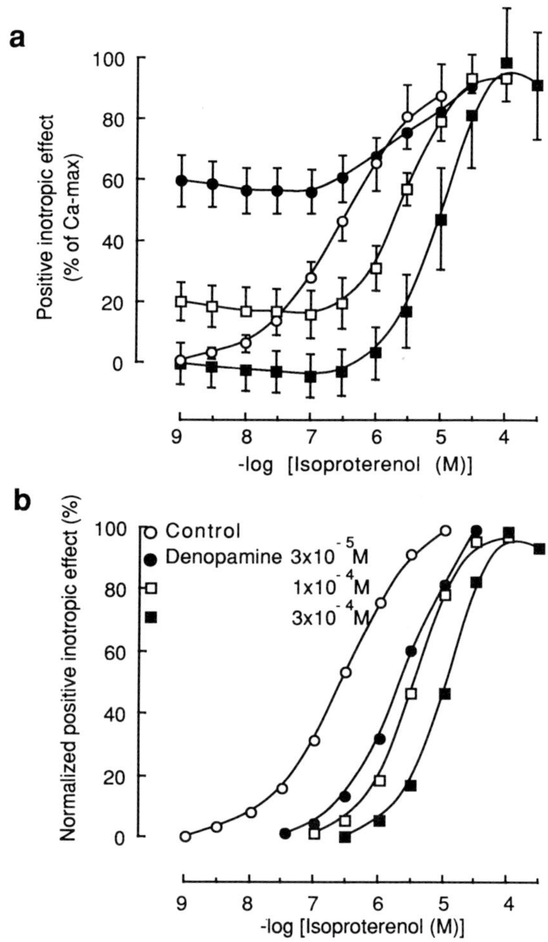

Computer-fitting to a two-component model of the control and the normalized concentration-effect curves of isoproterenol in the presence of cumulative concentrations of denopamine, with the assumption that the slope factor for the high-affinity β_1-receptors for isoproterenol is unity, revealed the following feature:

1. In the absence of denopamine, isoproterenol produced a positive inotropic effect by stimulating both the high- and the low-affinity β_1-receptors whose proportions are nearly half-and-half. The pD_2 value of isoproterenol was 7.21 ± 0.20 for the high-affinity and 6.17 ± 0.10 for the low-affinity β_1-receptors [23].
2. Denopamine antagonized the positive inotropic effect of isoproterenol more effectively due to stimulation of the high-affinity β_1-receptors rather than the low-affinity β_1-receptors.
3. The proportion of the high-affinity β_1-receptors decreased as cumulative concentrations of denopamine were raised.

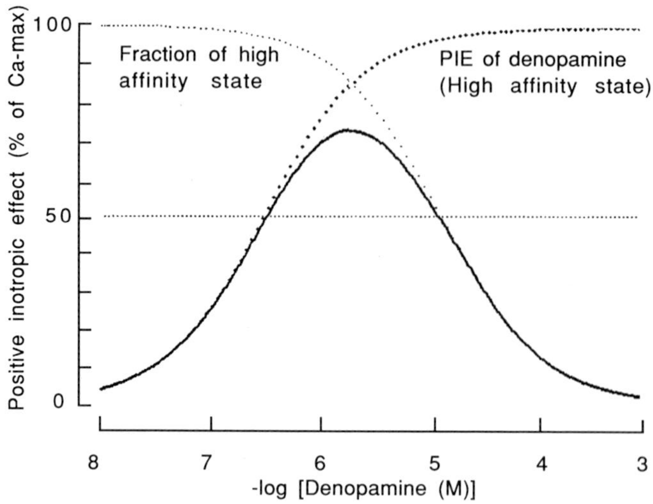

Fig. 6. Computer-simulation of the bell-shaped concentration-positive inotropic effect curve of denopamine. (From [23] with permission)

Schild analysis of the differential antagonism by denopamine of the positive inotropic effect of isoproterenol that was produced by stimulation of the two affinity β_1-receptors yielded two pA_2 values for denopamine: 6.59 ± 0.19 for the high-affinity and 5.05 ± 0.21 for the low-affinity β_1-receptors, respectively [23].

Computer Modeling of the Bell-shaped Concentration-effect Curves of Denopamine in the Cumulative-concentration Regimen

Denopamine can be described as a β_1-selective partial agonist which is able to antagonize the high-affinity β_1-receptors for isoproterenol, with a dissociation constant of $10^{-6.59}$ M, and the low-affinity β_1-receptors, with a dissociation constant of $10^{-5.05}$ M. By the definition of partial agonists, the pD_2 value of denopamine should be identical with its pA_2 value of 6.59 ± 0.19, which was indeed very close to 6.58 ± 0.21, a pD_2 value actually determined from the ascending limb of the bell-shaped curve [23]. The question arises about whether the bell-shaped concentration-effect curve of denopamine is a result of self antagonism. The bell-shaped curve of denopamine was well computer-simulated (Fig. 6) based on the following assumptions:

1. Denopamine produces a positive inotropic effect only when binding to the high-affinity receptors with a dissociation constant of $10^{-6.59}$ M. The positive inotropic effect of 10^{-x} M denopamine by this mechanism (PIE_H) is thus given by the following equation:

$$PIE_H = \frac{10^{-x}}{10^{-x} + 10^{-6.59}} \tag{1}$$

2. As denopamine binds to the low-affinity β_1-receptors, the fraction of the high-affinity β_1-receptors decreases. In other words, denopamine binds high-affinity β_1-receptors apparently in an irreversible fashion with a binding constant of $10^{-5.05}$. Thus, the remaining fraction of the high-affinity β_1-receptors (F_H) that can be stimulated by agonists in the presence of denopamine at a cumulative concentration of 10^{-x} M is given by the following equation:

$$F_H = 1 - \frac{10^{-x}}{10^{-x} + 10^{-5.05}} \tag{2}$$

where $10^{-5.05}$ is the dissociation constant with which denopamine binds to the low-affinity β_1-receptors. Therefore, the positive inotropic effect produced by denopamine at a cumulative concentration of 10^{-x} M (PIE) is given by the following equation:

$$\begin{aligned} \text{PIE} &= F_H \times \text{PIE}_H \\ &= \left(1 - \frac{10^{-x}}{10^{-x} + 10^{-5.05}}\right) \times \frac{10^{-x}}{10^{-x} + 10^{-6.59}} \end{aligned} \tag{3}$$

Equation (3) yielded 6.82 as a pD_2 value and 73.1% of the isoproterenol maximum at $10^{-5.82}$ M. These values were very close to the actual values obtained [22, 23].

Implication of Selective Stimulation of the High-Affinity β_1-Receptors and Occupation of the Low-Affinity β_1-Receptors by Denopamine in its Pharmacological Effects

As described previously, the smaller increase in cyclic AMP in myocardial cells with denopamine than with isoproterenol is thought to be responsible for the smaller increase in myocardial oxygen consumption and reduced arrhythmogenicity [20, 21]. The maximum increase in cyclic AMP produced by denopamine in canine ventricular muscle in the single-concentration regimen amounted to about half that produced by isoproterenol [22]. The increase was comparable to that produced by the β_1-selective full agonist T-1583 [10] at concentrations that produced the maximum positive inotropic effect. The concentration-positive inotropic effect curve of T-1583 had a slope factor of 1.16 [10], indicating that a homogeneous population of β_1-receptors, probably their high-affinity state alone or subtype, is involved. Thus, it is likely that the smaller increase in cyclic AMP with denopamine was due exclusively to selective stimulation of the high-affinity β_1-receptors but not due to its partial agonistic property. Unlike isoproterenol, tolerance scarcely develops with denopamine [18], and this property has been ascribed to denopamine's partial agonistic property [18]. The tolerance liability of isoproterenol has been ascribed to its full agonistic property, because no tolerance was induced by prenalterol, a β_1-selective partial agonist [24]. A biochemical explanation is that unoccupied or blocked β-receptors are not a substrate for β-receptor kinase, one of the protein kinases responsible for phosphorylation of β-receptors to desensitize [25, 26]. However, the possibility remains that stimulation of the low-affinity β_1-receptors is causally related to the development of tolerance, because high doses of isoproterenol more readily develop tolerance than low doses. As described in the previous section, denopamine stimulates only the high-affinity β_1-receptors, and at high doses it indeed is able to bind to the low-affinity β_1-receptors. However, as this binding is antagonistic, a chain of events leading to a positive inotropic effect does not follow, and tolerance does not develop.

Pharmacological Effects of Selective Stimulation of the High-Affinity β_1-Receptors

In a previous section we put forward the hypothesis that there exist two states or subtypes of β_1-receptors in canine ventricular muscle, i.e., the high-affinity and low-affinity β_1-receptors, and that isoproterenol produces a positive inotropic effect by stimulation of both high- and low-affinity β_1-receptors, whereas denopamine does so by stimulating the high-affinity but not the low-affinity β_1-receptors. Of course, isoproterenol is capable of producing some positive inotropy by stimulation of β_2-receptors in canine ventricular muscle [10]. However, the maximum positive inotropic effect produced by β_2-receptor stimulation remained about 10% of Ca-max and the increase in cyclic AMP accompanied also remained about 15% above the baseline level at most [10]. Therefore, according to this hypothesis, selective stimulation of the high-affinity β_1-receptors alone leads to positive inotropy with a small increase in cyclic AMP [10, 22]. In this section, we would like to explore the positive inotropic mechanisms of the two states or subtypes of β_1-receptors in relation to cyclic AMP metabolism [27].

T-0509 and T-1583 are β_1-Selective Full Agonists

The positive inotropic effects of T-0509 [27] and T-1583 [10] seems to be produced predominantly via stimulation of β_1-receptors for the reasons mentioned below. The cumulative concentration-response curves for the positive inotropic effect of T-0509 were shifted to the right by atenolol (10^{-8}–10^{-6} M). The pA_2 value of atenolol determined to be 7.53 was in the range of its pA_2 values in antagonizing β_1-receptors. The concentration-response curve for the positive inotropic effect of T-0509 was not shifted by 10^{-8} M ICI 118,551, but was shifted to the right by 10^{-6} M ICI 118,551. This shift gave a$-\log K_B$ of 6.90, which is nearly the same as the reported pA_2 value of ICI 118,551 in antagonizing β_1-receptors. Thus, it can be concluded that T-0509 is a β_1-selective full agonist in the concentrations we used (10^{-10}–10^{-5} M). The concentration-response curve for the positive inotropic effect of T-0509 was computer-fitted to a single component curve and the slope parameter was a little larger than unity, suggesting that T-0509 produced a positive inotropic effect by binding a single population of β_1-receptors. The slope of the Schild plot for antagonism

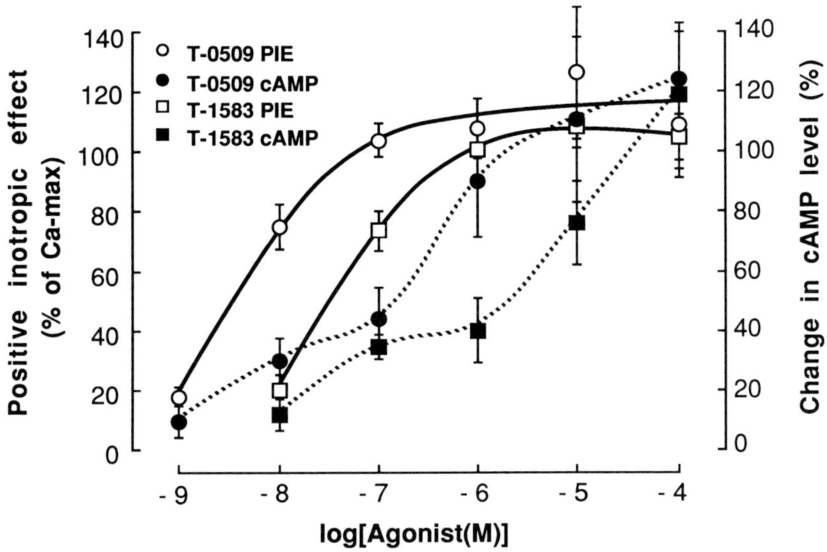

Fig. 7. Concentration-response curves for the positive inotropic effects and changes in cyclic AMP content produced by T-0509 and T-1583 in isolated canine right ventricular muscle. The curves were constructed with administration of single concentrations of T-0509 or T-1583 to single muscles. (From [27] with permission)

by atenolol of the effect of T-0509 being almost unity indicates competitive antagonism between T-0509 and atenolol on the same receptors. T-0509 and T-1583 also produced similar concentration-response curves for the positive inotropic effect when each preparation was subjected to only a single concentration of these two agonists. In these respects, the two agonists differed distinctly from denopamine, which behaved as a β_1-selective full agonist only when each preparation was exposed to a single concentration [22, 23].

Concentration-Response Curves for the Positive Inotropic Effect and Change in Cyclic AMP Level Caused by T-0509 and T-1583

To clarify the relationship between the positive inotropic effect and the increase in cyclic AMP produced by either T-0509 or T-1583, the concentration-response curves for these two variables were constructed from values obtained 5 min after administration of single concentrations of each agonist to single muscles. T-0509 (10^{-9}–10^{-4} M) and T-1583 (10^{-8}–10^{-4} M) gave monophasic concentration-response curves for the positive inotropic effect, reaching maxima with 10^{-7} M T-0509 and 10^{-6} M T-1583 (Fig. 7). The pD_2 values and slope factors of the curves were nearly the same as those constructed with cumulative administration. On the other hand, concentration-response curves for the increase in cyclic AMP produced by T-0509 and T-1583 were biphasic; the curves reached a plateau about 40% above the baseline levels with 10^{-7} M

T-0509 or 10^{-6} M T-1583. With increasing concentrations of either agonist, cyclic AMP again increased up to about 120% above the baseline levels attained with 10^{-5} M T-0509 or 10^{-4} M T-1583. It should be noted that their positive inotropic effects reached maxima at concentrations that produced about 40% increases in cyclic AMP above baseline levels. In several muscles, arrhythmic contractions occurred in the presence of 10^{-6}–10^{-4} M T-0509 and 10^{-5}–10^{-4} M T-1583, whereas no arrhythmic contractions occurred with 10^{-9}–10^{-7} M T-0509 and 10^{-8}–10^{-6} M T-1583. The arrhythmic contractions seemed to be due to the large increases in cyclic AMP content produced by higher concentrations of T-0509 or T-1583, because they were also able to be induced by isoproterenol especially at its medium and higher concentrations [27].

The Nature and Modification of Positive Inotropic Effects of Selective High-Affinity β_1-Receptor Agonists, T-0509 and T-1583

As were the cases with isoproterenol [28] and T-1583 [10], the positive inotropic effect and the concomitant increase in cyclic AMP produced by T-0509 were both inhibited by carbachol, a muscarinic receptor agonist, and enhanced by IBMX, a nonselective inhibitor of cyclic nucleotide phosphodiesterase, indicating that the positive inotropic effect is mediated by an increase in cyclic AMP. What most interested us in the present study was as follows: as described previously for T-1583 [10] or above for T-0509, the concentration-response curves for the positive inotropic effect were monophasic. However, the concentration-response curves for the increase in cyclic AMP measured simultaneously with those for positive inotropy were biphasic; cyclic AMP increased with increasing concentrations of T-0509 from 10^{-9}–10^{-7} M and T-1583 from 10^{-8}–10^{-6} M, and reached plateaux about 40% above the baseline levels with 10^{-7} M T-0509 and 10^{-6} M T-1583, respectively. At these concentrations, the positive inotropic effects of both agonists reached maxima. With further increasing concentrations of both agonists, cyclic AMP again increased and reached about 120% above the baseline levels at 10^{-5} M T-0509 and 10^{-4} M T-1583.

In the previous study with denopamine [22], cyclic AMP increased to about 40% above the baseline level at 10^{-6} M and the positive inotropic effect reached a maximum. However, even with further increases in concentration, cyclic AMP levels were not elevated further. In this respect, the selective β_1-full agonists T-0509 and T-1583 differed from denopamine. In the previous study [23], we hypothesized that denopamine produces a positive inotropic effect by stimulating only the high-affinity state of β_1-receptors, and that about 40% increases in cyclic AMP produced by this mechanism would be enough to produce a maximum positive inotropic effect. In analogy, it seems that T-0509 and T-1583 produced a maximum positive inotropic effect with an increase in cyclic AMP maximally about 40% above the baseline level by selective stimulation of high-affinity β_1-receptors. Unlike denopamine, however, T-0509 and T-1583 elevated cyclic AMP levels up to about 120% above the baseline with further increasing concentrations from 10^{-7} to 10^{-4} M, probably because they are full agonists of low-affinity β_1-receptors. Although an increase in the force of contraction produced by these high concentrations reached a ceiling, we hypothesize that the increase in cyclic AMP produced by stimulation of low-affinity β_1-receptors is not so closely coupled to positive inotropy as that produced by stimulation of high-affinity β_1-receptors.

The supposition described above can be reinforced by the results described below. The nearly maximum increase in the force of contraction (95% of Ca-max) produced by 3×10^{-8} M T-0509 was greatly reduced by 3×10^{-6} M carbachol *pari passu* with the increased cyclic AMP. Nevertheless, under these conditions, a slight increase in cyclic AMP seems to have produced a sizable increase in the force of contraction. The increases in the force of contraction and cyclic AMP produced by 10^{-5} M T-0509 were also reduced by 3×10^{-6} M carbachol. Under these conditions, the force of contraction produced by 10^{-5} M T-0509 was not as great as expected from the increase in cyclic AMP. T-0509 at 3×10^{-9} M produced an increase in the force of contraction amounting to about 40% of Ca-max, with a nearly undetectable increase in cyclic AMP. In the presence of 10^{-5} M IBMX, both effects were enhanced. Nevertheless, a large increase in the force compared with a small increase in cyclic AMP were still seen at this low concentration of T-0509. Similar findings have already been obtained with T-1583 [10]. To recapitulate, the increase in cyclic AMP produced by stimulation of low-affinity β_1-receptors does not seem to be coupled closely to positive inotropy. The increase in cyclic AMP produced by 10^{-9} to 10^{-7} M T-0509 which was at most about 40% above the baseline level was nearly eliminated by 10^{-6} M atenolol, and the positive inotropic effect produced by these concentrations were greatly reduced. However, most of the increase in cyclic AMP produced by 10^{-6}–10^{-5} M T-0509 was resistant to the blocking effect of 10^{-6} M atenolol. This may be due to stimulation of the low-affinity β_1-receptors.

The Low-Affinity β_1-Receptors in Cardiac Muscle may be Akin to β_3-Receptors in Rat Brown Adipocytes

A recent β_1-receptor binding study [29] has demonstrated that in rat ventricular myocytes there exist two forms of β_1-receptors with different affinities for bisoprolol, a selective β_1-antagonist, i.e., the high-affinity and the low-affinity form. However, no mention has been given as regards their functions [29]. Alternatively, the atypical β-receptor or β_3-receptor in rat brown adipocytes [30, 31], in the guinea-pig ileum [32] or heart [33] whose possible existence has recently been suggested is attractive. More recently, the primary structure of one of the human β_3-receptors from a human genomic library was determined [34]. All these putative β_3-receptors are not necessarily identical because interaction of some β-antagonists with these putative receptors is variable. In the previous study [23], we speculated that there are two states for β_1-receptors, i.e., the low-affinity and the high-affinity state, and that the two states are transformable. However, it is possible that the low-affinity state of β_1-receptors is a non-transformable subset of β_1-receptors, i.e., the low-affinity β_1-receptor or one of the putative β_3-receptors described above.

Implication of Selective Stimulation of High-Affinity β_1-Receptors in the Treatment of Mild Heart Failure

If there are positive inotropic agents which are able to reduce the generalized adrenergic activation by improving cardiac performance, they may be beneficial for the treatment of congestive heart failure. It has been reported that high-dose and long-duration β-adrenergic therapy with dobutamine is associated with higher β_1- and total β-receptor densities in hearts removed from cardiac transplant recipients [1]. If there is heterogeneity in the desensitization potential of catecholamines as has been suggested [35], the therapeutic use of an appropriate β-agonist could result in less receptor downregulation than might be produced by endogenous catecholamines.

In this article, we have demonstrated the possible existence of three subtypes of β-receptor in cardiac muscle, i.e., β_2-receptors, high-affinity β_1-receptors (so-called β_1-receptors) and low-affinity β_1-receptors (akin to β_3-receptors), which are coupled with increases in myocardial cyclic AMP content and positive inotropic effects. The endogenous catecholamines, noradrenaline and adrenaline, can more or less activate β_2-receptors, high-affinity and low-affinity β_1-receptors. Thus, the generalized activation of the sympathetic nervous system produces stimulation of all kinds of β-receptor subtypes, resulting in various adverse cardiac effects. The relationships between cyclic AMP and positive inotropic effects via these three β-receptor subtypes are different (Fig. 8). Cyclic AMP generated by activation of high-affinity β_1-receptors seems to be coupled with the positive inotropic effect much more effectively than that via β_2-receptors or low-affinity β_1-receptors. Since a large increase in cyclic AMP may result in phosphorylation of β-receptors by cyclic AMP-dependent protein kinase [26], stimulation of the low affinity state of β_1-receptor is causally related to the development of tolerance and to the adverse effects of nonselective β-full agonists, because high doses of isoproterenol more readily produce tolerance than low doses. It is conceivable that self- or cross-tolerance is hardly developed with denopamine [18], unlike isoproterenol, resulting from not only denopamine's partial agonistic property [18] but also its selectivity for high-affinity β_1-receptors. In accordance with such possibilities, selective stimulation of β_1-receptors by xamoterol involves incycling of β-adrenoceptors with different pathways utilized by isoproterenol [36]. It would be interesting to discover whether tolerance hardly develops with catechol-derivatives of denopamine, T-0509 and T-1583, as with denopamine, or whether it develops, as with isoproterenol.

Recently, there have been several lines of evidence that β-receptors are able to activate partly cardiac Ca^{2+} channels directly via G proteins, guanine nucleotide-binding proteins, and not via cyclic AMP pathways [37–39]. In our laboratory, selective stimulation of high-affinity β_1-receptors by T-1583 pre-

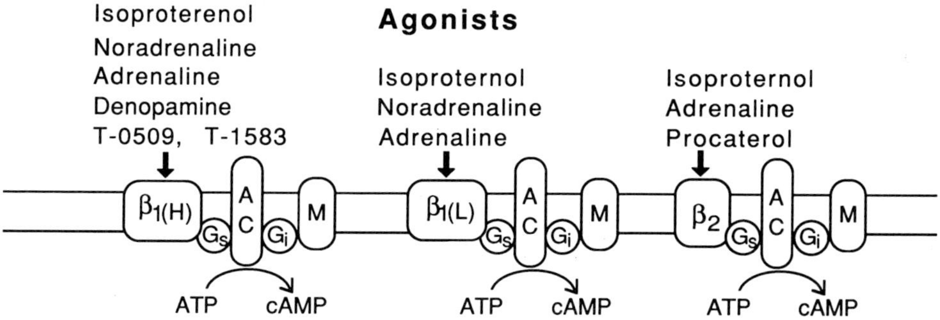

	β1(H)	β1(L)	β2
+ cAMP (%)	40%	80%	15%
PIE (%)	**100%**	**100%**	**10%**
Under stimulation of muscarinic receptors			
+ cAMP (%)	5%	50%	
PIE (%)	**20%**	**50%**	

Fig. 8. Relationship between cyclic AMP and positive inotropic effects via β-receptor subtypes. In cardiac muscle, there may be three kinds of β-receptor subtypes, i.e., β_2-receptors, high-affinity β_1-receptors (so-called β_1-receptors) and low-affinity β_1-receptors (akin to β_3-receptors), which are coupled with increases in myocardial cyclic AMP content and positive inotropic effects. Endogenous catecholamines, noradrenaline or adrenaline, and nonselective β-full agonist, isoproterenol, can more or less activate β_2-, high-affinity and low-affinity β_1-receptors. The relationships between cyclic AMP and positive inotropic effect via these three β-receptor subtypes is different. Such relationships are not modified even under the condition of stimulation of muscarinic receptors

ferentially increases Ca^{2+} current, whereas isoproterenol, a nonselective β-full agonist, equally and simultaneously increases both Ca^{2+} and delayed rectifier K^+ currents in single ventricular cells of guinea-pig hearts [40], in which only β_1-receptors exist [6]. Thus, it is possible that the high-affinity β_1-receptors are preferentially coupled with cyclic AMP-independent pathways and activate Ca^{2+} channels.

Whatever mechanisms of signal transduction are involved, selective stimulation of high-affinity β_1-receptors would be beneficial for the management of congestive mild heart failure. In contrast, stimulation of low-affinity β_1-receptors by endogenous catecholamines or nonelective β-agonists will contribute to deteriorating hemodynamic, symptomatic and prognostic consequences in patients with congestive heart failure.

Acknowledgments. These studies and this manuscript were partly supported by Grants-in-Aid for Scientific Research on Priority Areas (No. 01624001,

01641003) from the Ministry of Education, Science and Culture, Japan, and Research Grant for Cardiovascular Disease (1-A-1) from the Ministry of Health and Welfare, Japan. We are grateful to Tanabe Seiyaku Co., Ltd., Osaka, Japan for the generous supply of denopamine, T-0509 and T-1583 and to Imperial Chemical Industries PLC, Macclesfield, Cheshire, England, U.K. for ICI 118,551 and atenolol.

References

1. Bristow MR, Hershberger RE, Port JD, Gilbert EM, Sandoval A, Rasmussen R, Cates AE, Feldman AM (1990) β-Adrenergic pathways in nonfailing and failing human ventricular myocardium. Circulation 82(suppl I):I-12–I-25
2. Packer M (1990) Role of the sympathetic nervous system in chronic heart failure: a historical and philosophical perspective. Circulation 82(suppl I):I-1–I-6
3. The xamoterol in severe heart failure study group (1990) Xamoterol in severe heart failure. Lancet 336:1–6
4. Packer M (1990) Pathophysiological mechanisms underlying the effects of β-adrenergic agonists and antagonists on functional capacity and survival in chronic heart failure. Circulation 82(suppl I):I-77–I-88
5. Ruffolo RR Jr (1987) Review: the pharmacology of dobutamine. Am J Med Sci 294:244–248
6. Stiles GL, Caron MG, Lefkowitz RJ (1984) β-Adrenergic receptors: biochemical mechanisms of physiological regulation. Physiol Rev 64:661–743
7. Manalan AS, Besch HR Jr, Watanabe AM (1981) Characterization of $[^3H](\pm)$ carazolol binding to β-adrenergic receptors: application to study of β-adrenergic receptors subtypes in canine ventricular myocardium and lung. Circ Res 49:326–336
8. Brodde O-E, O'Hara N, Zerkowski H-R, Rohm N (1984) Human cardiac β-adrenoceptors: both β_1- and β_2-adrenoceptors are functionally coupled to adenylate cyclase in right atrium. J Cardiovasc Pharmacol 6:1184–1191
9. Liang BT, Molinoff PB (1986) *Beta*-adrenergic receptor subtypes in the atria: evidence for close coupling of *beta*-1 and *beta*-2 adrenergic receptors to adenylate cyclase. J Pharmacol Exp Ther 238:886–892
10. Yanagisawa T, Ishii K, Hashimoto H, Taira N (1989) Differential coupling to positive inotropic responses of cyclic AMP produced by stimulation of β_1- and β_2-adrenergic receptors. J Cardiovasc Pharmacol 13:64–75
11. Gille E, Lemoine H, Ehle B, Kaumann AJ (1985) The affinity of (-)-propranolol for β_1- and β_2-adrenoceptors for human heart: differential antagonism of the positive inotropic effects and adenylate cyclase stimulation by (-)-noradrenaline and (-)-adrenaline. Naunyn Schmiedebergs Arch Pharmacol 331:60–70
12. Ikezono K, Michel MC, Zerkowski H-R, Beckeringh JJ, Brodde OE (1987) The role of cyclic AMP in the positive inotropic effect mediated by β_1- and β_2-adrenoceptors in isolated human right atrium. Naunyn Schmiedebergs Arch Pharmacol 335:561–566
13. Kaumann AJ, Lemoine H (1987) β_2-Adrenoceptor-mediated positive inotropic effect of adrenaline in human ventricular myocardium: quantitative discrepancies with binding and adenylate cyclase stimulation. Naunyn Schmiedebergs Arch Pharmacol 335:403–411

14. Nagao T, Ikeo T, Murata S, Sato M, Nakajima H (1984) Cardiovascular effects of a new positive inotropic agent, (-)-(R)-(p-hydroxyphenyl)-2-[(3,4-dimethoxyphenyl)amino]-ethanol (TA-064) in the anesthetized dog and isolated guinea pig heart. Jpn J Pharmacol 35:415–423
15. Ikeo T, Nagao T (1985) Effects of denopamine (TA-064), a new positive inotropic agent, on myocardial oxygen consumption and left ventricular dimension in anesthetized dogs. Jpn J Pharmacol 39:179–189
16. Narita H, Yabana H, Kikkawa K, Miyazaki K, Ikeo T, Nagao T (1986) Weak arrhythmogenic property of the new cardiotonic agent denopamine in dogs: comparison with catecholamines. Jpn J Pharmacol 41:335–344
17. Sato T, Imanishi S, Arita M (1989) Comparative positive inotropic effects of TA-064 (denopamine), a new cardiotonic agent, and isoproterenol and ouabain on guinea pig ventricular muscles. J Cardiovasc Pharmacol 14:519–525
18. Yabana H, Naito K, Nagao T (1986) Effect of chronic administration of denopamine (TA-064), a new positive inotropic agent, on cardiac response of rats to denopamine. Jpn J Pharmacol 42:87–97
19. Carlsson E, Dahlöf C-G, Hedberg A, Persson H, Tångstrand B (1977) Differentiation of cardiac chronotropic and inotropic effects of β-adrenoceptor agonists. Naunyn Schmiedebergts Arch Pharmacol 300:101–105
20. Bing RJ, Sasaki Y, Burger W, Chemnitius JM (1984) Cardiac inotropic response of a new β-1-agonist (TA-064) with low sarcolemmal adenylate cyclase activation. Curr Ther Res 36:1127–1144
21. Chemnitius JM, Bing RJ (1985) Beta-1-adrenoceptor agonists with low adenylate cyclase activation: theoretical and clinical implications. Can J Cardiol 1:186–190
22. Yokoyama H, Yanagisawa T, Taira N (1988) Details of mode and mechanism of action of denopamine, a new orally active cardiotonic agent with affinity for β_1-receptors. J Cardiovasc Pharmacol 12:323–331
23. Yokoyama H, Ishii K, Yanagisawa T, Taira N (1989) An explanation of bell-shaped dose-positive inotropic effect curves for denopamine in canine ventricular muscle. J Cardiovasc Pharmacol 14:570–576
24. Hedberg A, Mattsson H, Nerme V, Carlsson E (1984) Effects of in vivo treatment with isoprenaline or prenalterol on beta-adrenoceptor mechanisms in the heart and soleus muscle of the cat. Naunyn Schmiedebergs Arch Pharmacol 325:251–258
25. Benovic JL, Strasser RH, Caron MG, Lefkowitz RJ (1986) β-adrenergic receptor kinase: identification of a novel protein kinase that phosphorylates the agonist-occupied form of the receptor. Proc Natl Acad Sci USA 83:2797–2801
26. Lohse MJ, Benovic JL, Caron MG, Lefkowitz RJ (1990) Multiple pathways of rapid β_2-adrenergic receptor desensitization: delineation with specific inhibitors. J Biol Chem 265:3202–3209
27. Kurosawa H, Satoh E, Yanagisawa T, Taira N (1990) Selective β_1-receptor full agonists, T-0509 and T-1583, increase the force monophasically and cyclic AMP biphasically in canine ventricular muscle. J Cardiovasc Pharmacol 16:646–653
28. Endoh M (1980) The time course of changes in cyclic nucleotide levels during cholinergic inhibition of positive inotropic actions of isoproterenol and theophylline in the isolated canine ventricular myocardium. Naunyn Schmiedebergs Arch Pharmacol 312:175–182
29. Mauz ABM, Pelzer H (1990) β-Adrenoceptor-binding studies of the cardioselective β blockers bisoprolol, H-I 42 BS, and HX-CH 44 BS to heart membranes and intact ventricular myocytes of adult rats: two β_1-binding sites for bisoprolol. J Cardiovasc Pharmacol 15:421–427

30. Arch JRS, Ainsworth AT, Cawthorne MA, Piercy V, Sennitt MV, Thody VE, Wilson C, Wilson S (1984) Atypical β-adrenoceptor on brown adipocytes as target for anti-obesity drugs. Nature 309:163–165
31. Arch JRS (1989) The brown adipocyte β-adrenoceptor. Proc Nutr Soc 48:215–223
32. Bond RA, Clarke DE (1988) Agonist and antagonist characterization of a putative adrenoceptor with distinct pharmacological properties from α- and β-subtypes. Br J Pharmacol 95:723–734
33. Kaumann AJ (1989) Is there a third heart β-adrenoceptor? Trends Pharmacol Sci 10:316–320
34. Emorine LJ, Marullo S, Briend-Sutren M-M, Patey G, Tate K, Delavier-Klutchko C, Strosberg AD (1989) Molecular characterization of the human β_3-adrenergic receptor. Science 245:1118–1121
35. Brodde O-E (1990) Physiology and pharmacology of cardiovascular catecholamine receptors: implications for treatment of chronic heart failure. Am Heart J 120: 1565–1572
36. Limas CJ, Limas C (1990) Effects of xamoterol on the reversible cycling of cardiac β-adrenoceptors. J Cardiovasc Pharmacol 16:945–951
37. Brown AM, Yatani A, Imoto Y, Codina J, Mattera R, Birnbaumer L (1989) Direct G-protein regulation of Ca^{2+} channels. Ann NY Acad Sci 560:373–386
38. Trautwein W, Hescheler J (1990) Regulation of cardiac L-type calcium current by phosphorylation and G proteins. Annu Rev Physiol 52:257–274
39. Brown AM (1990) Regulation of heartbeat by G protein-coupled ion channels. Am J Physiol 259:H1621–H1628
40. Iijima T, Imagawa J, Taira N (1990) Differential modulation by *beta*-adrenoceptors of inward calcium and delayed rectifier potassium current in single ventricular cells of guinea pig heart. J Pharmacol Exp Ther 254:142–146

13

Hemodynamic and Histopathological Consideration of Left Ventricular Assist System on Acute Myocardial Infarction: Experimental and Clinical Investigation

HISATERU TAKANO[1], TAKESHI NAKATANI[1]

Summary. A left ventricular assist system (LVAS) has been applied to treat the profound heart failure following acute myocardial infarction (AMI). The performance of our original automatic LVAS on AMI was evaluated experimentally and clinically. In chronic animal experiments, the LVAS earned time for the impaired heart to recover while maintaining normal circulation. Decompression of the left ventricle (LV) at the beginning of the LVAS support simultaneously prevented overextension of infarcted myocardium and accelerated scar formation. Gradual increase of LV work promoted the compensation mechanism of residual myocardium. Recovery from profound heart failure after use of the LVAS might have been due to increases in LV end-diastolic volume, left atrial pressure, and heart rate, hypertrophy of residual myocardium, and prevention of dyskinesis by solid scar formation. In clinical cases, the LVAS provided powerful circulatory assistance and maintained near normal circulation, and the heart showed recovery from profound heart failure. Many patients, however, died of multiple organ failure which was probably caused by prolonged ischemia before institution of the LVAS. For completely successful recovery from profound heart failure following AMI, the LVAS should be applied timely before major organs, including the heart, incur irreversible damage.

Key words: Acute myocardial infarction — Left ventricular assist system — Profound heart failure

Introduction

Intra-aortic balloon pumping (IABP) combined with potent medical therapy has improved the results for the treatment of acute myocardial infarction (AMI) [1–3]. Pump failure or rhythm disorders are the main causes of car-

[1]National Cardiovascular Center Research Institute, Suita, Osaka, 565 Japan

diogenic shock following AMI. Although mortality due to arrhythmia has been reduced by prompt pharmacologic and electrical means, mortality due to pump failure is still high, because of the limitation of the capability of IABP in cardiac assistance.

Recently, the left ventricular assist system (LVAS), which substitutes for cardiac pump function, has been used to treat profound heart failure patients [4–8]. LVAS appears to be effective in maintaining systemic circulation, although the results of treating these AMI patients are still unsatisfactory [9, 10]. To clarify the performance of LVAS on AMI, we have studied its effect on hemodynamics during profound left ventricular failure (LVF) and the actual recovering process of the natural heart from profound LVF in animal experiments and clinical cases [11–14].

In this paper, we review our experimental and clinical investigation of the performance of LVAS on AMI and the problems associated with the treatment of patients in cardiogenic shock due to AMI using LVAS.

Animal Experiments

Description of the LVAS

The LVAS, which was originally developed at our institute, consists of a blood pump and an automatic control drive unit (CDU) [8]. The temporary-use blood pump is an air-driven, diaphragm-type pump made of the segmented polyether polyurethane (TM series; Toyobo Co. Ltd., Japan). The stroke volume of the pump is 70 ml and maximum output is 7.0 l/min. The CDU alternately supplies compressed air and vacuum to drive the blood pump, triggered by an ECG detection mode or an independent internal mode. This CDU has a unique automatic level control (ALC) which can automatically regulate the bypass flow (BF) in response to changes in the systemic circulation evaluated by the left atrial pressure (LAP) and total systemic flow (TF: cardiac output (CO) + BF, or pulmonary flow) [15].

Materials and Methods

Fifteen adult goats weighing between 28 and 61 kg were used. After intramuscular injection of ketamine hydrochloride (10 mg/kg) and atropine sulfate (0.02 mg/kg), the goats were intubated and anesthesia was maintained with 1.0%–2.0% halothane and 50% nitrous oxide mixed with oxygen. Thoracotomy was performed through the left fifth costal bed. ECG, right atrial pressure (RAP), pulmonary arterial pressure (PAP), LAP, left ventricular pressure (LVP), aortic pressure (AoP) by pressure transducers, TF in the pulmonary artery, and BF through the LVAS by electromagnetic flow meters were continuously monitored. The pump was installed between the left atrium and the descending aorta and then placed paracorporeally on the chest wall.

Profound LVF following AMI was induced by intercepting blood supply to 50% of the LV free wall in five goats, 70%–80% in seven, and 80%–90%

in three. After confirming that the CO had decreased to less than 50% of the control level or that the heart had been in fibrillation, synchronous or asynchronous left heart bypass by our LVAS with ALC of LAP and TF were started. After the chest was closed, each goat was placed in a cage and extubated after awakening. An anticoagulant agent was used only during the pump implantation period, and no further anticoagulant was administrated during the entire postoperative course.

Left ventriculograpy (LVG) was performed in five goats after 70%–80% AMI during the LVAS assistance. Control LVG were obtained in four goats and LVG after removal of LVAS in three goats. Anesthesia was induced and maintained with halothane, administered through mask or endotracheal tube. The catheter tip transducer was introduced through the right or left carotid artery and its tip was positioned in the LV. LV volume was measured by area-length method.

Autopsies were performed when the goats were killed.

Results

Overall Results

Ventricular fibrillation (VF) occurred in 10 of 15 goats immediately after the induction of AMI or when the goat was placed in the cage. Adjustment of the circulating blood volume and electrolyte level and administration of anti-arrhythmic agents were performed in the same manner as in clinical patients. Defibrillation was successfully performed under LVAS pumping in all except one of the 50% AMI group and in all of the 80%–90% AMI group.

At the beginning of LVAS pumping, BF was maintained high to keep LAP at the low preset level of 0–5 mmHg and TF at the somewhat higher level of 100–130 ml/kg/min using the ALC. If TF could not be maintained at the preset level, volume loading was carried out. The recovering natural heart was able to decrease LAP gradually. Since LAP was set at a certain level, the ALC was used to decrease BF to maintain LAP at the preset level. During recovery from LVF, the preset level of LAP was gradually raised while checking the pulmonary function and the natural heart. When the natural heart output exceeded 100 ml/kg/min and at the same time LAP was below 18 mmHg, the pump was removed.

Four goats from the 50% AMI group recovered from LVF between 17 hours and 3 days after the onset of LVAS pumping, and all pumps were removed except in one goat that died of bleeding on the third day. One goat (case no.5) died of intractable VF when AMI was made. Seven goats from the 70%–80% AMI group recovered from profound LVF between the 6th and the 16th postoperative days (POD). In the 80%–90% AMI group, all three goats were unrecoverable because of intractable VF, but their circulation could be maintained for about 15 hours by LVAS alone.

A summary of the overall results is shown in Table 1.

Table 1. Overall results of chronic LVAS experiments in profound left ventricular failure following induced AMI in goats

No.	MI	VF	Duration	LVG	Results
1		–	17 hours		Recovered, pump removed
2		+	18 hours		Recovered, pump removed
3	50%	–	2 days		Recovered, pump removed
4		–	3 days		Recovered but died (bleeding)
5		+	6 hours		Died (defibrillation failed)
6		–	6 days		Recovered, pump removed
7		+	6 days	+	Recovered, pump removed
8	70%	+	7 days	+	Recovered, pump removed
9	~	+	13 days	+	Recovered, pump removed
10	80%	–	14 days	+	Recovered, pump removed
11		+	16 days	+	Recovered, pump removed
12		+	14 days		Recovered but died (sepsis)
13	80%	+	5 hours		Died (intractable VF, bleeding)
14	~	+	8 hours		Died (intractable VF)
15	90%	+	15 hours		Died (intractable VF)

MI, myocardial infarction; VF, ventricular fibrillation; LVG, left ventriculography

Hemodynamic Changes

Hemodynamic changes before, during, and after LVAS assistance for the 70%–80% AMI group were studied (Fig. 1). Immediately after AMI was produced or after defibrillation succeeded, LAP rose and TF markedly decreased. LVAS pumping could maintain LAP at around 5 mmHg and TF at over 90% of the control level. During the first several days, LAP was maintained at around 5 mmHg and TF was maintained at around 100 ml/kg/min. When the LVAS was temporarily stopped, heart rate and LAP increased, TF decreased, and the goats became uneasy. With the recovery of the failing heart, the preset level of LAP was gradually raised and BF was subsequently decreased so as to increase the preload for the natural heart. The heart rate gradually increased in spite of good hemodynamic conditions. When TF was maintained at around 100 ml/kg/min and LAP was kept below 18 mmHg by the natural heart alone, the LVAS was removed. Upon removal of the LVAS, TF was maintained at the control level, but LAP increased to a permissible level.

After removal of the pump, cardiac function was stable and improved slightly in most cases; heart rate gradually decreased, cardiac output increased, and LAP decreased gradually. However, mild heart failure (HF) persisted, depending upon the severity of the myocardial damage due to infarction.

In LVG, akinesis was observed around the LV apex. The LV pressure-volume curve of case No. 8 indicates that volume unloading of the LV is effective in reducing its stroke work with LA to Ao bypass (Fig. 2). After LVAS removal, the curve shifted to the right of the control curve. Stroke work after LVAS removal was 80% of the control on the 26th POD. The changes of left ventricular end-diastolic volume (LVEDV), ejection fraction (EF), stroke volume and stroke work are shown in Fig. 3. When LVAS was switched on,

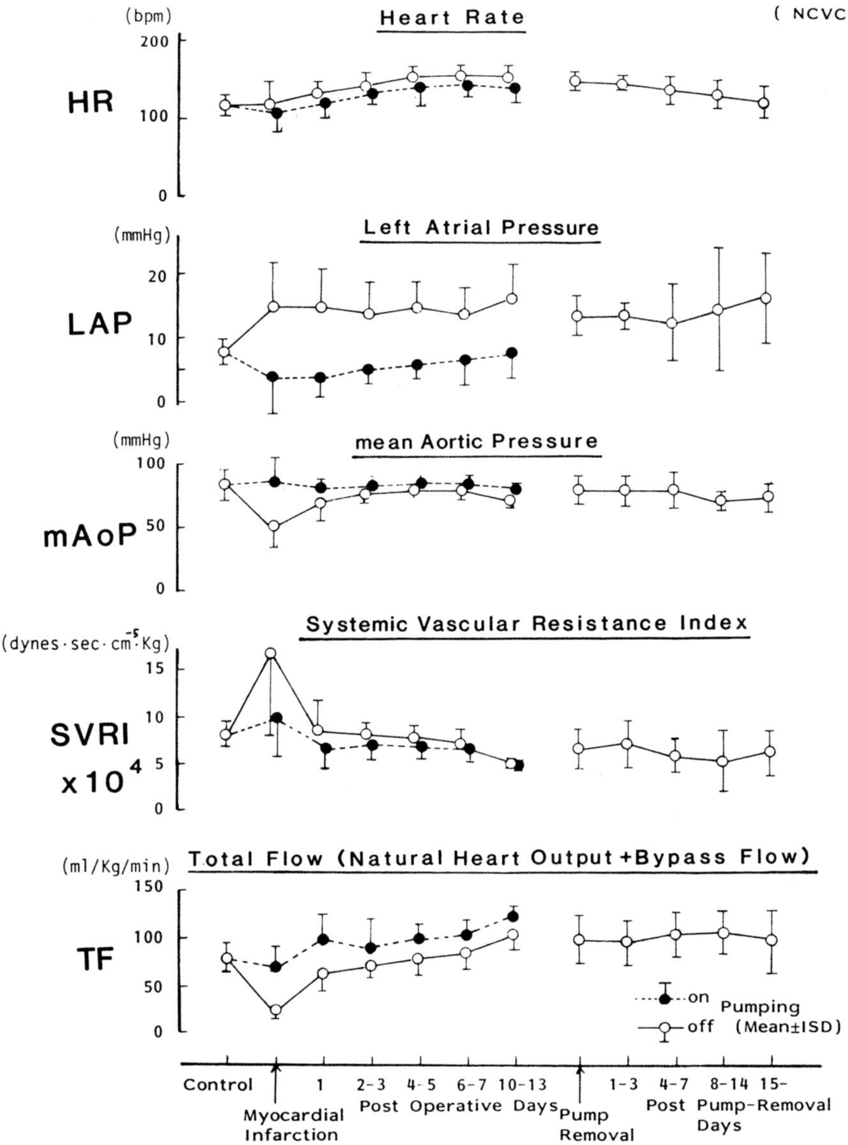

Fig. 1. Changes in heart rate (*HR*), left atrial pressure (*LAP*), total flow (*TF*), mean aortic pressure (*mAoP*) and systemic vascular resistance (*SVRI*) before, during, and after LVAS assistance for 70%–80% AMI group. (From [12] with permission)

LVEDV decreased to 80% of that with the LVAS off. After LVAS removal, LVEDV increased. EF decreased markedly after MI formation. After LVAS removal, EF did not improve and stayed lower than the control. When the LVAS was used, stroke volume decreased to 30% of the LVAS off value. After LVAS removal, stroke volume increased but did not reach the control

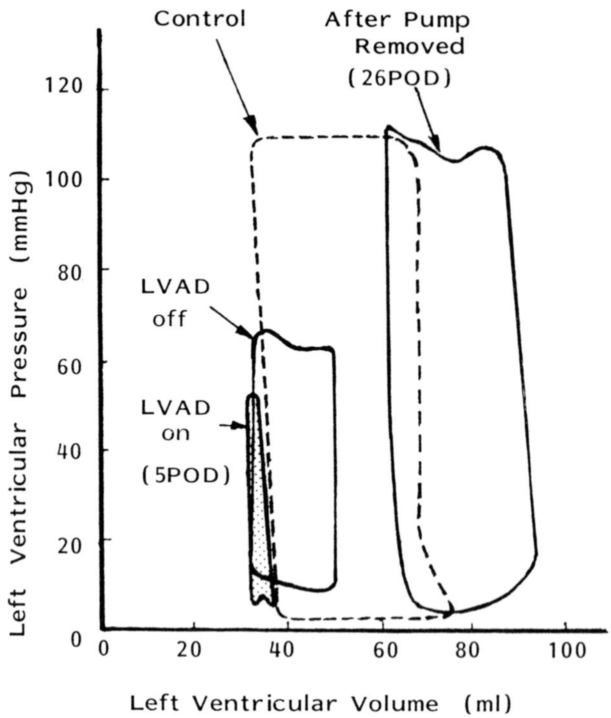

Fig. 2. Left ventricular pressure-volume curve (case No. 8). (From [11] with permission)

level. When the LVAS was on, stroke work decreased to 40% of the value with the LVAS off. After LVAS removal, stroke work increased, but did not reach the control value.

Pathological Findings

Autopsy was performed in eight goats between 8 and 15 days after the pump was removed and in three goats immediately after death. Figure 4 shows the ring slice of the heart of case No. 6. The infarcted area became a solid scar macroscopically and was completely replaced with connective tissue microscopically. In case No. 10, however, an area of MI was not solid but soft and was thin wall.

Residual myocardium became hypertrophic in comparison with normal heart muscle.

Clinical Cases

Outline of Patients

The major indications of LVAS application include: (1) cardiac index below $2.0\,l/min/m^2$, (2) LAP or pulmonary arterial wedge pressure over 18 mmHg,

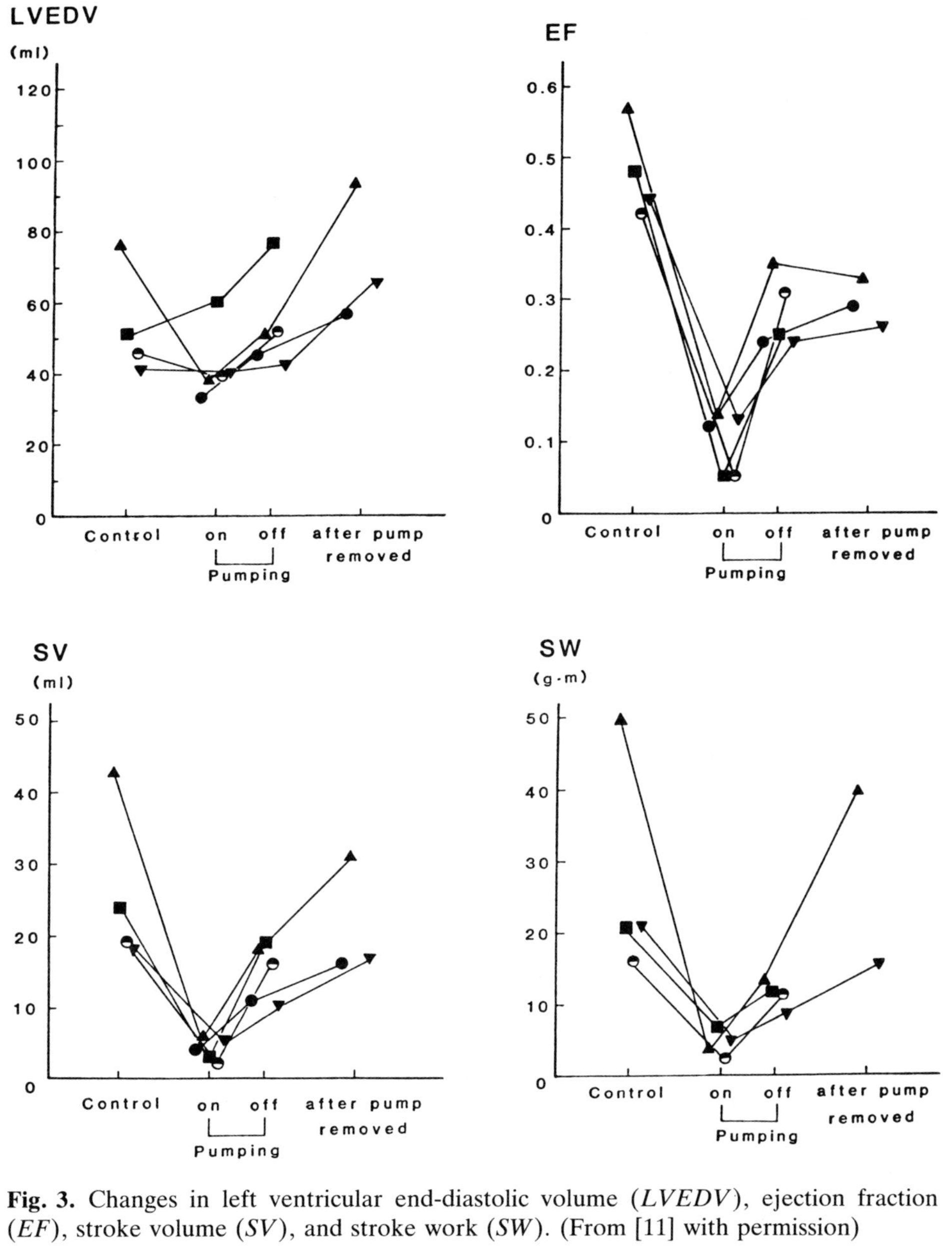

Fig. 3. Changes in left ventricular end-diastolic volume (*LVEDV*), ejection fraction (*EF*), stroke volume (*SV*), and stroke work (*SW*). (From [11] with permission)

(3) aortic pressure below 80 mmHg, or a potentially fatal arrhythmia in spite of antiarrhythmic drugs and IABP support. The patient in Killip 4th and Forrester 4th stage of cardiogenic shock is also considered as a candidate for the application of the LVAS. According to these indications, at our center, ten patients suffering from AMI had LVAS installed between the LA and the ascending aorta and placed on the epigastrium. These AMI patients were

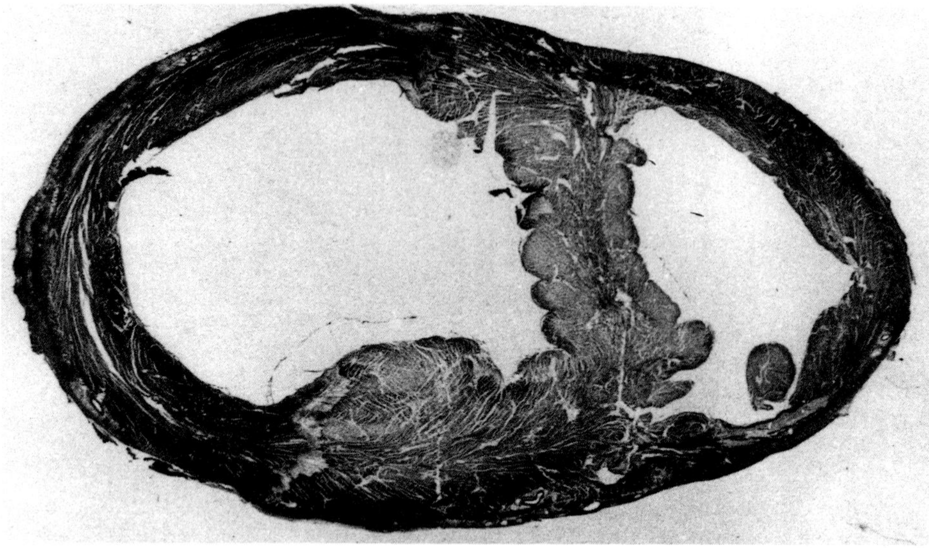

Fig. 4. Ring slice of the heart recovered from profound left ventricular failure following AMI (case No. 6) by the LVAS. (From [12] with permission)

divided into three groups. The first group (two cases) received no aorto-coronary bypass grafting (ACBG) because the patient in shock might be intolerant to prolonged surgery. In the second group (five cases), ACBG surgery was performed concomitantly with LVAS implantation. In the third group (three cases), ventricular septal perforation (VSP) occurred within 5–7 days after onset of AMI (Table 2).

Results

Clinical results are shown in Table 2 and 3. Appropriate, safe, and automatic circulatory control during HF was achieved by the automatic LVAS. Seven of the ten patients recovered from severe cardiogenic shock, allowing removal of the LVAS. However, four of seven patients were not long-term survivors.

Patient No. 2, without ACBG in group one, had ACBG surgery after removal of the LVAS. The other patient in group one could not be weaned from the LVAS because his general condition became critical, but his heart began to work.

Three patients out of five in the second group could be weaned from the LVAS. Two of them died of multiple organ failure which might have been caused by the prolonged low output condition before LVAS application. In patients No. 4 and 5, pathological examination showed that hemorrhagic necrosis had occurred in the bypassed infarcted area of myocardium although ACBG was performed at the right time. Only one survivor in the second group had applied the LVAS without delay. The systemic circulation of patient No. 6, who had broad left ventricular infarction, depended on the LVAS and

Table 2. Outline of patients to whom left ventricular assistance was applied for the treatment of acute myocardial infarction with cardiogenic shock

No.	Age	Sex	Diagnosis	Operation performed	Indication
Group I (without ACBG when LVAS implanted)					
1	69	M	AMI + Shock		Cardiogenic Shock
2	73	M	AMI + Shock		Cardiogenic Shock
Group II (ACBG performed when LVAS implanted)					
3	52	M	ASR, MSR AMI & VF during CAG	AVR, ACBG (1)	ECC dependent
4	66	M	OMI, AMI & VT during CAG	ACBG (2)	ECC dependent
5	60	M	AMI + Shock	ACBG (1)	Cardiogenic Shock ECC dependent
6	62	M	AMI + Shock during PTCR	ACBG (2)	Cardiogenic Shock
7	57	M	OMI + AP during PTCA	ACBG (3)	Cardiogenic Shock
Group III (with ventricular septal perforation-VSP)					
8	62	F	AMI + VSP	Patch closure of VSP Resection of LV infarcted area	ECC dependent
9	71	F	AMI + VSP	Patch closure of VSP	Elective use
10	73	F	AMI + VSP	Patch closure of VSP	ECC dependent

AMI, acute myocardial infarction; OMI, old myocardial infarction; VSP, ventricular septal perforation; ASR, aortic stenosis and regurgitation; MSR, mitral stenosis and regurgitation; VF, ventricular fibrillation; VT, ventricular tachycardia; AP, angina pectoris; CAG, coronary angiography; AVR, aortic valve replacement; ECC, extracorporeal circulation; ACBG, aorto coronary bypass grafting; LVAS, left ventricular assist system

several attempts at weaning from the LVAS failed. He finally died of multiple organ failure after 41 days pumping. Patient No. 3 had cardiac massage for over one hour and his peripheral vessels had already collapsed when LVAS was applied. In the third group, all LVASs were successfully removed. Although one patient died of cerebral hemorrhage 35 days after removal, the other two patients were discharged from hospital in satisfactory condition and have returned to their normal activities. They are doing well 5 and 4.5 years after LVAS application.

Description of a Representative Case

Case No. 8 was a cardiogenic shock patient with VSP after AMI. She underwent surgery for closure of the VSP and resection of 11 × 2 cm of infarcted LV wall, but could not be weaned from extracorporeal circulation because of reduced LV capacity. At this time the LVAS was used.

Table 3. Clinical results of the treatment

No.	Age	Sex	Pumping duration	Weaned	Result	Cause of death
Group I (without ACBG when LVAS implanted)						
1	69	M	12 days	No	Died	Respiratory failure
2	73	M	12 days	Yes	Hospital death	Infection & cerebral infarction: 149 days after removal
Group II (ACBG performed when LVAS implanted)						
3	52	M	4 hours	No	Died	Peripheral insufficiency
4	66	M	7 days	Yes	Died	MOF: 10 days after removal
5	60	M	14 days	Yes	Died	MOF & sepsis: 10 days after removal
6	62	M	41 days	No	Died	LVAS dependent MOF
7	57	M	7 days	Yes	Discharged	
Group III (with ventricular septal perforation-VSP)						
8	62	F	15 days	Yes	Hospital death	Cerebral bleeding: 35 days after removal
9	71	F	7 days	Yes	Discharged	
10	73	F	6 days	Yes	Discharged	

MOF, multiple organ failure; Weaned, Weaned from pump; LVAS, left ventricular assist sysytem; ACBG, aorto coronary bypass grafting

Hemodynamic changes during LVAS use are shown in Fig. 5. Although she had biventricular failure in the beginning of LVAS support, the LVAS alone could maintain normal circulation by keeping RAP at a level around 18 mmHg with the use of catecholamines. In the initial stage, BF was kept high to adequately reduce LV work and maintain LAP at 0–5 mmHg and TF at levels of 3.0–3.5 l/min/m^2. Total circulation was maintained by the LVAS alone during the first three days. From the fourth day, the preset level of LAP was gradually raised while checking the heart motion by echocardiography. ALC of LAP worked, and subsequently BF decreased with an increase in LV diastolic dimension and % of fractional shortening (Fig. 5). On the 11th day, cardiac output decreased due to excess tapering of the catecholamines, and the preset level of LAP was temporarily decreased to reduce LV load. When the cardiac index exceeded 2.5 l/min/m^2, the patient was weaned from LVAS and switched to IABP, successfully. The natural heart recovered enough to discontinue IABP on the 20th day. However, peritoneal dialysis was required because of oliguria, and several plasma exchanges were performed for correction of high bilirubin levels. The patient suddenly died of cerebral bleeding on the 35th day after weaning.

Hemodynamic Considerations

Figure 6 shows hemodynamic changes before, during, and after LVAS assistance. Most cases were associated with right ventricular failure, but the LVAS

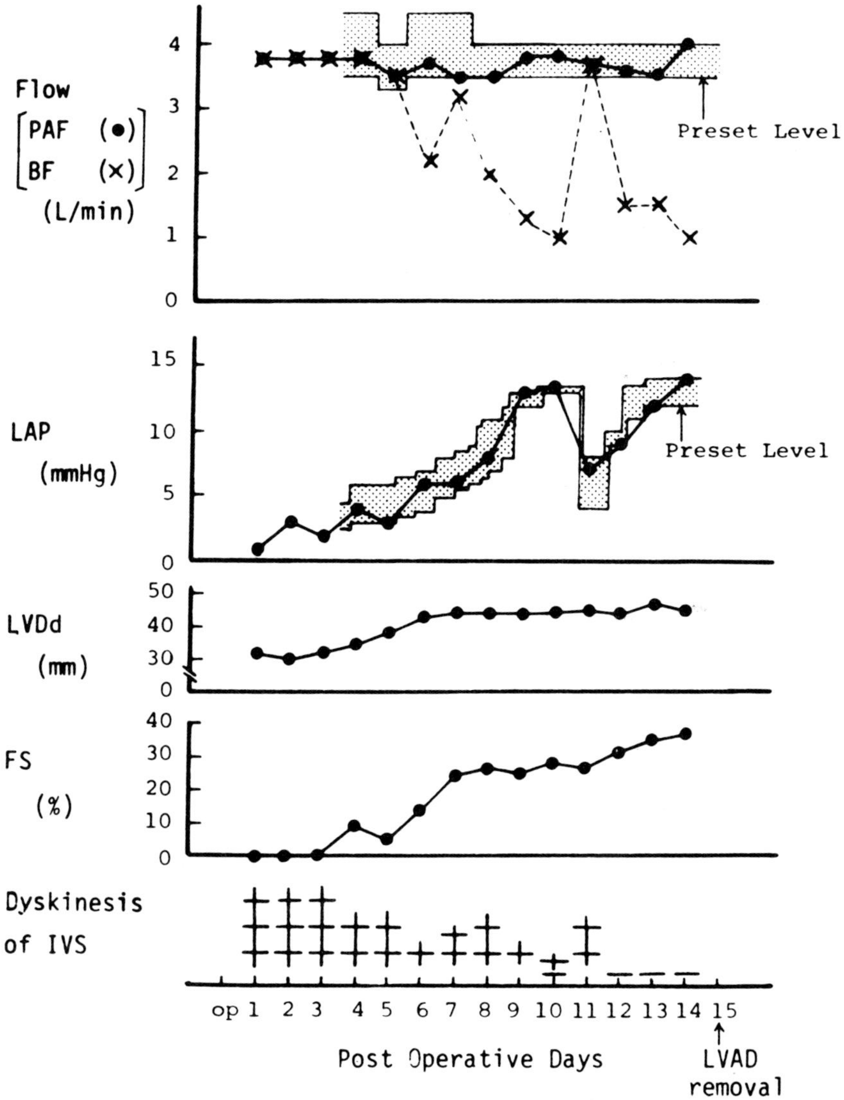

Fig. 5. Hemodynamic responses during LVAS assistance under automatic level control in case No. 8. *PAF*, pulmonary arterial flow; *BF*, bypass flow; *LAP*, left atrial pressure; *LVDd*, left ventricular diastolic dimension; *FS*, fractional shortening; *IVS*, intraventricular septum. (From [13] with permission)

alone maintained normal circulation when RAP was kept at a level more than 15 mmHg and catecholamines were used. Right ventricular failure recovered within 1–3 days, but in some cases, RAP remained higher than normal. Initially, LAP was intentionally kept low at 0–5 mmHg to reduce LV work sufficiently while maintaining TF at a somewhat higher level of 3.0–3.5 l/min/m^2

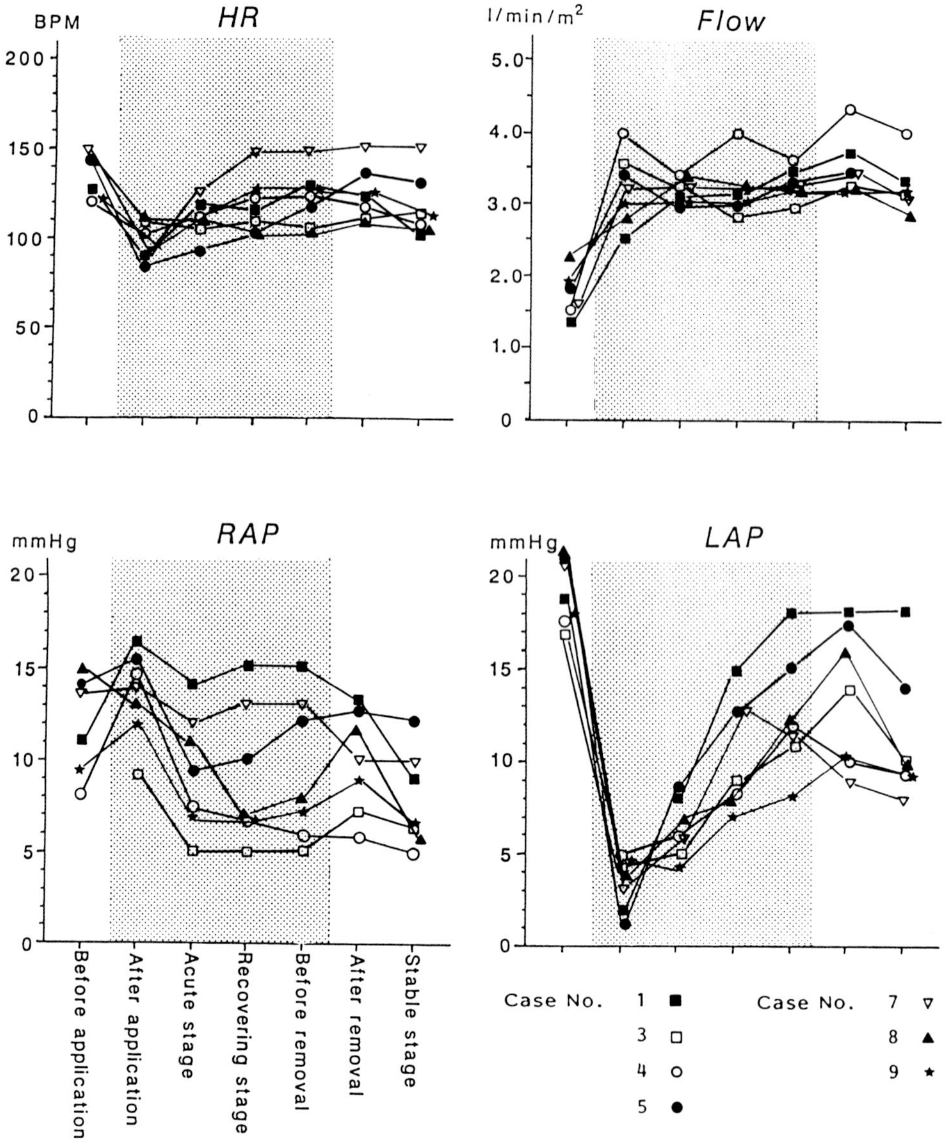

Fig. 6. Hemodynamic changes before, during and after LVAS assistance. *HR*, heart rate; *RAP*, right atrial pressure; *LAP*, left atrial pressure

to promote recovery of damaged organs due to hypoperfusion before LVAS application. During the recovery stage, the preset level of LAP was gradually raised. Thus, ALC of LAP worked as expected and BF decreased according to the natural heart function. Heart rate decreased while on LVAS, and increased as LV preload was increased.

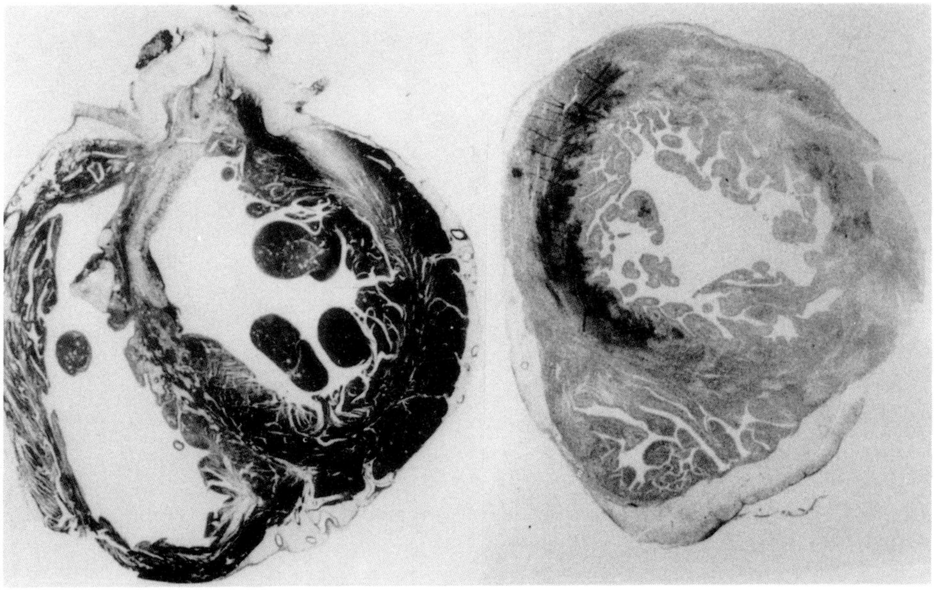

Fig. 7. Ring slices of the hearts: *left*, the heart which recovered from profound heart failure; *right*, the heart which did not recover from profound heart failure shows extensive hemorrhagic necrosis. (From [13] with permission)

The patients' circulations were well maintained over a period of 7–15 days. The failing heart gradually recovered, and the LVAS was successfully removed when the cardiac index exceeded 2.5–2.7 l/min/m^2. After removal of the LVAS, heart rate, RAP, and LAP were still higher than normal, but tended to decrease gradually with time.

Pathological Findings

Autopsies were performed on all the patients who died. Generally, infarcted myocardium changed either into granulation tissue in the patients who died in the early post AMI period or was replaced with fibrous tissue and had become solid scar in the patients who survived longer than 1 month after AMI. In addition, residual myocardium became hypertrophic when compared with normal myocardium. Findings in case No. 8, of AMI with VSP, disclosed that the reduced LV capacity following resection of the infarcted wall had returned to almost normal size (Fig. 7; left). Emergency ACBGs were done in cases No. 4 and 5. However, hemorrhagic infarction into the AMI area was noticed (Fig. 7; right).

Although seven patients were weaned from the LVAS, four patients eventually died because of delay in its application. Figure 8 shows microscopic findings in major organs, such as lung, liver, and kidney. Patchy fibrosis was scattered throughout otherwise normal tissues.

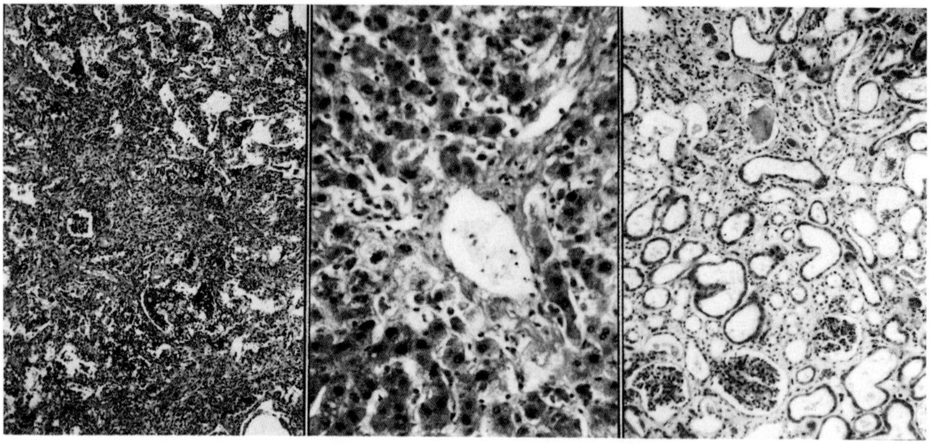

Fig. 8. Pathological findings of the major organs (case No. 8). (From [13] with permission)

Discussion

AMI may cause profound heart failure, which is beyond the limit of IABP capability. Since the VAS is a blood pump which can take over heart function, its heart assist capability is powerful. The purpose of using VAS for profound heart failure is to maintan normal circulation and to help the failing heart recover. For these reasons, VAS should be controlled to increase or decrease BF effectively, depending upon the level of severity of heart failure or recovery from heart failure, to prevent pulmonary congestion and regulate preload levels appropriately. In addition, it is desirable that control of the circulation should be achieved appropriately, safely, and automatically.

Control of Bypass Flow

In profound heart failure, it is particularly important to keep LAP low, since an elevated LAP will cause overload of impaired LV, resulting in extension of myocardial damage. High LAP will also give rise to pulmonary congestion, resulting in deterioration of gas exchange, which in turn will deteriorate the general condition. We usually keep LAP around 5 mmHg in the initial stage (Fig. 9). Even when LAP is maintained at the preset level, TF may be less than the preset level in some cases. In such cases, ALC of TF takes effect to increase BF, although LAP may become less than the preset level [8]. Since hypovolemia may exist under such circumstances, volume loading is mandatory and actually is very effective. Conversely, hypervolemia causes a high TF to maintain LAP at the preset level. Although the influence of excessive output is not clear, readjustment of TF by volume control is probably desirable. In the

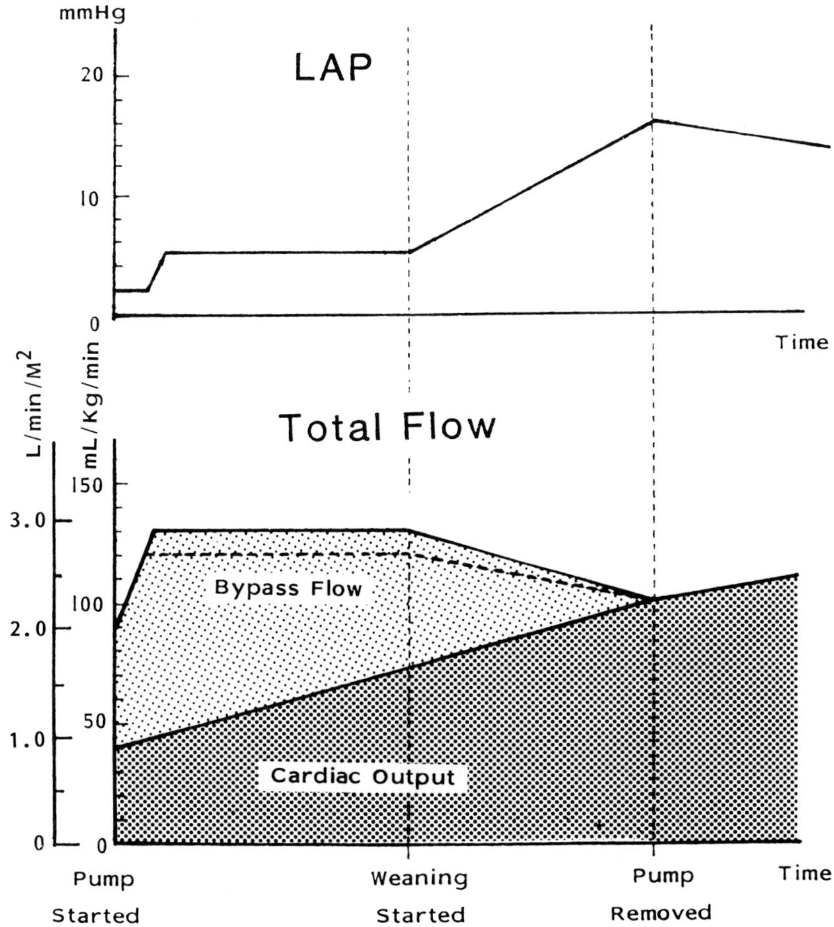

Fig. 9. Scheduled reference values of left atrial pressure (*LAP*) and total flow (*TF*) during LVAS pumping and expected increase in cardiac output. (From [12] with permission)

initial stage, we usually intended to keep TF between 120 and 130 ml/kg/min in goats and between 2.5 and 3.0 l/min/m^2 in patients (Fig. 9).

Since excessive assist may delay the recovery of the failing heart, while insufficient assist causes deterioration of the failing heart and the general condition, BF should be altered according to cardiac function. In LA to Ao bypass, the natural heart and LVAS compete with each other at the atrial level. Therefore, BF was high in the beginning of LVAS pumping but gradually decreased as the heart recovered. In the recovery stage, the heart continuously increased its stroke volume, hence lowering LAP. However, since LAP was preset at a certain level, the ALC of LAP began functioning in order to decrease BF and maintain LAP at the preset level.

When myocardial contraction did not recover readily, inotropic agents were successfully administered in order to avoid LVAS dependency [16]. During the actual weaning procedure, LAP was gradually raised while pulmonary function and cardiac function were carefully monitored (Fig. 9). In the treatment of profound heart failure, LVAS was discontinued when cardiac output exceeded the control level of 90–100 ml/kg/min in goats and 2.3 l/min/m^2 in patients, even though LAP was higher than normal levels but less than 18 mmHg (Fig. 9).

Although the LVAS can maintain normal circulation regardless of synchronization, pumping during the diastolic phase has the advantage of augmenting coronary blood flow as well as decreasing afterload [16]. In our experimental and clinical studies, synchronization modes were selected to promote recovery of the failing heart.

Coexistence of Right Ventricular Failure

When right ventricular failure (RVF) exists, pulmonary venous return decreases and LAP drops [17]. In such cases, the LVAS alone can maintain normal circulation if the RAP is kept at a higher level. In cases of poor myocardial protection during anoxic arrest and in other studies [18], including cases of cardiac arrest, the LVAS alone could keep TF within the normal range if the RAP was kept around 14–18 mmHg. When the pulmonary vascular resistance is high, biventricular assist may be necessary [5, 6, 17]. It has been reported that isoproterenol improves RVF during LVAS assistance [17]. In our clinical series, all the patients were considered for biventricular assistance at the application of the LVAS. However, in all but one patient who had high pulmonary vascular resistance, the right VAS was not necessary. High RAP and administration of epinephrine was effective.

Recovery from Profound LVF

The severely impaired heart cannot maintain normal circulation without LVAS assistance. However, the heart that has recovered from LVF with the LVAS can maintain almost normal circulation. Pathologic studies of the heart have shown that the necrotic myocardium is replaced with fibrous tissue that eventually becomes a scar, while the residual myocardium becomes hypertrophic (Fig. 4). Removal of overload and decompression of the LV at the beginning of LVAS pumping will prevent overextension of the impaired myocardium and accelerate scar formation, which does not cause dyskinetic movement. Gradual increase of LV work will promote compensation by the residual myocardium [19].

Continuous LVAS assistance can earn time for the impaired heart to recover, while maintaining the normal circulation. Time required for recovery depends upon the severity of myocardial damage, and was 7–15 days in our cases.

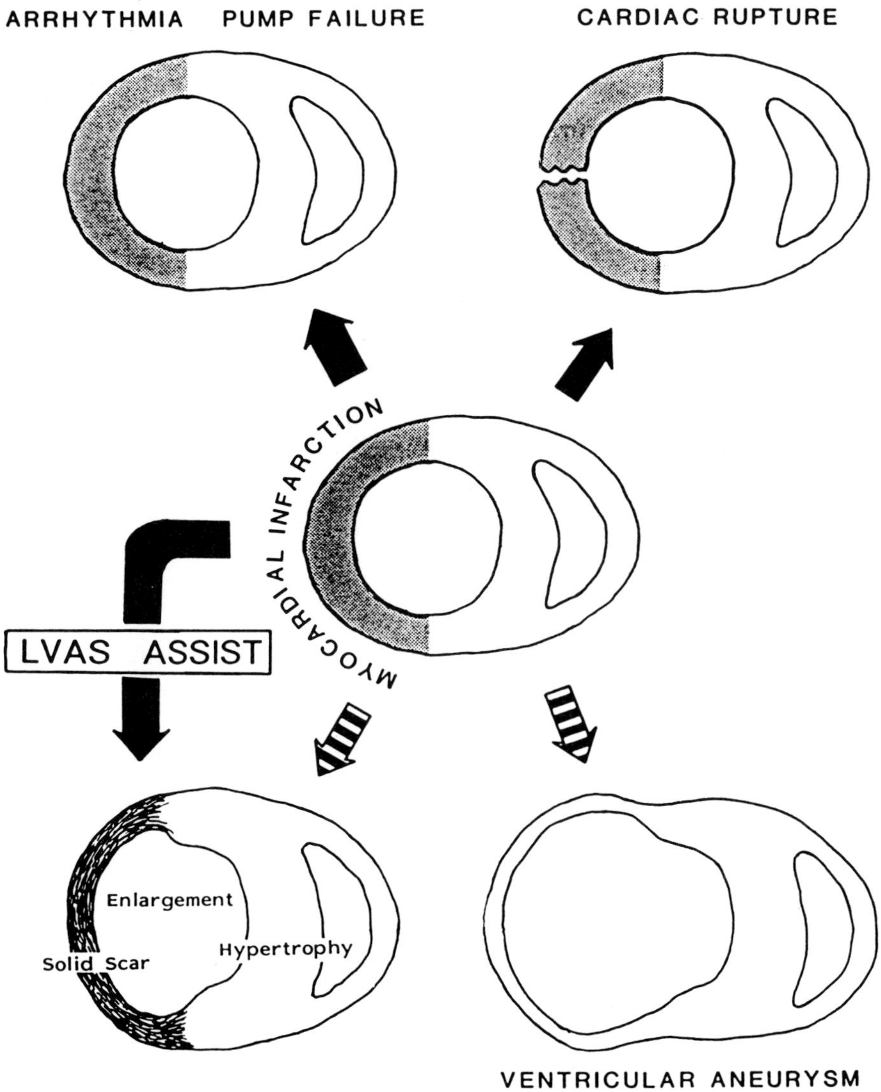

Fig. 10. Recovery mechanism from extensive myocardial infarction

In extensive myocardial infarction, pump failure, arrhythamia and cardiac rupture are the main causes of death. Overload to impaired myocardium may result in large left ventricular aneurysm, which may complicate patient management. These complications can be avoided by application of the LVAS. According our study, the recovery mechanism from profound LVF appears to be affected by increases in LVEDV, LAP and heart rate, and hypertrophy of heart muscle and prevention of dyskinesis by solid scar formation are thought to help maintain the impaired myocardial function (Fig. 10). From the standpoint of limitation of recovery, if 50% of LV free wall were damaged, salvation of the heart was difficult [20]. However, application of the LVAS could restore as much as 70–80% of LV free wall in the damaged heart as shown in our study. For salvaging the heart with severe damage exceeding 80%–90% of LV free wall, future investigation is necessary.

Surgery with Concomitant LVAS Application

In our patients with cardiogenic shock after AMI, heart surgery such as ACBG, closure of a VSP, and excision of infarcted myocardium were all performed concomitantly with LVAS application. Use of the LVAS has proved effective after closure of a VSP and excision of infarcted tissue because it allows for reduction of the LV wall tension. However, ACBG, when performed 6 h after an AMI, causes hemorrhagic infarction. Although the influence of this hemorrhagic infarction is not clear, we think that the LVAS alone should be used to support the patient in cardiogenic shock at 6 h post-AMI, and ACBG should be considered only after recovery from the shock.

Multiple Organ Failure (MOF)

In spite of a high weaning rate from the LVAS, only three patients could leave the hospital. Four other patients recovered from profound LVF, but most of them needed dialysis or plasma exchange and did not survive for long. Their biochemical profiles showed malfunction of the major organs, and microscopic studies of the major organs revealed areas of patchy fibrosis scattered within the normal tissues. These findings indicate that the major organs were damaged during prolonged ischemia before LVAS assistance. Ineffective cardiac massage and/or a low output state were in place for many hours before the LVAS was used in our cases. A close relationship was seen between the severity of complication and delayed application of the LVAS. If the use of the LVAS is delayed, sequelae in major organs will follow, even though the heart may recover from profound heart failure. Since hemodynamic derangement will promptly progress in the case of AMI, it should be kept in mind that the decision to use the LVAS should not be delayed, as it should be applied before major organs, including the heart itself, are irreversibly damaged.

Systematic Use of the LVAS

Richenbacher et al. [21] reported that early hemodynamic stabilization with the LVAS minimized the risks of hypoperfusion and sequelae. Our clinical experience suggested two basic concepts to established the best way of LVAS application for AMI. The first is that in the treatment of AMI with cardiogenic shock, the use of the LVAS should be contemplated. Since hemodynamic derangement will promptly progress in the case of AMI, the LVAS should be applied before major organs are irreversibly damaged. The second concept is how to make a decision for or against the ACBG operation at the time of

LVAS implantation. The life-saving effect of emergency ACBG surgery still remains uncertain because the patient in shock is occasionally intolerant to major surgery. Bypass of the infarcted myocardium may not only be ineffective as regards recovery of heart function but may even result in hemorrhagic necrosis of the ischemic myocardium in patients with shock.

We had two clinical cases with massive myocardial infarction, but ACBG surgery was not performed. Although both patients died of complications, their heart function recovered, and in one case the heart recovered enough to be weaned from the LVAS. This suggests that the LVAS alone may be enough to support the patient in cardiogenic shock, and ACBG can be considered after recovery from the shock.

It is important to establish a way of systematically introducing the LVAS into the treatment of AMI. AMI patients in shock should be treated always bearing in mind the possibility of the LVAS.

Conclusions

The LVAS is powerful and effective in treatment of profound heart failure after an AMI that is beyond the capability of IABP. Appropriate, safe, and automatic circulation control during heart failure and subsequent recovery from profound left ventricular failure can be achieved by our automatic LVAS.

Decompression of the LV at the beginning of LVAS pumping will prevent overextension of infarcted myocardium and simultaneously accelerate scar formation. Gradual increase of LV work will promote compensation by the residual myocardium. Continuous LVAS assist can earn time for the imparied heart to recover while maintaining normal circulation. Recovery from profound LVF using the LVAS might have been due to increase in LVEDV, LAP and heart rate, hypertrophy of residual myocardium and prevention of dyskinesis by solid scar formation.

In clinical cases, many patients later died of MOF, although the heart recovered, which was probably caused by prolonged ischemia before institution of the LVAS. For completely successful recovery from profound heart failure, the decision to use the LVAS should not be delayed. The LVAS should be applied promptly before major organs, including the heart itself, incur irreversible damage.

References

1. Scheidt S, Wilner G, Mueller H, Summers D, Lesch M, Wolff G, Krakauer J, Rubenfire M, Flemming P, Noon G, Oldham N, Killip T, Kantrowitz A (1973) Intra-aortic balloon counterpulsation in cardiogenic shock. Report of a co-operative clinical trial. N Engl J Med 288:979–984
2. McEnany MT, Kay HR, Buckley MJ, Dagget WM, Erdmann AJ, Mundth ED, Rao RS, de Toeuf J, Austen WG (1978) Clinical experience with intra-aortic balloon pump support in 728 patients. Circulation 58(SupplI):I124–I132

3. Bregham D (1982) Percutaneous intra-aortic balloon pumping. A time for reflection. Chest 82:397–398
4. Wolner E, Deutsch M, Losert U, Stellweg F, Thoma H, Unger F, Polzer K, Navratil J (1978) Clinical application of the ellipsoid left heart assist device. Artif Organs 2:268–272
5. Bernhard WF, Berger RL, Stetz JP, Carr JG, Calo NA, MaCormick JR, Fishbein MC (1979) Temporary left ventricular bypass: factors affecting patient survival. Circulation 60(SupplI):I131–I141
6. Pae WE, Rosenberg G, Donachy JH, Landis DL, Phillips WM, Parr GVS, Prophet GA, Pierce WS (1980) Mechanical assistance for postoperative cardiogenic shock: a three year experience. Trans Am Soc Artif Intern Organs 26:256–261
7. Turina M, Bosio R, Senning A (1978) Clinical application of paracorporeal uni- and biventricular artificial heart. Trans Am Soc Artif Intern Organs 24:625–631
8. Takano H, Taenaka Y, Nakatani T, Akutsu T, Manabe H (1985) Successful treatment of profound left ventricular failure by automatic left ventricular assist system. World J Surg 9:78–88
9. Pae WE, Cynthia AM, Pierce WS (1989) Combined registry for the clinical use of mechanical ventricular assist pumps and the total artificial heart: third official report — 1989. J Heart Transplant 8:277–280
10. Takano H, Taenaka Y, Noda H, Kinoshita M, Yagura A, Tatsumi E, Sekii H, Sasaki E, Umezu M, Nakatani T, Kyo S, Omoto R, Akutsu T, Manabe H (1989) Multi-institutional studies of the National Cardiovascular Center Ventricular Assist System: use in 92 patients. Trans Am Soc Artif Intern Organs 35:541–544
11. Nakatani T, Takano H, Taenaka Y, Umezu M, Tanaka T, Yutani C, Matsuda T, Iwata H, Noda H, Nakamura T, Takatani S, Seki J, Hayashi K, Akutsu T, Manabe H (1984) Therapeutic effect of left ventricular assist device on induced profound left ventricular failure: evaluation by left ventriculography. Trans Am Soc Artif Intern Organs 30:533–538
12. Takano H, Nakatani T, Taenaka Y, Umezu M (1985) Development of the ventricular assist pump system: experimental and clinical studies. In: Akutsu T (ed) Artificial Heart-1 Springer, Tokyo pp 141–151
13. Takano H, Nakatani T, Noda H, Umezu M, Fukuda S, Tanaka T, Matsuda T, Iwata H, Takatani S, Taenaka Y, Kinoshita M, Kumon K, Kito Y, Yutani C, Fujita T, Akutsu T, Manabe H (1986) Clinical consideration of a left ventricular assist system for acute myocardial infarction with cardiogenic shock. Trans Am Soc Artif Intern Organs 32:467–473
14. Noda H, Takano H, Taenaka Y, Nakatani T, Umezu M, Kinoshita M, Tatsumi E, Yagura A, Sekii H, Kito Y, Ohara K, Tanaka K, Kumon K, Hiramori K, Yutani C, Beppu S, Fujita T, Akutsu T, Manabe H (1989) Treatment of acute myocardial infarction with cardiogenic shock using left ventricular assist device. Int J Artif Organs 12:175–179
15. Nakatani T, Umezu M, Takano H, Taenaka Y, Tanaka T, Iwata H, Matsuda T, Noda H, Adachi S, Fukuda S, Nakamura T, Seki J, Takatani S, Hayashi K, Akutsu T (1985) Evaluation of automatic level control system for left ventricular assist device (LVAD) in circulatory support to profound left ventricular failure. Jpn J Artif Organs 14:1231–1234
16. Takano H, Hayashi K, Umezu M, Taenaka Y, Nakamura T, Matsuda T (1981) Hemodynamic effects of partial artificial heart on cardiac performance of failed heart. Jpn J Artif Organs 10:647–650

17. Laks H, Berger RL, Parr GVS, Penningon DG (1982) Panel conference. Acute cardiac faulure: the importance of the right ventricle. Trans Am Soc Artif Intern Organs 28:678–680
18. Takano H, Taenaka Y, Nakatani T, Umezu M, Iwata H, Tanaka T, Noda H, Matsuda T, Takatani S, Akutsu T, Manabe H (1985) Circulatory maintenance with a single artificial heart. Trans Am Soc Artif Intern Organs 30:550–555
19. Swan HJ, Forrester JS, Diamond G, Chatterjee K, Parmley WW (1972) Hemodynamic spectrum of myocardial infarction and cardiogenic shock. A conceptual model. Circulation 45:1097–1110
20. Shiozawa T (1978) Experimental and clinical studies on the effect of intra-aortic balloon pumping for cardiogenic shock due to acute myocardial infarction. J Jpn Assoc Thorac Surg 26:1501–1517
21. Richenbacher WE, Dash H, Buick MK, Pierce WS (1984) Utilization of left ventricular assistance in patients with acute myocardial infarction and cardiogenic shock. ASAIO Journal 7:32–40

14

Therapeutic Effects of the Left Ventricular Assist System on Myocardial Ischemia

TAKESHI NAKATANI[1], HISATERU TAKANO[1], HIROYUKI NODA[1], MASAYUKI KINOSHITA[1]

Summary. Left ventricular assist systems (LVAS) are a powerful means of cardiac assistance. The therapeutic effects of the LVAS in acute myocardial ischemia were evaluated from the standpoint of ischemic size, myocardial free fatty acid (FFA) metabolism and myocardial energy balance in acute animal experiments using mongrel dogs. In the study using magnetic resonance imaging (MRI) with gadolinium-DTPA, the LVAS decreased effectively both the ischemic area and degree of myocardial ischemia. 3-Beta-methyl-iodophenyl-pentadecanoic-acid (BMIPP)-imaging indicating tissue FFA metabolism was compared with thallium-201 chloride (TL) imaging to indicate tissue perfusion during LVAS assistance. LVAS pumping not only improved BMIPP and TL uptake in the ischemic myocardium, but also preserved the normal myocardium as evaluated by the FFA metabolism. High energy phosphate in myocardium and plasma catecholamine levels, which influenced cardiac energy metabolism, were evaluated under LVAS pumping. High energy phosphate levels showed no change in the normal myocardium by LVAS pumping. LVAS pumping reserved high energy phosphate concentrations in the ischemic myocardium and prevented the rise of catecholamine levels in profound heart failure.

Key words: Left ventricular assist system — Acute myocardial ischemia — Magnetic resonance imaging — Free fatty acid metabolism — High energy phosphate — Catecholamine

Introduction

Acute pump failure remains one of the main causes of death in patients with acute myocardial infarction (AMI) in spite of various pharmacological therapies and intra-aortic balloon pumping (IABP). Left ventricular assist

[1] National Cardiovascular Center Research Institute, Suita, Osaka, 565 Japan

systems (LVAS) have been applied for the treatment of patients with profound pump failure to provide better mechanical support [1].

Several studies have shown that LVAS maintained the systemic and the coronary circulation of patients with profound heart failure while decompressing the left ventricle (LV) and increasing the tissue blood flow [2–5]. These effects salvage ischemic myocardium, prevent enlargement of the infarcted area and promote replacement of the infarcted area by solid scar, which prevents dyskinesis [6]. In addition, the LVAS is expected to improve impaired cardiac function [7]. Recovery of impaired myocardium, however, depends not only upon myocardial blood supply but also myocardial cell function. There have been a few studies in which therapeutic effects of LVAS were evaluated from this aspect.

As image intensity of magnetic resonance imaging (MRI) is sensitive to the early changes in water content and to T1 and T2 relaxation times in the infarcted tissue, MRI has the potential to identify and quantify the infarcted area noninvasively [8]. Fatty acid myocardial imaging is promising to estimate the viability of myocardium because myocardial free fatty acid (FFA) metabolism plays an important role in myocardial energy metabolism and is affected by myocardial ischemia or hypoxia [9]. In addition, measurement of myocardial energy levels reflects myocardial energy metabolism which is affected by tissue perfusion and work [10].

In this paper, we describe the therapeutic effects of the LVAS in acute myocardial ischemia from the standpoint of ischemic size evaluated by MRI, myocardial free fatty acid metabolism and myocardial energy balance.

Ischemic Size Evaluated by Magnetic Resonance Imaging

Materials and Methods

Six mongrel dogs weighting 27–31 kg were starved for over 12 h and premedicated by ketamine hydrochloride (10 mg/kg) with atropine sulfate (0.02 mg/kg). After intrathoracheal intubation, anesthesia was maintained with pentobarbital sodium (10 mg/kg). The dogs were ventilated with a pressure controlled respirator (Bird respirator: model Mark 7), and the blood oxygen partial pressure was maintained above 100 mmHg by controlling the inspired oxygen fraction. The left femoral vein was cannulated for infusion of lactated Ringer's and sorbitol solution. The heart was exposed through a left thoracotomy, and the pericardium was opened. AMI was induced by a ligature immediately distal to the first diagonal branch of the left anterior descending artery (LAD). Terminal branches of the circumflex (Cx) and right coronary arteries (RCA) extending to the apex of the heart were also ligated. Lidocaine (1 mg/kg) was administered to prevent ventricular arrhythmias before ligation and thereafter continuous administration was performed at 1 mg/kg/h. The wound was covered with moistened gauze.

Our own air-driven, diaphragm-type LVAS [1] was installed between the left atrium and descending aorta and set in the fixed rate mode (pump rate: 60 to

70 beats/min). LVAS pumping was continued for 6–11 h after the induction of an AMI, then 0.5 mmoles/kg of gadolinium-diethylaminetriaminepentaacetic acid (Gd-DTPA) was injected intravenously to enhance the infarcted area. After 10–100 min, MRI was performed with and without LVAS pumping.

MRI was carried out with a Magnetom (1.5 Tesla, superconductive type, Siemens Company, Ltd.). Nonferromagnetic ECG leads were placed on the left trunk, and electrocardiographically-gated MRIs were obtained of 10-mm slices at two adjacent levels of the heart during end-diastole. Two spin-echo signals (first and second signal intensity) were taken with an echo delay time of 35 and 70 msec at both the infarcted and the normal myocardium. The operator defined the regions of interest using a CRT display. The MR signal intensity was proportional to the T2 relaxation time and tissue hydrogen density and was inversely proportion to the T1 relaxation time. The percent difference in signal intensity between the infarcted and the normal myocardium (MR contrast) was defined as infarcted myocardial image intensity (I) minus normal myocardial image intensity (N) divided by normal myocardial intensity. The following formula expresses the MR contrast: MR contrast $= (I - N)/N \times 100(\%)$

To evaluate the effect of Gd-DTPA on the MR images, seven experiments were performed in the same manner on 10–31 kg adult mongrel dogs with induced AMIs. Four dogs were placed on the LVAS, and three dogs had no mechanical assistance. After 11–12 h from induction of the AMI, 0.5 mmoles/kg Gd-DTPA was administered intravenously, and 30 min later the hearts were stopped by potassium chloride infusion. After cardiectomy, the heart was placed in a box at room temperature, and MRI was performed at three contiguous 5-mm-thickness sites with MR signal intensity and T1 and T2 relaxation times.

In these dogs, 10–15 mCi of ^{99}mTc-pyrophosphate was administered 4–6 h after AMI induction. Scintigrams were taken of the same slices that underwent MRI to re-examine the infarcted area.

All data were expressed as mean ± SD. The statistical significance of the differences between two populations was calculated using Student's two-tailed *t* test.

Results

Since the first echo signal had high signal intensity and the images were clear, as compared with the second echo, the evaluation was done on the first echo signal image. Technically satisfactory first-echo image studies were carried out on five of the six dogs.

With the LVAS on, enhancement of the location and signal intensity of the infarcted area decreased as compared with the LVAS off (Fig. 1). MRI contrasts were 23%–75% (49 ± 22%) with the LVAS on, and they increased significantly to 55%–189% (116 ± 58%) with the LVAS off ($P < 0.05$).

In the control experiments, signal intensity of the ischemic area increased, and MRI contrast varied according to the degree of ischemia. The T1 relaxa-

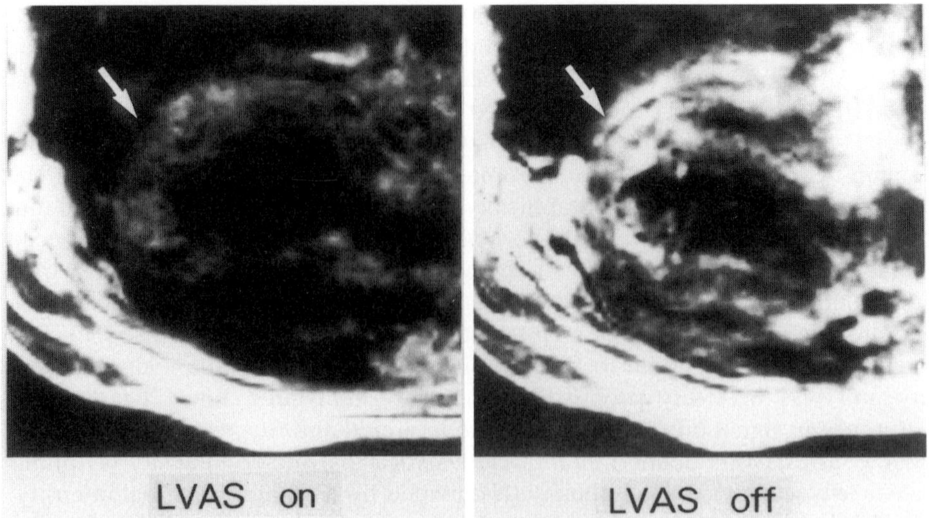

Fig. 1. Electrocardiographically-gated magnetic resonance images with and without *LVAS* pumping (*arrows* indicate the enhanced ischemic area by Gd-DTPA)

tion time of the infarcted area was short, and the T2 relaxation time was long. The mean values of MRI contrast were as high as 109% ($P < 0.002$). The mean value for the T1 relaxation time of the infarcted myocardium (212 ± 73 ms) was significantly shorter than the value for the normal myocardium (393 ± 82 ms) ($P < 0.001$). The mean value for the T2 relaxation time of the infarcted myocardium (38 ± 7 ms) was significantly greater than that of the normal myocardium (30 ± 3 ms) ($P < 0.05$).

The area enhanced on MRI agreed with the area that was seen after autoradiopgaphy.

Myocardial Tissue Perfusion and Free Fatty Acid Metabolism

Materials and Method

Characteristics of BMIPP

Two radioactive agents were employed for evaluation of the effects of the LVAS on blood flow and tissue FFA metabolism. One was thallium-201 chloride (TL) which has been a clinically available and well-known tracer for myocardial imaging which reflects myocardial blood flow. The other was 3-beta-methyl-iodophenyl-pentadecanoic acid (BMIPP) which was developed as a radiographic probe of metabolic processes in myocardial FFA metabolism. BMIPP was designed to defuse into myocytes from blood serum by the same pathway of natural free fatty acids [11, 12]. Since the methyl group of BMIPP inhibits its catabolism in the beta cycle in FFA metabolism, BMIPP is supposed to be trapped in the triglyceride pool [11–14]. The trapped BMIPP is frozen on the radiological imaging. The separation on the radioactivity imaging of these tracers is easy because the photopeak of iodine-123 on BMIPP is 159 keV while that of TL is 80 keV.

Experimental Procedure

Eighteen mongrel dogs weighting 10–12 kg were anesthetized with halothane and mixed oxygen under mechanical ventilation. Left thoracotomies were performed in all animals to insert a left atrial line for injection of both tracers. The LVAS was implanted between the left atrium and the descending aorta to the groups of circulatory assist.

The dogs were divided into four groups. The first myocardial infarction model group (MI group) consisted of three dogs whose LAD and major collateral branches from the Cx or RCA were ligated for 6 h. Three other dogs with MI caused by same procedure were supported by a LVAS throughout the experiment (MI+LVAS group). Nine other dogs received occlusions of the LAD for 3 h at the same segment as that of the MI group, and the coronaries were reperfused for 1 h (Rp group). The last three dogs received the same procedure as the Rp group, and the LVAS was used throughout the experiment (Rp+LVAS group).

At the end of the experiment, the heart was excised and sliced for static tissue radioactivity counting of both tracers. The result of tissue counting was analyzed by the circumferential method using a RI data processing system (DEC, POP 11/60).

Results

In analysis by the circumferential method, the counting numbers in each sampling pixel was presented as a percentage against the peak counting in the pixel. In the MI group, the BMIPP and TL uptake equally and dynamically decreased in the infarction area compared to the normal area. Transition of BMIPP and TL uptake increased gradually from the infarction area to the normal. In the MI + LVAS group, BMIPP and TL uptakes decreased in the infarction area as much as was seen in the MI group, while transition from the infarction area toward the normal was dynamic. In the Rp group, BMIPP and TL uptakes in the infarction area were kept higher than those in the MI group. The value of BMIPP uptake was higher than that of TL in the infarction area. The normal area both in the MI and Rp group showed no difference in the uptake of both tracers. In the Rp + LVAS group, the uptakes of both tracers were improved and there was no discrepancy between both images in the infarcted and/or ischemic area. In the normal areas of MI + LVAS and Rp + LVAS, the uptake of BMIPP was less than that of TL. The data of these four groups are summarized in Table 1 and the typical results in each groups obtained by circumferential analysis are displayed in Fig. 2.

Table 1. Comparison of BMIPP and TL uptake in left ventricular segments

		Infarct/Ischemic (anterior)			Marginal (septal)			Normal (posterior)			Marginal (lateral)		
Experiment	N	BM > TL	BM = TL	BM < TL	BM > TL	BM = TL	BM < TL	BM > TL	BM = TL	BM < TL	BM > TL	BM = TL	BM < TL
MI	3	2	1	–	–	3	–	–	3	–	2	1	–
MI + LVAS	3	–	2	1	1	–	2	–	3	–	–	–	3
Rp	9	4	4	1	1	8	–	1	6	2	2	6	1
Rp + LVAS	4	2	2	–	–	3	1	–	3	1	–	1	3

BMIPP, three-beta-methyl-iodophenyl-pentadecanoic acid; TL, thalliun chloride; MI, Myocardial infarction group; Rp, Reperfusion group; LVAS, Left ventricular assist system
(From [9] with permission)

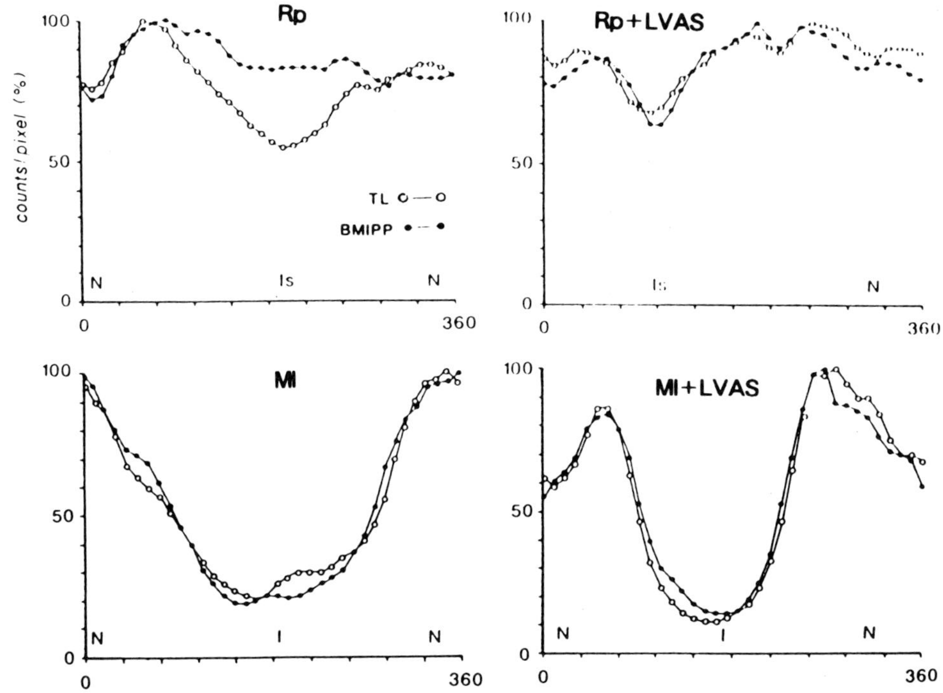

Fig. 2. Myocardial tissue analysis by isotopic counting of BMIPP by the circumferential method. *BMIPP*, three-beta-methyl-iodophenyl-pentadecanoic acid; *TL*, thallium chloride; *MI*, myocardial infarction group; *Rp*, reperfusion group; *LVAS*, left ventricular assist system; *I*, infarcted and/or ischemic area of the left ventricle; *N*, residual normal area of the left ventricle; *Is*, ischemic area of the left ventricle. (From [9] with permission)

Energy Balance

Methods

Twenty mongrel dogs weighing 18–27 kg were used and divided into three groups. In the normal heart group (group 1, 3 dogs), the LVAS was implanted between the left atrium and descending aorta, and dogs were assisted with the maximal flow of the LVAS to unload the left ventricle using a fixed rate. In 17 other dogs, myocardial ischemia was caused by ligation immediately distal to the first diagonal branch of the LAD, branches of the first and second diagonal artery, terminal branches of the LAD and the marginal branch. Immediately after ischemia, LVAS pumping was begun in six dogs (group 2). The LVAS was not used in 11 dogs and ventricular fibrillation occurred in six of these. In the five others without ventricular fibrillation, the following studies were performed (group 3): full-thickness left ventricular biopsies were performed with a biopsy drill for assessment of myocardial high energy phosphates (CrP, ATP,

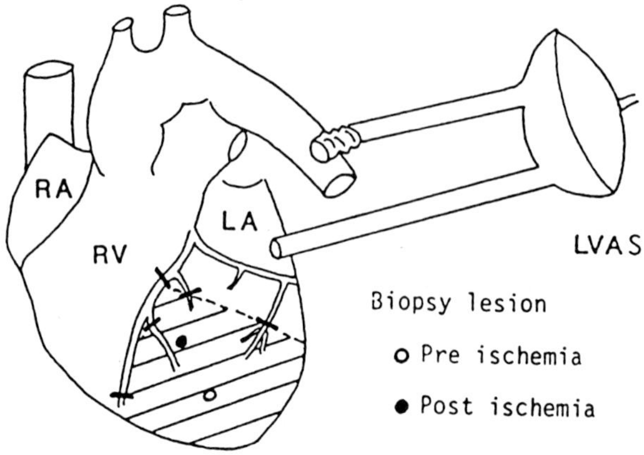

Fig. 3. Schema of experiment. *Hatched area*, ischemic area

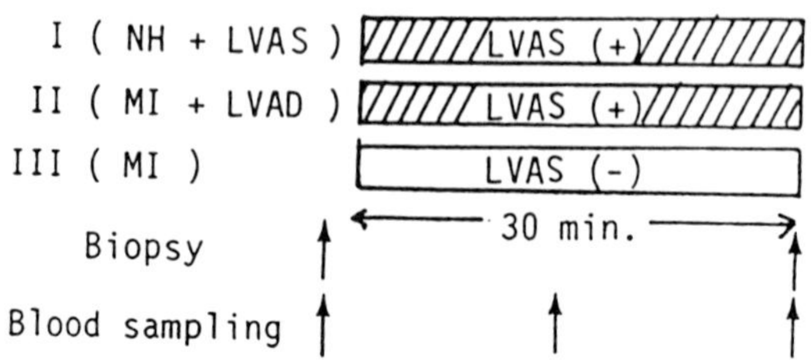

Fig. 4. Schema of sampling points. *NH*, normal heart; *MI*, myocardial infarction

ADP and AMP). The control samples were obtained from the left ventricular apex. Other myocardial samples were obtained 30 min after the start of LVAS pumping in group 1, 30 min after ligation in group 2 and 3 from the area surrounding the main LAD, the first and the second diagonal branches (Fig. 3).

High energy phosphates were determined by high-performance liquid chromatography. Plasma catecholamine (adrenaline and noradrenaline) levels were measured before the procedure, 15 and 30 min after ischemia by high-performance liquid chromatography [15]. Sampling points of myocardial biopsies and blood are shown in Fig. 4.

Results

Myocardial High Energy Phosphate Levels

In group 1, CrP showed no significant change before and after LVAS pumping. In group 2 and group 3, CrP decreased significantly after ligation (Fig. 5). Normalized CrP levels (values 30 min after procedure/control value × 100%) were significantly low in group 3 ($P < 0.01$).

ATP showed no significant changes in the control and 30 min after LVAS pumping (group 1) or ischemia with LVAS pumping (group 2). In group 3, the ATP level 30 min after ischemia decreased significantly compared with that of

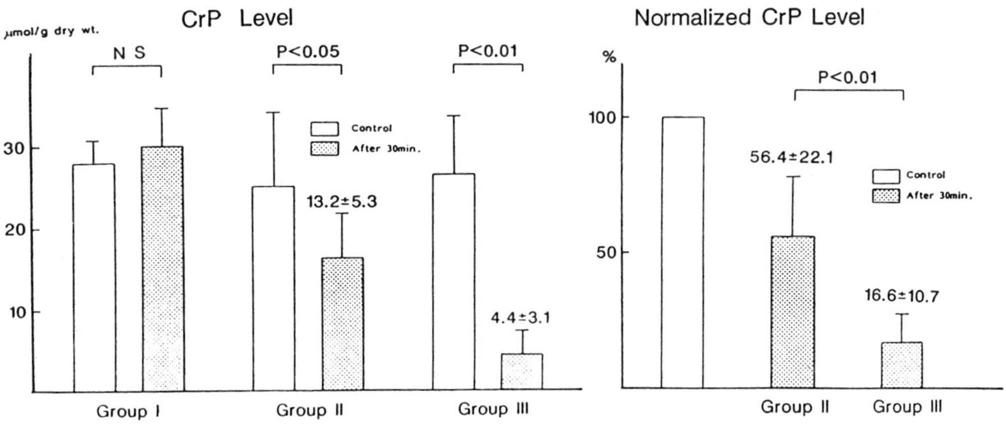

Fig. 5. CrP and normalized CrP levels. *Group* I, normal heart + LVAS; *Group* II, myocardial infarction + LVAS; *Group* III, myocardial infarction

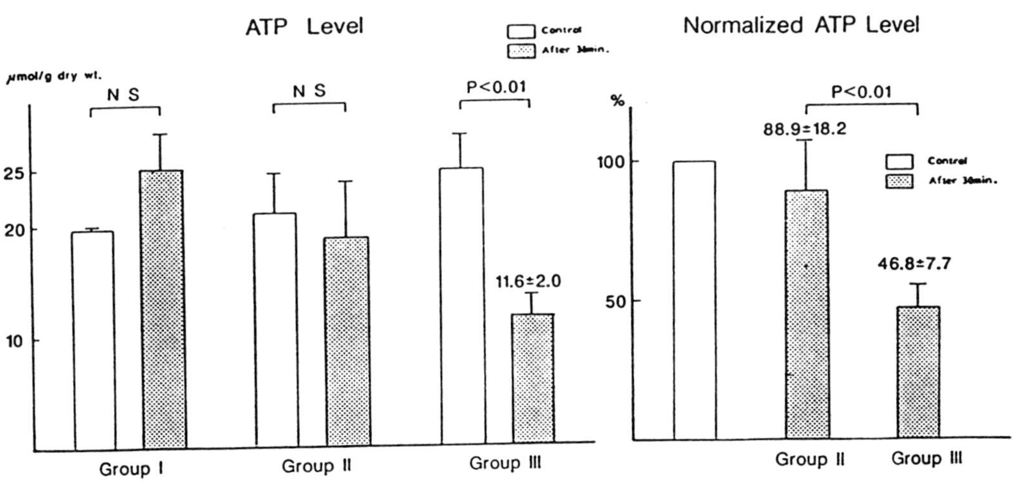

Fig. 6. ATP and normalized ATP levels

the control level (Fig. 6). In addition, normalized ATP levels were significantly low in group 3 ($P < 0.01$). The ATP/ADP ratio, which is an indicator of energy balance and mitochondrial function, showed significantly in group 3 ($P < 0.01$) (Fig. 7).

Plasma catecholamine levels

Plasma adrenaline and noradrenaline levels of control, 15 and 30 min after ischemia showed no changes in group 2. In group 3, these levels of 15 and 30 minutes after ischemia increased markedly (Figs. 8, 9).

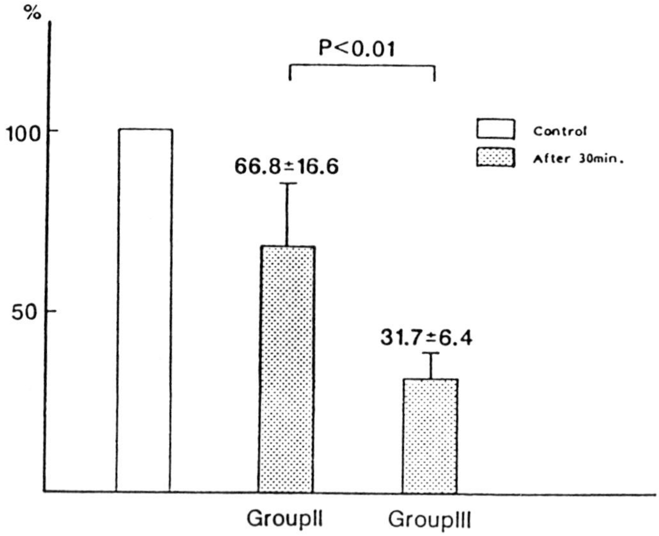

Fig. 7. Normalized ATP/ADP levels

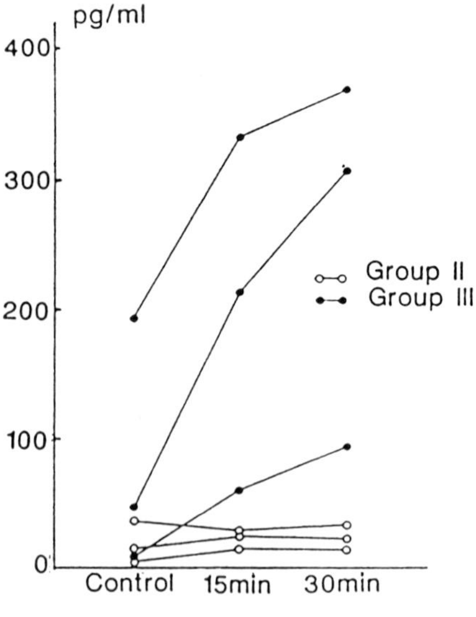

Fig. 8. Plasma adrenaline levels

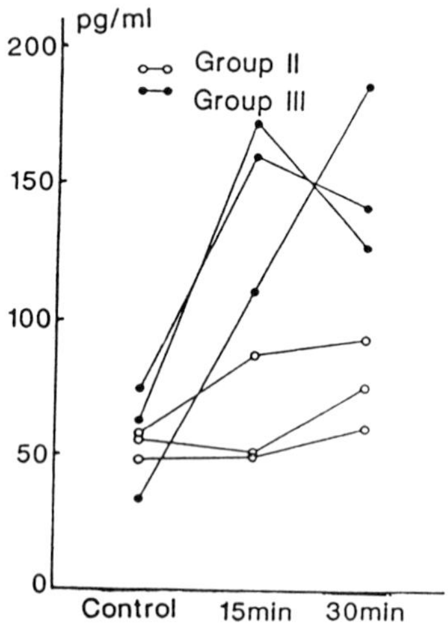

Fig. 9. Plasma noradrenaline levels

Discussion

Infarcted Size Evaluated by MRI

MRI is a noninvasive means of depicting high-resolution tomographic and three-dimensional images of vital organs. The signal intensity of the structures delineated in the MRI is sensitive to several biophysical properties of tissues including water content and T1 and T2 relaxation times. Since the water content of the injured myocardium in AMI is increased in comparison with the normal myocardium, AMI can be identified by MRI [16–18].

In our ex vivo study, MRI contrast of the first signal echo was of great value, since T1 values were markedly decreased and T2 values increased in the infarcted area, suggesting that we can evaluate the ischemic area, and possibly its degree, using MRI with Gd-DTPA. In another study, Gd-DTPA showed significant contrast enhancement of the infarcted area because of greater shortening and the extent of Gd-DTPA contrast enhancement expressed the infarct size precisely [19].

Gd-DTPA is a marker of blood flow in the early phases, and a possible marker of tissue edema, only after the agent has been cleared from normal tissue [18–19]. Gd-DTPA is slowly absorbed into the ischemic, and especially the jeopardized, myocardium through residual flow in collateral vessels ("wash-in") and is then slowly eliminated ("wash-out"), while in normal myocardium, Gd-DTPA is quickly absorbed and eliminated. These wash-in and wash-out patterns may be affected by the degree of neovascularization, collaterals and myocardial necrosis at the infarcted area [20, 21]. These differences influence the signal intensity and T1 and T2 values of the infarcted and the normal myocardium, and the Gd-DTPA enhancement pattern may be valuable for evaluating myocardial tissue characterization at the infarcted and ischemic area [22].

In this study, the area enhanced by Gd-DTPA decreased, as did the signal intensity of injured myocardium with LVAS pumping. MRI signal intensity is arbitrary, and attenuation of the signal level varied from animal to animal, making signal intensity values of little use when comparing different animals. However, the percent differences in values between normal and ischemic myocardium were useful. In this study, MR contrast decreased with the LVAS on. It is thought that LVAS assistance decreases both the ischemic area and the degree of ischemic change of the myocardium. Increase of collateral flow to the injured area by the LVAS may also cause these changes.

Myocardial Tissue Perfusion and Free Fatty Acid Metabolism

TL is well known as a clinically available tracer for myocardial imaging, giving information on myocardial perfusion. However, in the impaired myocardium, such as the MI, where the blood flow is disturbed, TL image cannot display the viability of the tissue. On the other hand, FFA plays a great part in energy production in ischemic areas. Thus, investigation of FFA metabolic processes in myocardium becomes important in diagnosis of heart disease. For this purpose, several FFA analogues have been developed and investigated to prove their usefulness as myocardial tracers indicating FFA metabolic processes. Methylated FFA analogues, one of which is BMIPP, are designed not to be catabolized in the beta cycle in mitochondria, and to be retained in the cell for a period long enough to make a radiographical image [14, 23].

BMIPP is transferred by the circulating blood to the cytoplasma as TL is, and it is possible that BMIPP simply diffuses into the cell cavity while TL is taken up by the sodium-potassium pump of the cell membrane. The BMIPP image may be frozen by being trapped mainly in the triglyceride pool. Thus, the image obtained by BMIPP may show the preservation in FFA metabolic processes. The discrepancy seen in the Rp group may be explained by a hypothesis that FFA, which diffuses into cytoplasm, cannot be catabolized in the beta-cycle because of metabolic injury, and accumulates in the myocardial cell. Reske et al. [23] also reported the discrepancy between excess myocardial blood flow (over 200 ml/min per 100 g) and unmethylated fatty acid uptake. Detailed biological behavior of BMIPP is still unclear as van der Wall mentioned [14], but metabolic imaging technique using BMIPP can be useful for evaluation of myocardial fatty acid metabolism.

LVAS has been proved to maintain systemic circulation in cardiogenic shock and to reduce left ventricular work [6, 7]. In our study, the LVAS was proved to preserve the cell function of the impaired myocardium from the view point of FFA metabolism. A rapid increase of BMIPP uptake, paralleled to TL uptake, was observed in the marginal area which may be mainly constructed of stunned myocardium in the MI + LVAS group. This result supported the reports that the improvement of tissue perfusion in the marginal area of MI may prevent the expansion of MI with the use of the LVAS [4, 5]. In the normal area, BMIPP uptake was decreased compared with TL uptake, while the BMIPP disappearance rate was maintained at a normal level. This result should be caused by a reduction of ventricular work when the LVAS assisted the systemic circulation. Thus the LVAS was proved to preserve the normal myocardium of the ischemic heart from the point of view of FFA metabolism.

Energy Balance

Myocardial Energy Balance

The LVAS can decrease left ventricular volume loading and work by reducing LV preload [6, 7]. The LVAS can maintain not only the systemic flow but also the coronary circulation. These effects may improve the myocardial energy balance. Energy balance has been studied from energy supply such as myocardial tissue flow [4] and energy demand such as myocardial oxygen consumption [24]. In this study, we measured high energy phosphate in the myocardium directly and evaluated the effect of LVAS from the energy balance.

In group 2 (MI + LVAS), the levels of CrP, ATP, and ATP/ADP, which is an indicator of energy balance, were higher than those in group 3 (MI). These suggest that the LVAS may reduce ischemic injury and salvage the damaged myocardium by a decrease in consumption of high energy phosphate. In the infarcted area, blood supply was interrupted and no further energy was supplied, so high energy phosphate was exhausted finally in spite of unloading effect of LVAS. In ischemic, especially jeopardized, myocardium, however, a decrease in consumption of high energy phosphate by LVAS may reduce the expansion of the infarcted area and salvage the ischemic area with an increase of flow in collateral vessels.

In group 1 (normal heart + LVAS), high energy phosphate showed no change with or without LVAS pumping. This indicates that the normal myocardium unloaded by the LVAS maintained a normal energy balance. From this, it is considered that LVAS pumping may preserve the energy balance of the residual myocardium and prevent expansion of ischemic injury in cardiogenic shock following AMI.

Plasma Catecholamine Levels

In AMI, plasma catecholamine levels were raised by stimulation of the adrenal glands. Raised catecholamine levels increased myocardial oxygen consumption by raising afterload by systemic vasoconstriction, increasing heart rate and inotropic action [25]. Raised plasma catecholamines also have metabolic effects, including glucose intolerance and the raise in FFA, which will induce cardiac injury. In our study, group 2 showed no raise of catecholamine levels after AMI induction. In cardiogenic shock, maintenance of systemic circulation with the LVAS is considered to be effective to prevent hormonal and energy balance abnormalities.

Conclusion

The LVAS is a powerful means of cardiac assistance. Some therapeutic effects of the LVAS have been clarified through our studies: (a) the LVAS effectively decreased both the ischemic area and degree, and myocardial ischemia, (b) the LVAS improved cell function from FFA metabolism, (c) high energy phosphate showed no change in the normal myocardium with LVAS pumping, and (d) LVAS pumping preserved high energy phosphate concentrations in the ischemic myocardium and prevented raise of catecholamine levels in profound heart failure. The therapeutic effects of the LVAS on AMI has yet to be sufficiently clarified. Future study is needed to establish an effective strategy for salvaging profound heart failure following AMI.

References

1. Takano H, Taenaka Y, Nakatani T, Akutsu T, Manabe H (1985) Successful treatment of profound left ventricular failure by automatic left ventricular assist system. World J Surg 9:78–88
2. LeGal YM, Rideout SC (1983) Reduction of myocardial infarct size: a comparison of the effectiveness of intra-aortic balloon pumping and transapical left ventricular bypass. Trans Am Soc Artif Intern Organs 26:593–598
3. Mickleborough LL, Rebeyka I, Wilson GL, Gray G, Desroiers A (1987) Comparison of left ventricular assist and intra-aortic balloon counterpulsation during early reperfusion after ischemic arrest of the heart. J Thorac Cardiovasc Surg 93:597–608

4. Noda H, Nakatani T, Takano H, Fukuda S, Kinoshita M, Akutsu T (1985) The effect of LVAD on myocardial regional blood flow. Life Support System 4:35–40
5. Grossi EA, Krieger KH, Cunningham JN, Laschinger JC, Weiss MR, Nathan IM, Hunter CE, Spencer FC (1986) Time course of effective interventional left heart assist for limitation of evolving myocardial infarction. J Thorac Cardiovasc Surg 91:624–629
6. Nakatani T, Takano H, Taenaka Y, Umezu M, Tanaka T, Yutani C, Matsuda T, Iwata H, Noda H, Nakamura T, Takatani S, Seki J, Hayashi K, Akutsu T, Manabe H (1984) Therapeutic effect of left ventricular assist device on induced profound left ventricular failure — evaluation by left ventriculography. Trans Am Soc Artif Intern Organs 30:533–538
7. Nakamura T, Hayashi K, Seki J, Nakatani T, Noda H, Fukuda S, Takano H, Akutsu T (1990) Effects of cardiac assist on the bulk and regional mechanics of the ischemic left ventricle in dogs. Artif Organs 14:57–68
8. Nakatani T, Takano H, Noda H, Fukuda S, Nishimura T, Yamada Y, Kozuka T, Akutsu T (1986) Therapeutic effect of a left ventricular assist device on acute myocardial infarction evaluated by magnetic resonance imaging. Trans Am Soc Artif Intern Organs 32:201–206
9. Noda H, Nishimura T, Kinoshita M, Taenaka Y, Kihara K, Sago M, Hayashi M, Takano H, Akutsu T (1988) Myocardial free fatty acid metabolism of the ischemic heart treated by left ventricular assist device. Trans Am Soc Artif Intern Organs 34:294–296
10. Kinoshta M, Taenaka Y, Nakatani T, Noda H, Tatsumi E, Yagura A, Sekii H, Takano H, Akutsu T (1988) The effect of left ventricular assist device (LVAD) on the myocardial energy balance. Jpn J Artif Organs 17:919–922
11. Knapp FF, Ambrose KR, Goodman MM (1986) New radioiodinated methyl-balanced fatty acids for cardiac studies. Eur J Nucl Med 12:539–544
12. Dudezak R, Schmoliner R, Angelberger P, Knapp EF, Goodman MM (1986) Structurally modified fatty acids: clinical potential as tracers of metabolism. Eur J Nucl Med 12:45
13. Otto CA, Brown LE, Scott AM (1985) Radioiodonated branched-chain fatty acids: substrates for beta oxidation? J Nucl Med 25:75–80
14. van der Wall EE (1986) Myocardial imaging with radiolabeled free fatty acids: application and limitation. Eur J Nucl Med 12:511–515
15. Watanabe F, Hashimoto T, Tagawa K (1985) Energy-independent protection of the oxidative phosphorylation capacity of mitochondria against anoxic damage by ATP and its nonmetabolizable analogs. J Biochem 97:1229–1234
16. Higgins CB, Herfkens R, Lipton MJ, Sheldon P, Kaufman L, Crooks LE (1983) Nuclear magnetic resonance imaging of acute myocardial infarction in dogs: alterations in magnetic relaxation times. Am J Cardiol 52:184–188
17. Wesbey GE, Higgins CB, Lauzer P, Botvinick E, Lipton MJ (1984) Imaging and characterization of acute myocardial infarction in vivo by gated magnetic resonace. Circulation 69:125–130
18. Pflugfelder PW, Wisenberg G, Prato F, Carroll SE, Turner KL (1985) Early detection of canine myocardial infarction by magnetic resonace imaging in vivo. Circulation 71:587–594
19. Nishimura T, Yamada Y, Hayashi M, Kozuka T, Nakatani T, Noda H, Takano H (1989) Determination of infarcted size of acute myocardial infarction in dogs by magnetic resonance imaging and gadolinium-DTPA: comparison with indium-111 antimyosin imaging. Am J Physiol Imag 4:83–88

20. Tsholakoff D, Higgins CB, Sechtem U, McNamara MT (1986) Occlusive and reperfused myocardial infarcts: effect of Gd-DTPA on ECG-gated MR imaging. Radiology 160:515–519
21. McNamara MT, Tscholakoff D, Revel D, Soulen R, Schechtmann N, Botvinick E, Higgins CB (1986) Differentiation of reversible and irreversible myocardium injury by MR imaging with and without gadolinium-DTPA. Radiology 158:765–769
22. Wesbey GE, Higgins CB, McNamara MT, Engelstad BL, Sievers R, Lipton MJ, Ehman RL, Lovin J, Brasch RC (1984) Effect of gadolinium-DTPA on the magnetic relaxation times of normal and infarcted myocardium. Radiology 153:165–169
23. Reske SN, Schöen S, Schmitt W, Machulla HJ, Knopp R, Winkler C (1986) Effect of myocardial perfusion and metabolic interventions on cardiac kinetics of phenylpentadecanoic acid (IPPA) I 123. Eur J Nucl Med 12:527–531
24. Wei CM, Imura M, Hattori R, Saito K, Fukuyama M, Yada I, Yuasa H, Kusagawa M (1986) The effect of left heart bypass on canine myocardial hemodynamics and metabolism. Jpn J Artif Organs 15:596–599
25. Norris RM (1982) Metabolic sequelae of myocardial infarction. In: Myocardial infarction. Churchhill Livingstone, Edinburgh, pp 89–96

Index